Nebraska Symposium on Motivation

Volume 65

Series editor

Debra A. Hope, Lincoln, NE, USA

More information about this series at http://www.springer.com/series/7596

Debra A. Hope • Rick A. Bevins
Editors

Change and Maintaining Change

Springer

Editors
Debra A. Hope
Department of Psychology
University of Nebraska–Lincoln
Lincoln, NE, USA

Rick A. Bevins
Department of Psychology
University of Nebraska–Lincoln
Lincoln, NE, USA

ISSN 0146-7875
Nebraska Symposium on Motivation
ISBN 978-3-030-07272-8 ISBN 978-3-319-96920-6 (eBook)
https://doi.org/10.1007/978-3-319-96920-6

This Springer imprint is published by the registered company Springer Nature Switzerland AG
The registered company address is: Gewerbestrasse 11, 6330 Cham, Switzerland

Preface

We are pleased to offer this volume from the 65th Nebraska Symposium on Motivation.

This year the volume is edited by myself and Rick Bevins. After several years of dreaming of co-chairing a Nebraska Symposium on behavioral change, we were thrilled to bring together the esteemed scholars for a stimulating meeting and an excellent series of papers on change and maintaining change from neuroscience to public policy across a wide range of important public health challenges. I would like to express my appreciation to Prof. Bevins for partnering with me on this endeavor.

This Symposium series is supported by funds provided by the Chancellor of the University of Nebraska-Lincoln, Harvey Perlman, and by funds given in memory of Professor Harry K. Wolfe to the University of Nebraska Foundation by the late Professor Cora L. Friedline. Given Chancellor Perlman's retirement in 2016, we honored his longstanding generous support by naming the poster session and reception in his honor. We are also grateful for the University of Nebraska Foundation's support via the Friedline bequest. This symposium volume, like those in the recent past, is dedicated to the memory of Professor Wolfe, who brought psychology to the University of Nebraska. After studying with Professor Wilhelm Wundt in Germany, Professor Wolfe returned to this, his native state, to establish the first undergraduate laboratory in psychology in the nation. As a student at Nebraska, Professor Friedline studied psychology under Professor Wolfe.

Lincoln, NE, USA Debra A. Hope

Acknowledgments

The nature of the publication process forces us to have an authorship and editorship order. Alas, we have met current publication conventions and selected an order for each. However, we want to make the reader aware that the entire process, from the inception of the idea for this volume to the writing of the introduction to the chapters, reflects a fully collaborative partnership.

DAH was partially funded by grant MH108897 from the National Institute of Mental Health and RAB was partially funded by grant DA034389 from the National Institute on Drug Abuse while writing this Introduction.

Contents

Contributors

Dolores Albarracín Department of Psychology and Department of Business Administration, Gies College of Business, University of Illinois at Urbana–Champaign, Champaign, IL, USA

Chloe E. Bird RAND Corporation, Santa Monica, CA, USA

Wenhao Dai Department of Psychology, University of Illinois at Urbana–Champaign, Champaign, IL, USA

Danielle R. Davis Vermont Center on Behavior and Health, Departments of Psychiatry and Psychological Science, University of Vermont, Burlington, VT, USA

Stephen T. Higgins Vermont Center on Behavior and Health, Departments of Psychiatry and Psychological Science, University of Vermont, Burlington, VT, USA

George F. Koob National Institute on Alcohol Abuse and Alcoholism, National Institutes of Health, Bethesda, MD, USA

Allison N. Kurti Vermont Center on Behavior and Health, Departments of Psychiatry and Psychological Science, University of Vermont, Burlington, VT, USA

Martha E. Lang Providence College, Providence, RI, USA

Gregory J. Madden Department of Psychology, Utah State University, Logan, UT, USA

Edward Wile Maibach Department of Communication and Center for Climate Change Communication, George Mason University, Fairfax, VA, USA

Joseph Price Department of Economics, Brigham Young University, Provo, UT, USA

Connie Roser-Renouf Center for Climate Change Communication, George Mason University, Fairfax, VA, USA

Aashna Sunderrajan Department of Psychology, University of Illinois at Urbana–Champaign, Champaign, IL, USA

Heidi Wengreen Department of Nutrition Dietetics and Food Science, Utah State University, Logan, UT, USA

Introduction

Ways for Making and Maintaining Behavior Change

Changing and maintaining that change are fundamental to the motivational processes the founders of the Nebraska Symposium on Motivation (NSM) had in mind when they established this historic series. In this 66th Volume, we focus on processes by which behavior change occurs and how this change may or may not be maintained. This topic is quite timely as researchers across many domains seek a fundamental understanding to guiding and maintaining behavior change in areas of significant societal importance (e.g., Higgins, 2014).

As a way of illustration, consider the probable but hypothetical story of Jessica, a 26-year-old single mom, who smoked her first cigarette at 12 years old, a cigarette snuck from the pack that always sat on her mother's nightstand.

> Jessica has been sitting restlessly in this small pale blue aseptic room waiting for hours to hear from the surgeons. Her mother, recently diagnosed with lung cancer, was in their care. They thought stage 2, but the doctors could not be certain until the surgery. With a rerun of Seinfeld droning in the background, her thoughts darted to and from the half unsmoked pack of cigarettes in her worn denim handbag. "Just one more, then I will quit," she tells herself. Propelled by such thoughts as this so many times before, she leaned over the chair and reached into the handbag on the floor to grab her cigarettes and lighter. As the tips of her fingers touched the Marlboro Menthol® pack, her resolve suddenly stiffened, "I must stop now. I can't follow the fate of so many of my loved ones." That resolve brought Jessica's thoughts to her father, also a smoker, who died of lung cancer 8 years ago, never meeting his granddaughter. With sadness she implored, "Be a better role model for Sofia! What would happen to her if I die? Throw away the pack and never…" Her thoughts interrupted by the surgeon entering the room. It was worse than they had thought.

In various forms, this scenario has played out too many times in reality. Jessica is an individual with a long history of unhealthy behavior. Namely, she experimented with smoking at 12 years of age and, over time, developed into a chronic smoker dependent on nicotine. In addition, she has additional risk factors. Such factors include social modeling and a family history of smoking that spans generations. Also, once smoking, females are more likely to become dependent and relapse after a quit attempt (Perkins, 2009). Of course, life stressors such a very sick parent and the demands of being a single parent also contribute to the tenacity of the addiction, the pattern of unhealthy behaviors, and the difficulty sustaining a quit attempt.

Although the eminent speakers at this year's Symposium describe research conducted at different levels of analysis (i.e., synapse to society) and on different critical social issues (e.g., addiction, unhealthy eating, climate change), we can learn a lot from them about how we can help Jessica quit smoking, sustain that cessation, and not relapse even after years of abstinence. They also provide us with general principles and guidelines for effective prevention and intervention approaches at the individual and societal level. For instance, Koob has made us consider the role of stress, withdrawal, and negative reinforcement in the drug dependence and treatment process. Higgins, Kurti, and Davis focus our attention to reinforcement history and the use of reinforcement principles to treat individuals with chronic unhealthy behavior patterns. Relatedly, Madden, Price, and Wengreen, within the context of healthy food choices in children, lead us to consider how to structure early childhood environments in order to reinforce desired behaviors. Albarracín, Sunderrajan, and Dai, as well as Roser-Renouf and Maibach, bring critical ideas of how to effectively communicate messages around prevention and intervention to increase their efficacy and impact. Finally, Lang and Bird help us recognize and remediate local, state, and/or federal policies that can serve as barriers to improving outcomes for individuals.

The Chapters

The tenacity of addiction and associated dependence requires us to consider more than reward processes if long-term change is to be affected. Koob describes his allostatic model of compulsive drug seeking. From this perspective, chronic drug use leads to dysfunctional regulation of reward systems along with withdrawal and strong negative affect. Removal of such aversive stimuli (i.e., negative reinforcement) is a strong motivator of drug seeking and compulsive use. Koob provides a thoughtful review of known neurobiological processes mediating such controlling factors and outlines future directions of research to further understand negative reinforcement and its contribution to addiction and treatment.

In the chapter by Higgins, Kurti, and Davis, they focus on approaches in vulnerable populations (e.g., lower socioeconomic status) that encourage long-term behavior change to decrease unhealthy behaviors that contribute to chronic diseases and premature death. Importantly, these very same reinforcement processes that produce unhealthy behavior patterns can be used strategically to reinforce and sustain healthy behaviors (e.g., contingency management), thus decreasing the risk of chronic disease and premature death. Higgins, Kurti, and Davis conclude that such a strategy can be employed across a wide domain of unhealthy behaviors and their associated diseases.

A physician may discuss a smoking cessation program with their patient but whether the patient will attempt to quit smoking or maintain abstinence is highly variable. In their chapter, Albarracín, Sunderrajan, and Dai address the mechanisms that can improve the likelihood that recommendations for behavior change will be effective. The structure of the recommendation for behavior change (e.g., how many changes are requested), the context in which the recommendation occurs, and behavioral, affective and cognitive engagement all influence the effectiveness of the communication. Interventions that are highly *actionable* have a number of characteristics that increase their impact. Albarracín, Sunderrajan, and Dai conclude their chapter with a series of recommendations that are broadly applicable in improving health as well as many other spheres in which persuasive communication is utilized.

Developing eating habits that are healthy early in life has enormous benefit to the individual and society in terms of health, well-being, and financial costs. Madden, Price, and Wengreen review the behavioral and economic literature researching factors that may improve fruit and vegetable intake of children within schools. Also in this chapter, they describe their innovative research program that includes the use of a relatively inexpensive game-based program to incentivize healthier eating. Madden, Price, and Wengreen conclude with a set of policy recommendation aimed at producing substantive and sustained change in the food choice children make in schools.

In the health care system in the United States, the change in question is patient adherence to treatment to help ensure good clinical outcomes. Using the example of compliance with antiviral medication for cisgender women living with HIV, Lang and Bird describe how decisions made at the level of family, workplace, community, and governmental policy can create barriers to initiating and maintaining medication adherence. The authors nicely demonstrate the range of forces that come to bear on an individual making daily decisions about taking medication, leading a healthy lifestyle, and engaging in needed medical care. Lang and Bird outline how local, state, and federal policies can reduce these barriers and improve clinical outcomes and reduce societal costs of HIV.

The final chapter in this volume addresses change at a global level. Roser-Renouf and Maibach describe the work at the Center for Climate Change Communication at George Mason University. The mission of the Center is to develop and apply social science insights to help society make informed decisions that will reduce climate change. Through a careful program of research that identifies the most effective messages and messengers, they have developed a three-pronged approach of messaging through television weathercasters, improving understanding of the human health effects of climate change, and targeted messages to create a narrative about climate change that appeals to conservatives. Their work demonstrates how research can be leveraged to create behavior and policy change to address one of the most important global challenges of our time.

In Closing

The diversity of approaches, topics, and levels of analyses seen across these chapters illustrate an interdisciplinary approach that is required to address society's most pressing public health challenges. On the one hand, these chapters can be discouraging in that the authors portray the complexities of the processes of change and maintaining change. On the other hand, the authors also identify how small achievable changes can have profound impact. Modest incentives for healthy eating can improve children's nutrition. Local weather broadcasters mentioning climate change can impact societal attitudes. It is our hope that this volume benefits readers as they better understand the push and pull of forces ranging from neurons to institutional policies that can inform research and policymaking as we tackle key public health challenges.

A Note of Appreciation

The success of endeavors such as organizing the annual Nebraska Symposium on Motivation depends on a strong team. We the editors are very grateful for Brady Thompson, Scott Barrett, and Jennifer Murray for their assistance in making the Symposium a success. Pam Waldvogel provided outstanding logistical support and helped keep everyone on track at each step for both the conference and the volume. Pam's professionalism, sense of humor, and attention to detail are much appreciated. Finally, we would like to thank Morgan Ryan and Sara Yanny-Tillar at Springer Science+Business media for their editorial guidance.

University of Nebraska–Lincoln Rick A. Bevins
Lincoln, NE, USA Debra A. Hope

References

Higgins, S. T. (2014). Behavior change, health, and health disparities: An introduction. *Preventive Medicine, 68*, 1–4. https://doi.org/10.1016/j.ypmed.2014.10.007

Perkins, K. A. (2009). Sex difference in nicotine reinforcement and reward: Influences on the persistence of tobacco smoking. In R. A. Bevins & A. R. Caggiula (Eds.), *The motivational impact of nicotine and its role in tobacco use: The 55th Nebraska Symposium on Motivation* (pp. 143–169). New York, NY: Springer Science+Business Media.

Chapter 1
Motivating Change in Addiction via Modulation of the Dark Side

George F. Koob

Introduction

Reward and stress are intimately linked. Some levels of stress can actually be rewarding, and excess reward can lead to stress. I began my research career at John Hopkins University (JHU) where I initiated studies that explored this relationship under the mentorship of Dr. Zoltan Annau who had trained with Dr. James Olds, one of the co-discoverers (with Dr. Peter Milner) of brain stimulation reward. However, framing the background of my education at JHU were towering figures in physiology and psychology: W. Horsley Gantt and Joseph V. Brady, who both indirectly and directly influenced my thinking on emotion and motivation and how they are linked, particularly in the domain of reward and stress (Fig. 1.1).

Reward can be defined as a stimulus that increases the probability of a response and has some positive hedonic connotation. Stress can be defined as anything that causes alterations of psychological homeostatic processes (Burchfield, 1979). Early work in my career focused on the ways in which stress influences reward (Koob & Annau, 1973) and later moved me to try to understand the ways in which reward influences stress (Kreek & Koob, 1998). Drs. Gantt and Brady provided the conceptual framework for understanding the interaction between reward and stress and ultimately provided me with a foundation that would later move me to the construct of the "dark side" of addiction (Koob & Le Moal, 2005; Schulteis & Koob, 1994), defined here as the negative emotional state that is observed during drug abstinence that drives negative reinforcement in addiction (see below).

Horsley Gantt and Joseph Brady shared a conceptual framework about the motivational power of negative motivational states from two different but parallel

G. F. Koob (✉)
National Institute on Alcohol Abuse and Alcoholism, National Institutes of Health, Bethesda, MD, USA
e-mail: george.koob@nih.gov

D. A. Hope, R. A. Bevins (eds.), *Change and Maintaining Change*, Nebraska Symposium on Motivation 65, https://doi.org/10.1007/978-3-319-96920-6_1

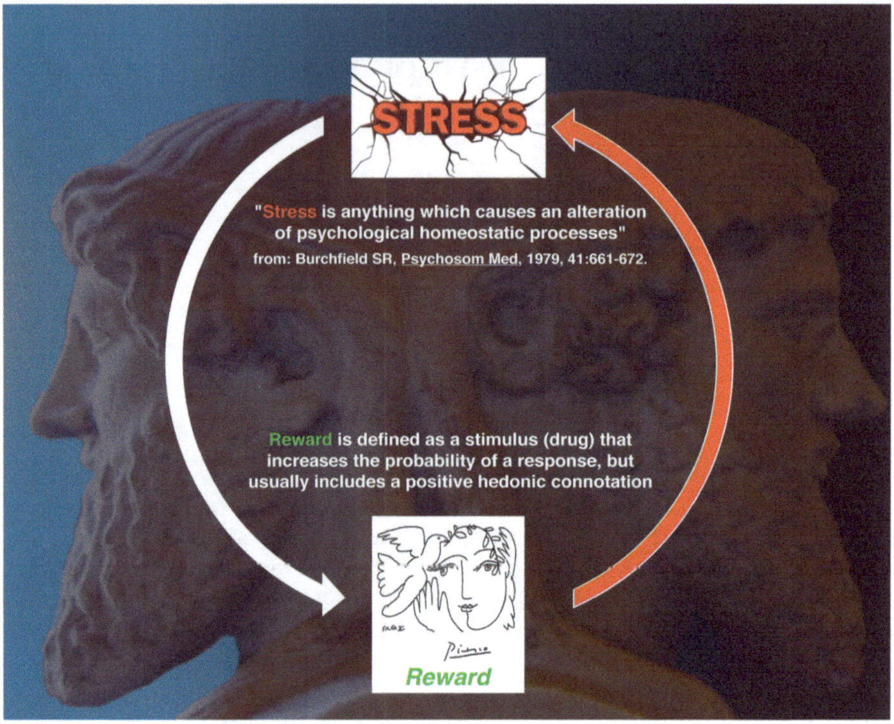
STRESS
"Stress is anything which causes an alteration of psychological homeostatic processes"
from: Burchfield SR, Psychosom Med, 1979, 41:661-672.
Reward is defined as a stimulus (drug) that increases the probability of a response, but usually includes a positive hedonic connotation
Reward

Fig. 1.1 Stress and reward: the two faces of Janus. Janus was the god of doors, passages, and transitions, and his two faces look to the future and to the past. Reward and stress represent different components of transitions in our brain emotional systems that lead to and perpetuate addiction. Stress can be rewarding in small or intense doses, possibly mediated by glucocorticoids that act on brain reward systems (see text). However, excessive engagement of the reward systems can produce chronic stress that is aversive and contributes to negative emotional states that drive negative reinforcement in addiction (see text)

psychological traditions: classical conditioning and operant conditioning (Koob, 2017). Dr. Horsley Gantt was a student of Ivan Pavlov, and as such, he was well trained in the study of classical conditioning (Pavlov & Gantt, 1941). Pavlov defined classical conditioning and demonstrated its fundamentals, whereby the stimulus that is to become the signal in a conditioned reflex must overlap in a point of time with the action of an unconditioned stimulus and begin to operate before the unconditioned stimulus comes into action (Pavlov, 1927). Gantt carried work on conditioned reflexes to the domain of negative emotional states by describing the emotional response of an animal when a conflict situation is introduced, generating what he described as "experimental neurosis." He first elicited a conditioned response to a conditioned stimulus for food in a hungry animal that reflected strong "excitation" but then elicited an inhibitory process that elicited a signal that was similar to the first signal but failed to reinforce it with food (Gantt, 1942). A conflict situation was then introduced, in which he used "two tones (as signals for the signal for food and no food) so close together in pitch that the nervous systems is physically incapable of discriminating" (Gantt, 1942, p. 476). This resulted in:

> [the production of a chronic anxiety-like neurosis] is expressed in his general behavior (restlessness, etc.), by a loss of equilibrium between all the CRs (changing the relative intensities, e.g. over-reacting to some, under-reacting to others), and finally, as we have been able to show recently by records of the heart rate and respiration, in emotional changes (Gantt, 1942, p. 476).

In a parallel history, derived from the operant behaviorist tradition engaged by B. F. Skinner, an almost identical framework was developed for the motivational power of negative emotional states. Here, early on, researchers showed that responding for food can be suppressed by a cue that is paired with an aversive stimulus, a phenomenon he termed "conditioned suppression" (Estes & Skinner, 1941). Dr. Joseph Brady, another one of my mentors and chairman of my thesis committee at JHU, showed that reserpine reversed conditioned suppression, and amphetamines potentiated conditioned suppression (Brady, 1956), providing some of the early neuropharmacological mechanisms for conditioned suppression. These early observations that conflict and aversive stimuli can result in emotional-like responses and behavioral changes led to my interest in how aversive stress can alter reward. In my thesis work, I observed that hypoxic stress can facilitate brain stimulation reward (Koob & Annau, 1973). Much subsequent work showed that glucocorticoids facilitated initial drug-seeking behavior, and high glucocorticoid activity can form an initial vulnerability to excessive drug seeking (Piazza & Le Moal, 1997).

Thus, as part of the rich tradition of the study of reinforcement, from both classical and operant conditioning perspectives, Drs. Horsley Gantt and Joseph Brady laid the conceptual groundwork for motivation and emotion that resonated in my brain and prepared me to recognize that the converse could also be true: excess reward can engage homeostatic-like mechanisms in response, and these attempts of the brain to return to motivational homeostasis generate another source of motivation. In particular, a conceptual thesis, termed the "behavioral universe" and outlined by Joseph Brady at an early Nebraska Symposium on Motivation, provided a guiding framework for how interactions of reinforcers with the brain, both from the classical conditioning and operant conditioning traditions, can generate emotional states of motivational significance (Brady, 1975; Fig. 1.2). To quote Brady:

> Indeed, the characterization of identity relationships between distinguishable physiological and behavioral participants, on the one hand, and the rather arbitrary "feelings" and "emotional behavior" dichotomy on the other, is of course both over simplified and somewhat artificial. Some heuristic value can be expected to derive, however, from an account of emotion events which proceeds by defining the properties of identifiable constituents and examining in detail the interrelationships between external behavioral interactions and the broader patterning or balance of biochemical and physiological processes which in concert regulate the internal milieu (Brady, 1975).
>
> Even the 'hedonic' characteristics of motivational functions can be accommodated within the empirical framework of this conceptual analysis by appealing to the experimentally based distinctions between 'positive' and 'negative' reinforcement operations. The evident byproducts (e.g., 'euphoria') of 'appetitive' consequating relations which increase the likelihood of behavior, on the one hand, and the 'dysphoric' accompaniments of 'aversive' consequences which weaken behavior (or strengthen escape and avoidance

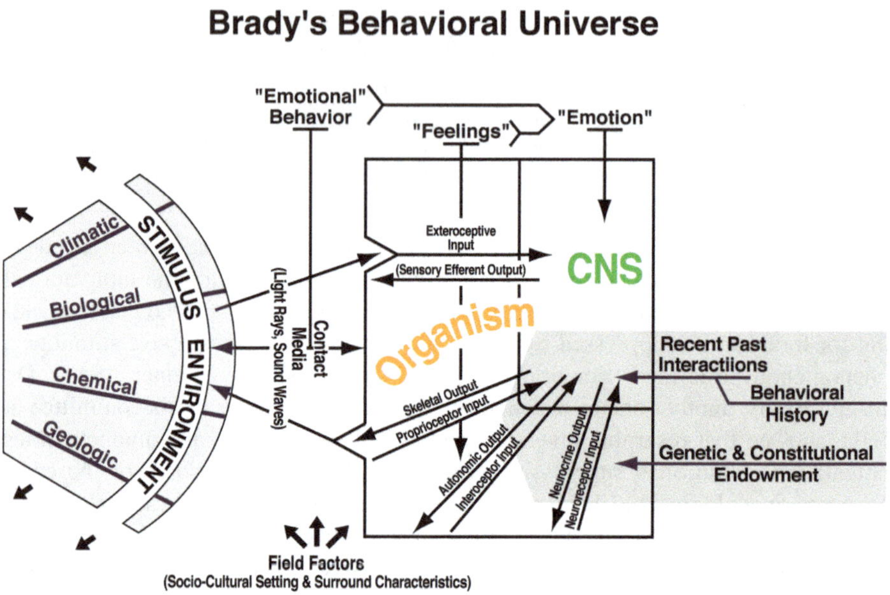

Fig. 1.2 Diagrammatic representation of a 'behavioral universe' emphasizing organism–environmental interactions. 'Emotional behavior' is represented at the interface between organism and environment, whereas 'feelings' are localized within the reacting organism. The generic reference to the term 'emotion' with its suggestive arrow into the central nervous system is meant simply to imply a conceptual creation of the brain, not the existence of a resident entity [Taken with permission from Brady, 1975]

> performances), would seem to provide a fruitful point of departure for the experimental analysis of this eudaemonic dimension (Brady & Emurian, 1978, p. 83).

Indeed, in the past 40 years, Richard Solomon's opponent-process theory, combined with an overlay of Sterling and Eyer's allostasis theory, allowed the gradual unveiling of the neurocircuitry of negative emotional states that were described by Gantt and Brady.

Addiction as a Motivational Disorder

Drug addiction is often defined as a compulsion to seek and take a drug and loss of control in limiting intake, but I also added to the definition, "the emergence of a negative emotional state when access to the drug is prevented" (Koob & Le Moal, 1997; Russell, 1976). Addiction has been conceptualized in a heuristic framework as a three-stage cycle: *binge/intoxication*, *withdrawal/negative affect*, and *preoccupation/anticipation* (Koob & Le Moal, 1997). These stages have been hypothesized to represent dysregulation in three functional domains (incentive salience/habits, negative emotional states, and executive function) that are mediated by three major neurocircuitry elements (basal ganglia, extended amygdala, and prefrontal cortex, respectively) and feed into each other, become more intense, and ultimately lead to the pathological state known as addiction (Fig. 1.3). Two primary sources of reinforcement, positive and negative reinforcement, have been hypothesized to contribute to the compulsion to seek drugs. Positive reinforcement is defined as the process by which the presentation of a stimulus increases the probability of a response. Negative reinforcement is defined as the process by which the removal of an aversive stimulus (or an aversive, negative emotional state of withdrawal in the case of addiction) increases the probability of a response. The early studies of Gantt and Brady found that aversive stimuli generate emotional behavior. These studies, combined with my early work that showed that hypoxic stress facilitated reward, ultimately led to my conceptualization that excessive engagement in reward activity engages an anti-reward system that produces a negative emotional state that contributes to motivational drive. However, in the case of addiction, this motivational drive sets up a powerful negative reinforcement process rather than punishment (Koob & Le Moal, 2008).

The overall hypothesis is that a key part of addiction involves long-term, persistent dysregulation of the activity of neural circuits that mediate anti-reward motivational systems that derive from two sources: a decrease in the function of brain reward systems that normally mediate natural rewards and recruitment of brain stress systems that drive aversive states (Koob & Le Moal, 2008). Such anti-reward derives from an opponent-process concept that is triggered by the excessive activation of brain reward systems that forms a general feature of biological systems (Solomon, 1980).

I should emphasize that the symptoms defined herein as a negative emotional state, manifested as a withdrawal syndrome in the *withdrawal/negative affect* stage, do not represent the classical physical signs of withdrawal as described in the early work on dependence after the removal of chronic drug administration (Himmelsbach, 1943). For the purposes of this chapter, withdrawal is defined in terms of motivational aspects of dependence, such as the emergence of a negative emotional state (e.g., dysphoria, anxiety, and irritability) when access to the drug is prevented (Koob & Le Moal, 2001), but can also include physical signs of dependence, such as pain. In fact, some have argued that the development of such a negative affective state can define dependence as it relates to addiction:

> The notion of dependence on a drug, object, role, activity or any other stimulus-source requires the crucial feature of negative affect experienced in its absence. The degree of dependence can be equated with the amount of this negative affect, which may range from mild discomfort to extreme distress, or it may be equated with the amount of difficulty or effort required to do without the drug, object, etc. (Russell, 1976).

Opponent Process as a Motivational Construct in Addiction

Motivation is a construct that is often described as the guiding behavior in relation to changes in the environment. The temporal dynamics of motivation for drug seeking was inextricably linked with hedonic, affective, or emotional states in

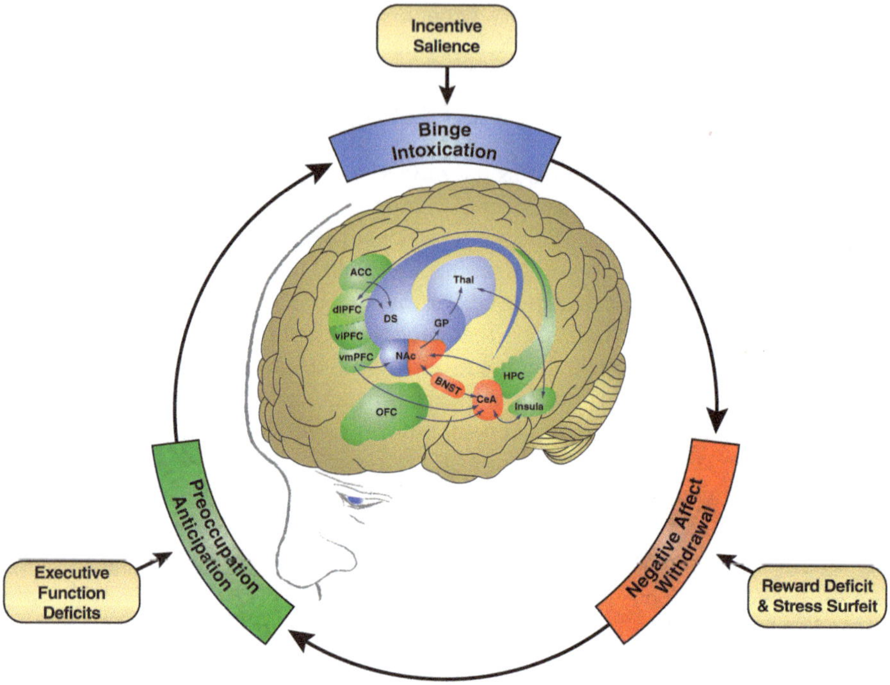

Fig. 1.3 Conceptual framework for the neurobiological basis of addiction. In the *binge/intoxication* stage, reinforcing effects of drugs may engage reward neurotransmitters and associative mechanisms in the nucleus accumbens shell and core and then engage stimulus-response habits that depend on the dorsal striatum. Two major neurotransmitters that mediate the rewarding effects of drugs of abuse are dopamine and opioid peptides. In the *withdrawal/negative affect* stage, the negative emotional state of withdrawal may engage activation of the extended amygdala. The extended amygdala is composed of several basal forebrain structures, including the bed nucleus of the stria terminalis, central nucleus of the amygdala, and possibly a transition zone in the medial portion (or shell) of the nucleus accumbens. Major neurotransmitters in the extended amygdala that are hypothesized to function in negative reinforcement are corticotropin-releasing factor, norepinephrine, and dynorphin. There are major projections from the extended amygdala to the hypothalamus and brainstem. The *preoccupation/anticipation* (craving) stage involves the processing of conditioned reinforcement in the basolateral amygdala and the processing of contextual information by the hippocampus. Executive control depends on the prefrontal cortex and includes the representation of contingencies, the representation of outcomes, and their value and subjective states (i.e., craving and, presumably, feelings) associated with drugs. The subjective effects termed "drug craving" in humans involve activation in functional imaging studies of the orbital and anterior cingulate cortices and temporal lobe, including the amygdala. A major neurotransmitter that is involved in the craving stage is glutamate that is localized in pathways from frontal regions and the basolateral amygdala that project to the ventral striatum. *ACC* anterior cingulate cortex, *BNST* bed nucleus of the stria terminalis, *CeA* central nucleus of the amygdala, *DS* dorsal striatum, *dlPFC* dorsolateral prefrontal cortex, *GP* globus pallidus, *HPC* hippocampus, *NAC* nucleus accumbens, *OFC* orbitofrontal cortex, *Thal* thalamus, *vlPFC* ventrolateral prefrontal cortex, *vmPFC* ventromedial prefrontal cortex [Modified from Koob & Volkow, 2010]

addiction by the opponent-process theory of motivation by Solomon and Corbit (1974). Here, positive hedonic states, once initiated, are automatically modulated by mechanisms that reduce the intensity of hedonic feelings, presumably mediated by the central nervous system, resulting in both affective or hedonic habituation (or tolerance) and affective or hedonic withdrawal (abstinence). Solomon defined two processes: the *a-process* and *b-process*. The *a-process* could consist of either positive or negative hedonic responses (but in the case of addiction, the *a-process* was a positive hedonic response) and occur shortly after the presentation of a stimulus, correlate closely with the stimulus intensity, quality, and duration of the reinforcer, and show tolerance. In contrast, the *b-process* appears after the *a-process* has terminated, is sluggish in onset, is slow to build up to an asymptote, is slow to decay, and gets larger with repeated exposure (Fig. 1.4). Thus, as argued by Solomon (1980) and particularly relevant to our understanding of addiction from the perspective of compulsivity, the affective dynamics of opponent-process theory generate new opportunities for motivating drug-seeking behavior.

More specifically, from a drug-taking perspective, Solomon and Corbit (1974) hypothesized that the initial acute, positive hedonic effects of a drug were opposed or counteracted by homeostatic changes in brain systems. An affect control system was conceptualized to serve as a single negative feedback (or opponent) loop that opposes the stimulus-aroused affective state (Poulos & Cappell, 1991; Siegel, 1975; Solomon & Corbit, 1974). Affective states (in the case of drugs, highly pleasurable states) were hypothesized to be automatically opposed by centrally mediated mechanisms that reduce the intensity of these affective states. In the context of the development of drug dependence, Solomon argued that the first few self-administrations of an opiate drug produce a pattern of motivational changes that are similar to those of an *a-process* or euphoria, followed by a decline in intensity. After the drug's effects wear off, an opposing, aversive negative emotional state emerges, termed the *b-process* (Fig. 1.4). Certain systems in the brain were hypothesized to suppress or reduce departures from hedonic neutrality (Solomon & Corbit, 1974).

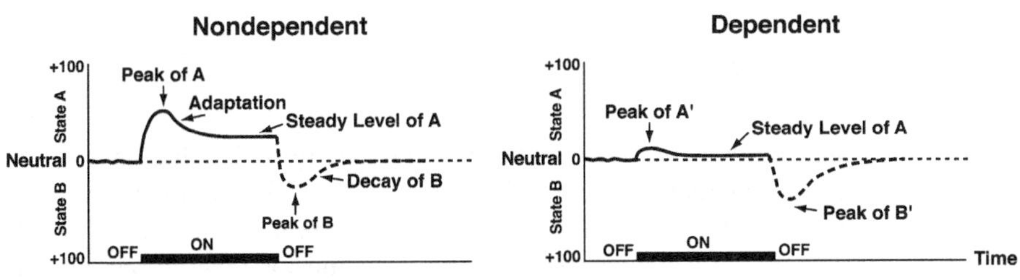

Fig. 1.4 Standard pattern of affective dynamics produced by novel and repeated unconditioned stimuli. See text for details [Taken with permission from Solomon, 1980]

Animal Models of the Dark Side of Addiction

Key to my research on the dark side of addiction was to develop animal models that reflect the hypothetical construct of the opponent process. Dr. Athina Markou and I tested the hypothesis that chronic cocaine self-administration may result in an opposite effect on brain stimulation reward thresholds (i.e., a measure of hedonic activity in the brain), namely an elevation of brain stimulation reward thresholds (Markou & Koob, 1991). Rats were allowed to self-administer cocaine intravenously for long periods of time, and reward thresholds were monitored during the course of cocaine withdrawal (Markou & Koob, 1991). The rats were allowed to self-administer cocaine for different periods of time (3, 6, 12, 24, and 48 h using a within-subjects design). Intracranial self-stimulation (ICSS) thresholds were determined at various time points after termination of the self-administration session (0, 1, 3, 6, 12, 24, 48, and 72 h). Cocaine withdrawal elevated brain stimulation reward thresholds compared with pre-drug baseline levels and compared with thresholds in control animals. The magnitude and duration of the elevation of reward thresholds was proportional to the amount of cocaine self-administered (i.e., the duration of the self-administration session). This elevation of reward thresholds was hypothesized to reflect an anhedonic state, or perhaps more accurately a hypohedonic state, and as such was purported to be homologous to anhedonia or hypohedonia that is reported by human cocaine users (Gawin & Kleber, 1986). The effects of cocaine withdrawal on ICSS thresholds were opposite to those of acute cocaine (Kornetsky & Esposito, 1981), suggesting that during the course of a cocaine self-administration bout and withdrawal, the drug can dramatically alter substrates in the medial forebrain bundle that mediate brain stimulation reward. Subsequent studies showed that the elevation of brain reward thresholds that was associated with withdrawal from chronic administration of drugs of abuse is a common element of all drugs of abuse, including cocaine (Markou & Koob, 1991), amphetamine (Paterson, Myers, & Markou, 2000), opioids (Schulteis, Markou, Gold, Stinus, & Koob, 1994), cannabinoids (Gardner & Vorel, 1998), nicotine (Epping-Jordan, Watkins, Koob, & Markou, 1998), and alcohol (Schulteis, Markou, Cole, & Koob, 1995; Fig. 1.5).

Negative Reinforcement in Addiction

More compelling for the thesis of anti-reward, compulsivity, and addiction was our later work that showed that animal models of prolonged access to intravenous cocaine self-administration, combined with measures of brain stimulation reward, provided key evidence of negative reinforcement mechanisms that are involved in the transition from drug use to compulsive-like drug use. Elevations of baseline reward thresholds were temporally and highly correlated with the escalation of

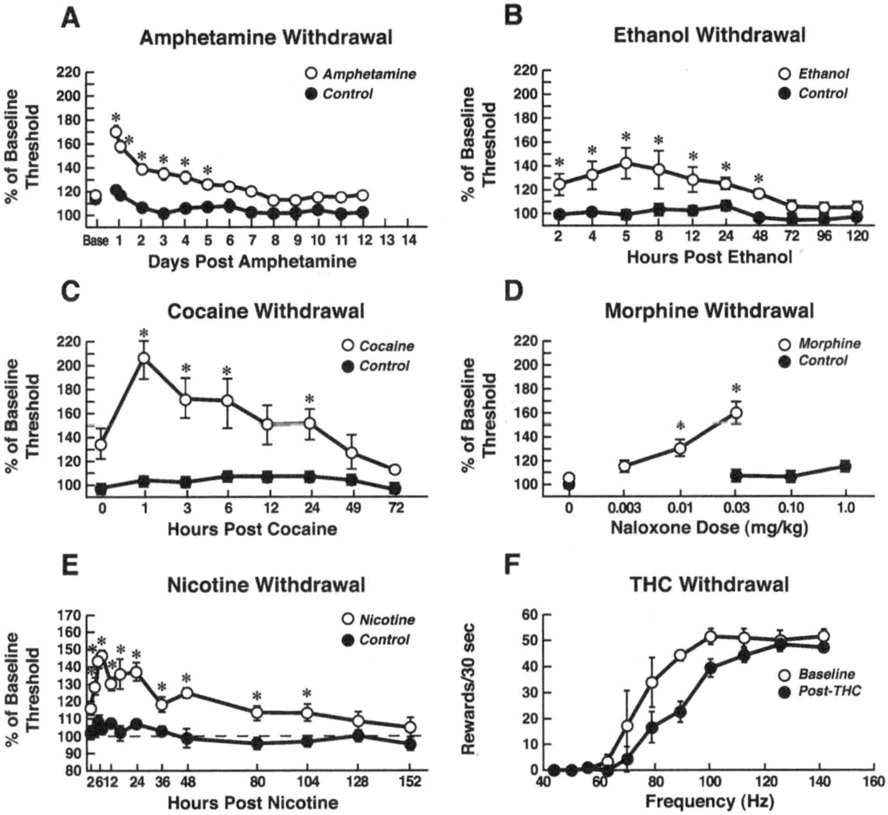

Fig. 1.5 (**a**) Mean intracranial self-stimulation (ICSS) reward thresholds (±SEM) in rats during amphetamine withdrawal (10 mg/kg/day for 6 days). The data are expressed as a percentage of the mean of the last five baseline values prior to drug treatment. (**b**) Mean ICSS thresholds (±SEM) in rats during ethanol withdrawal (blood alcohol levels achieved: 197.29 mg%). Elevations of thresholds were time-dependent. (**c**) Mean ICSS thresholds (±SEM) in rats during cocaine withdrawal 24 h following the cessation of cocaine self-administration. (**d**) Mean ICSS thresholds (±SEM) in rats during naloxone-precipitated morphine withdrawal. The minimum dose of naloxone that elevated ICSS thresholds in the morphine group was 0.01 mg/kg. (**e**) Mean ICSS thresholds (±SEM) in rats during spontaneous nicotine withdrawal following surgical removal of osmotic minipumps that delivered nicotine hydrogen tartrate (9 mg/kg/day) or saline. (**f**) Mean ICSS thresholds (±SEM) in rats during withdrawal from an acute 1.0 mg/kg dose of Δ^9-tetrahydrocannabinol (THC). Withdrawal significantly shifted the reward function to the right (indicating lower reward). Figures taken with permission from Paterson et al. (2000), Schulteis et al. (1994, 1995), Markou and Koob (1991), Epping-Jordan et al. (1998; figure adapted from data), and Gardner and Vorel (1998). Note that because different equipment systems and threshold procedures were used in the collection of the above data, direct comparisons among the magnitude of effects induced by these drugs cannot be made. *$p < 0.05$, significant difference from saline control group

cocaine intake, and post-session elevations of reward thresholds failed to return to baseline levels before the onset of each subsequent cocaine self-administration session, thereby deviating progressively more from control levels (Ahmed, Kenny, Koob, & Markou, 2002). Similar results have been observed with extended access to heroin (Kenny, Chen, Kitamura, Markou, & Koob, 2006) and methamphetamine (Jang, Whitfield, Schulteis, Koob, & Wee, 2013; Fig. 1.6).

These observations supported the hypothesis that opponent processes may be a viable framework for negative emotional states, the avoidance of which engage another source of motivation for drug seeking, namely the removal of the negative emotional state or negative reinforcement. Accompanying the increase in intake observed in the extended-access group, the observation that animals will work harder for the drug on a progressive-ratio schedule of reinforcement suggests enhanced motivation to seek cocaine or enhanced efficacy of cocaine reward (Paterson & Markou, 2003; Wee, Mandyam, Lekic, & Koob, 2008). Such increases in progressive-ratio responding for drug self-administration in animals have now been demonstrated with cocaine, methamphetamine, nicotine, heroin, and alcohol (Barbier et al., 2013; Cohen, Koob, & George, 2012; Walker & Koob, 2007; Wee et al., 2008; Wee, Wang, Woolverton, Pulvirenti, & Koob, 2007). Similarly, extended access to drugs increases drug taking in the presence of aversive consequences. Rats with extended access to cocaine did not suppress drug seeking in the presence of an aversive conditioned stimulus or punishment (Deroche-Gamonet, Belin, & Piazza, 2004; Vanderschuren & Everitt, 2004).

Opponent processes (or drug-opposite responses) have long been hypothesized to occur even with a single injection of a drug and contribute to tolerance (Siegel, 1975). In the domain of reward function, rapid acute tolerance and opponent-process-like effects in response to the hedonic effects of cocaine have been reported in human studies of smoked coca paste (Van Dyke & Byck, 1982; Fig. 1.7).

The onset and intensity of the "high" are very rapid via the smoked route of administration, and rapid tolerance is present, even after a single smoking session. The "high" decreases rapidly, despite blood cocaine levels that remain significantly elevated. Even more intriguing for the "dark side" hypothesis is that human subjects also actually report "dysphoria," despite high blood levels of cocaine. In human laboratory studies, intravenous cocaine produced patterns of a rapid "rush" followed by an increased "low" (Breiter et al., 1997; Fig. 1.8).

In animal models of intravenous cocaine self-administration, similar observations have been quantified in the context of the extended-access model of intravenous cocaine self-administration (Kenny, Gasparini, & Markou, 2003). Here, elevations of reward threshold begin rapidly and can be observed within a single session of self-administration (Kenny et al., 2003; Fig. 1.9), bearing a striking resemblance to human subjective reports. These results demonstrate that the elevation of brain reward thresholds following prolonged access to cocaine failed to return to baseline levels between repeated, prolonged exposure to cocaine self-administration (i.e., residual hysteresis), thus creating a progressively greater elevation of "baseline" ICSS thresholds. These data provide compelling evidence of brain reward dysfunction in escalated cocaine self-administration that parallels the increased motivation to take drug under conditions of extended access.

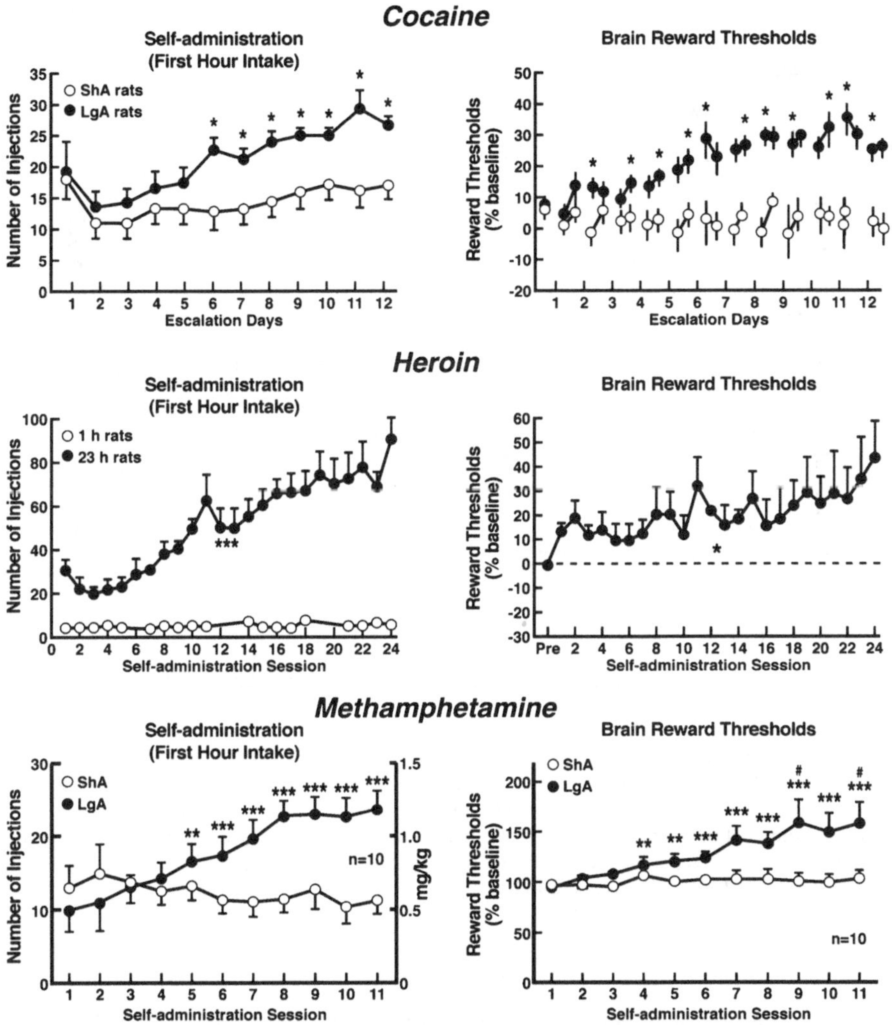

Fig. 1.6 (**a**) Relationship between elevation of ICSS reward thresholds and cocaine intake escalation. (*Left*) Percent change from baseline response latencies (3 h and 17–22 h after each self-administration session; first data point indicates 1 h before the first session). (*Right*) Percent change from baseline ICSS thresholds. *$p < 0.05$, compared with drug-naive and/or ShA rats (tests for simple main effects) [Taken with permission from Ahmed et al., 2002]. (**b**) Unlimited daily access to heroin escalated heroin intake and decreased the excitability of brain reward systems. (*Left*) Heroin intake (±SEM; 20 μg per infusion) in rats during limited (1 h) or unlimited (23 h) self-administration sessions. ***$p < 0.001$, main effect of access (1 or 23 h). (*Right*) Percent change from baseline ICSS thresholds (± SEM) in 23 h rats. Reward thresholds, assessed immediately after each daily 23 h self-administration session, became progressively more elevated as exposure to self-administered heroin increased across sessions. *$p < 0.05$, main effect of heroin on reward thresholds [Taken with permission from Kenny et al., 2006]. (**c**) Escalation of methamphetamine self-administration and ICSS in rats. Rats were daily allowed to receive ICSS in the lateral hypothalamus 1 h before and 3 h after intravenous methamphetamine self-administration with either Fig. 1.6 (continued) 1- or 6-h access. (*Left*) Methamphetamine self-administration during the first hour of each session. (*Right*) ICSS measured 1 h before and 3 h after methamphetamine self-administration. *$p < 0.05$, **$p < 0.01$, ***$p < 0.001$, compared with session 1; $^{\#}p < 0.05$, compared with LgA 3 h after [Taken with permission from Jang et al., 2013]

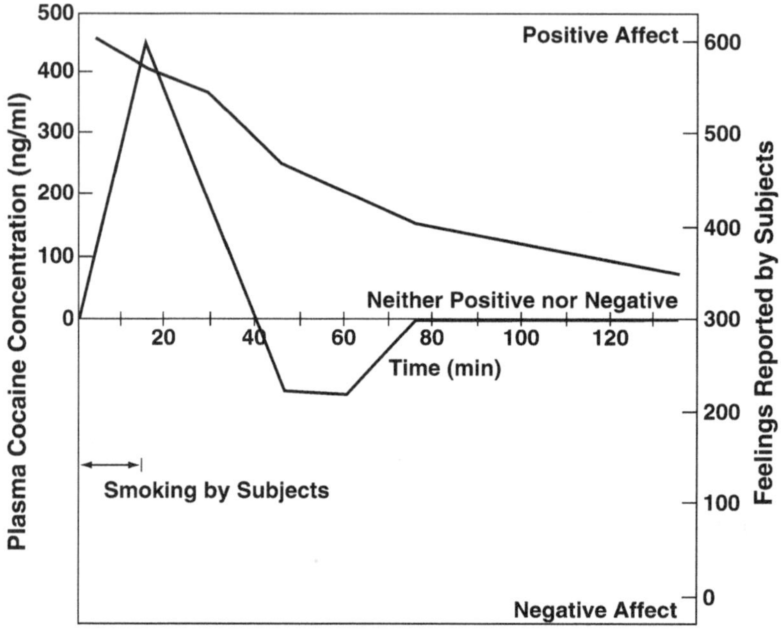

Fig. 1.7 Dysphoric feelings followed the initial euphoria in experimental subjects who smoked cocaine paste, although the plasma concentration of cocaine remained relatively high. The dysphoria is characterized by anxiety, depression, fatigue, and a desire for more cocaine. The peak feelings for the subjects were probably reached shortly before the peak plasma concentration, but the first psychological measurements were made later than the plasma assay. Therefore, the temporal sequence of the peaks that are shown in the figure cannot be regarded as definitive [Taken with permission from Van Dyke & Byck, 1982]

Similar results have been observed with dysphoria-like responses that accompany acute opioid and alcohol withdrawal (Liu & Schulteis, 2004; Schulteis & Liu, 2006). Naloxone administration following single injections of morphine elevated brain stimulation reward thresholds, and threshold elevations increased further with repeated experience with morphine administration and naloxone-precipitated withdrawal (Liu & Schulteis, 2004). Similar results were observed during repeated acute withdrawal from alcohol (Schulteis & Liu, 2006).

Neurobiological Bases for the Dark Side of Addiction

Clear evidence of an opponent-process-like elevation of reward thresholds and establishment of an aversive motivational state with extended access to drugs in animal models led to the challenge of investigating the neurobiological bases for

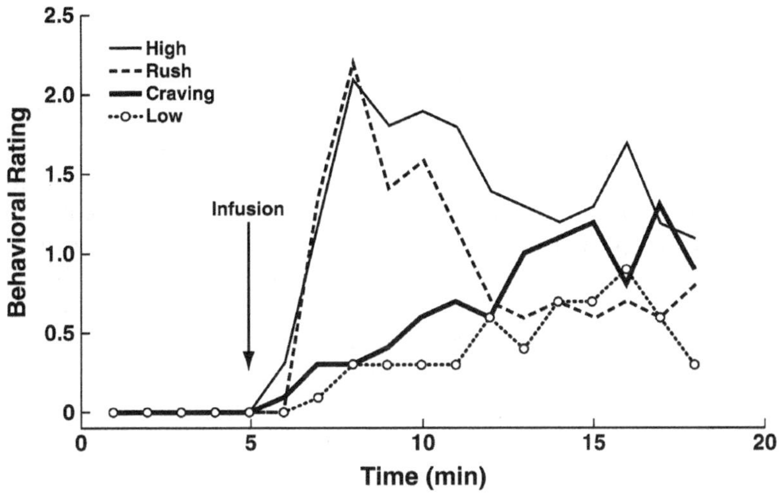

Fig. 1.8 Average behavioral ratings after an infusion of cocaine (0.6 mg/kg over 30 s; $n = 9$). The rush, high, low, and craving ratings were averaged within each category for the subjects who had interpretable cocaine functional magnetic resonance imaging data after motion correction and behavioral ratings time-locked to the scanner. Both peak rush and peak high occurred 3 min post-infusion. Peak low (primary reports of dysphoria and paranoia) occurred 11 min post-infusion. Peak craving occurred 12 min post-infusion. No subject reported effects from the saline infusion on any of the four measures. Ratings obtained for rush, high, low, and craving measures were higher in subjects blinded to the 0.6 mg/kg cocaine dose compared with subjects unblinded to a 0.2 mg/kg cocaine dose [Taken with permission from Breiter et al., 1997]

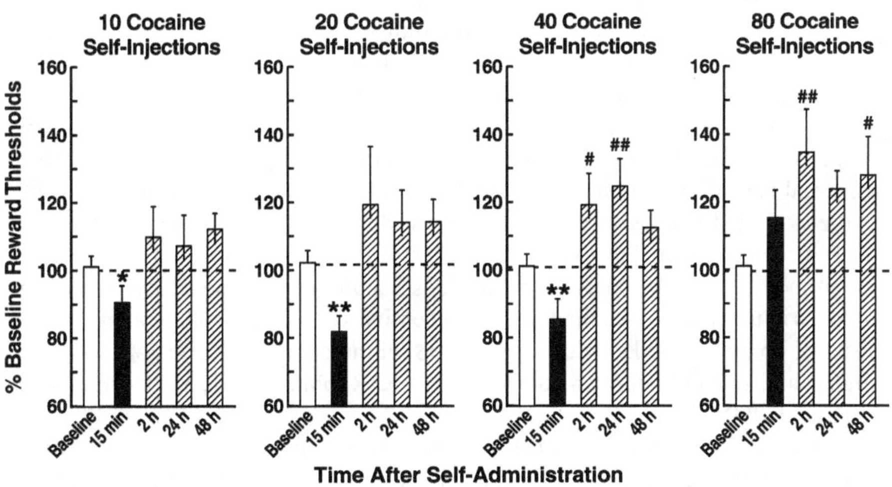

Fig. 1.9 Rats ($n = 11$) were allowed to self-administer 10, 20, 40, and 80 injections of cocaine (0.25 mg per injection), and intracranial self-stimulation reward thresholds were measured 15 min and 2, 24, and 48 h after the end of each intravenous cocaine self-administration session. The horizontal dotted line in each plot represents 100% of baseline levels. All data are presented as mean + SEM percentage of baseline reward thresholds. $^{*}p < 0.05$, $^{**}p < 0.01$, compared with baseline (paired t-test); $^{\#}p < 0.05$, $^{\#\#}p < 0.01$, compared with baseline (Fisher's least significant difference test after a statistically significant effect in the repeated-measures analysis of variance) [Taken with permission from Kenny et al., 2003]

such hypothesized counteradaptive hedonic states. Two mechanisms were proposed: within-system neuroadaptations and between-system neuroadaptations (Koob & Bloom, 1988). Within-system neuroadaptations were defined as the process by which the primary cellular response element to the drug (circuit A) adapts to neutralize the drug's effects. Persistence of the opposing effects after the drug disappears produces adaptation. A between-system neuroadaptation was defined as a circuitry change, in which circuit B (i.e., stress or anti-reward circuits) is activated by circuit A (i.e., the reward circuit). Clearly, within-system neuroadaptations can also dynamically interact with between-system neuroadaptations, in which circuit B (i.e., the anti-reward circuit) is activated either in parallel or in series to suppress the activity of circuit A. Substantial data have been marshalled to argue for chronic deviation of the reward set point that is fueled by both the decreased activity of reward circuits (within-system change) and the recruitment of brain and hormonal stress responses (between-system change).

As noted above, the presence of motivational signs of withdrawal in humans, observed during the *withdrawal/negative affect* stage, includes chronic irritability, physical pain, emotional pain, malaise, dysphoria, alexithymia, and the loss of motivation for natural rewards, a general hypersensitivity to a negative emotional state termed "hyperkatifeia" (Shurman, Koob, & Gutstein, 2010). The neuranatomical substrates for the motivational signs of withdrawal derive largely from animal studies but can be argued to be mediated largely by the neurocircuitry of a neuroanatomical construct known as the "extended amygdala."

The extended amygdala is composed of the bed nucleus of the stria terminalis, the central nucleus of the amygdala, and a transition zone in the medial subregion of the nucleus accumbens (shell of the nucleus accumbens). These regions have cytoarchitectural similarities and similar neuroanatomical connections. Furthermore, these regions of the extended amygdala receive numerous afferents from limbic structures, such as the basolateral amygdala and hippocampus, and send efferents to the medial part of the ventral pallidum and lateral hypothalamus, thus further defining the extended amygdala as a brain region that interfaces classic limbic (emotional) structures with the extrapyramidal motor system (Alheid, De Olmos, & Beltramino, 1995). The shell of the nucleus accumbens is also a key part of the ventral striatum and as such mediates the incentive salience-pathological habit component of compulsive-like behavior via neuro circuits that comprise corticostriatal, pallidal, and thalamic-cortical loops (Everitt & Robbins, 2005; Haber, Fudge, & McFarland, 2000).

From a within-system framework, decreases in dopaminergic transmission in the ventral striatum (nucleus accumbens) during drug withdrawal have been systematically observed with most drugs of abuse. Measures include decreases in extracellular dopamine in the nucleus accumbens as measured by in vivo microdialysis during withdrawal from drugs of abuse (Parsons & Justice, 1993; Weiss, Markou, Lorang, & Koob, 1992) and also decreases in the firing of dopaminergic neurons in the ventral tegmental area (Diana, Pistis, Carboni, Gessa, & Rossetti, 1993; Diana, Pistis, Muntoni, & Gessa, 1995; Grieder et al., 2012; Tan, Bishop, Lauzon, Sun, &

Laviolette, 2009). Human imaging studies of individuals with addiction during withdrawal or protracted abstinence have generated results that are consistent with animal studies, suggesting decreased presynaptic release (Ashok, Mizuno, Volkow, & Howes, 2017). There are decreases in dopamine D_2 receptors (hypothesized to reflect hypodopaminergic functioning), hyporesponsiveness to dopamine challenge (Volkow, Fowler, & Wang, 2003), and hypoactivity of the orbitofrontal-infralimbic cortex system (Volkow et al., 2003).

At the molecular level, within-system changes include the perturbation of intracellular signal transduction pathways. Many of these are drug-specific changes, such as an increase in the sensitivity of opioid receptor transduction mechanisms in the nucleus accumbens during opioid withdrawal (Stinus, Le Moal, & Koob, 1990), a decrease in γ-aminobutyric acid (GABA)-ergic transmission, and increase in *N*-methyl-D-aspartate (NMDA) glutamatergic transmission during alcohol withdrawal (Davidson, Shanley, & Wilce, 1995; Morrisett, 1994; Roberts, Cole, & Koob, 1996; Weiss et al., 1996), and differential regional changes in nicotinic receptor function (Collins, Bhat, Pauly, & Marks, 1990; Dani & Heinemann, 1996).

Other molecular changes within the incentive salience-reward circuitry that may be common to all drugs of abuse include upregulation of a postsynaptic G_s/cyclic adenosine monophosphate (cAMP)/protein kinase A signaling pathway in the nucleus accumbens that is central to establishing and maintaining the addicted state (Edwards & Koob, 2010). Transcription factors, such as cAMP response element binding protein (CREB), and downstream ΔFosB, nuclear factor κB, and CDK5, can also change gene expression and produce long-term changes in protein expression and thus neuronal function (Nestler, 2005) and even structural changes in the cytoskeleton of neurons via actions on actin (Russo et al., 2010). Thus, within-system molecular changes may form a significant mechanism by which genetic/epigenetic factors influence the vulnerability to negative emotional states that are associated with excessive drug use.

In the domain of between-system neuroadaptations, the hypothesis is that neurobiological systems that are involved in arousal and stress become engaged to overcome the chronic presence of the perturbing drug and restore normal function despite the presence of drug (Koob, 2008). Neurobiological systems that are currently implicated in such between-system neuroadaptations include corticotropin-releasing factor (CRF), dynorphin, norepinephrine, hypocretin, vasopressin, glucocorticoids, and neuroinflammatory factors.

Two neuropeptides, CRF and dynorphin, have been long known to be activated in stress and produce aversive effects in animals. CRF and dynorphin are recruited in the extended amygdala and are hypothesized to contribute to negative emotional states (hyperkatifeia) of drug withdrawal. Both the hypothalamic–pituitary–adrenal (HPA) axis and extrahypothalamic brain stress systems that are mediated by CRF are dysregulated by chronic administration of all major drugs with dependence or abuse potential, with a common response of elevated adrenocorticotropic hormone, corticosterone, and amygdala CRF during acute withdrawal (Delfs, Zhu, Druhan, & Aston-Jones, 2000; Koob, 2009; Koob, Heinrichs, Menzaghi, Pich, & Britton, 1994;

Merlo-Pich et al., 1995; Olive, Koenig, Nannini, & Hodge, 2002; Rasmussen et al., 2000; Rivier, Bruhn, & Vale, 1984; Roberto et al., 2010). Indeed, activation of the HPA axis may be an early dysregulation that is associated with excessive drug taking that ultimately "sensitizes" extrahypothalamic CRF systems (Koob & Kreek, 2007; Vendruscolo et al., 2012). Both high-dose chronic glucocorticoids and high-dose chronic alcohol exposure downregulate the HPA axis by blunting the expression of CRF in the paraventricular nucleus of the hypothalamus but drive an increase in CRF expression in the central nucleus of the amygdala (Fig. 1.10). Via this mechanism, activation of the CRF stress axis (pituitary adrenal and extrahypothalamic CRF systems) may partially mediate the negative emotional responses that are associated with acute and protracted abstinence for all major drugs of abuse. These negative emotional states can be reversed by CRF receptor antagonists during acute withdrawal and protracted abstinence from all major drugs of abuse (Koob, 2015). For example, neuropharmacological studies showed that a CRF_1 receptor antagonist reversed the elevation of brain stimulation reward thresholds associated with alcohol and nicotine withdrawal (Bruijnzeel et al., 2010, 2012; Bruijnzeel, Prado, & Isaac, 2009; Bruijnzeel, Zislis, Wilson, & Gold, 2007).

Providing evidence of the direct relevance of activation of the CRF system to the construct of negative reinforcement, CRF receptor antagonists selectively blocked

Fig. 1.10 (continued) which in turn stimulates adrenocorticotropic hormone release from the pituitary, which results in enhanced release of glucocorticoids from the adrenal gland. High levels of glucocorticoids through negative feedback decrease CRF synthesis at the level of the PVN but activate CRF activity at the level of the central nucleus of the amygdala. Extrahypothalamic CRF stress system: Stressful stimuli also activate CRF systems in the basal forebrain, notably the bed nucleus of the stria terminalis and the central nucleus of the amygdala, to help mediate behavioral responses to stressors and mediate sympathetic activation associated with stressors. Glucocorticoids, instead of exerting a feedback suppression of CRF synthesis in the central nucleus of the amygdala, actually increase the synthesis of CRF, providing a means for extending the contribution of the brain stress systems to allostasis. *ACTH* adrenocorticotropic hormone, *AMYG* amygdala, *BNST* bed nucleus of the stria terminalis, *CRF* corticotropin-releasing factor, *HPC* hippocampus, *NE* norepinephrine, *PIT* pituitary gland, *PFC* prefrontal cortex, *PVN* paraventricular nucleus. (**b**) Chronic corticosterone exposure produces a blunted HPA axis vs. sensitized central nucleus of the amygdala. CRF mRNA hybridization levels in the (Left) dorsal part of the lateral bed nucleus of the stria terminalis (BSTLD) and (Right) ventral part induced by corticosterone pellet (200 mg) implantation over 2 weeks. Control rats (n = 12) were obtained from the pool of rats that were sacrificed at the same time points as the experimental groups (n = 7 for each time point). The data are expressed as mean ± SEM. $*p < 0.05$, vs. control [Taken with permission from Makino, Gold, & Schulkin, 1994]. (**c**) Chronic alcohol exposure produces a blunted HPA axis vs. sensitized central nucleus of the amygdala. (Left) CRF mRNA was significantly decreased in the pPVN in alcohol-dependent animals compared with alcohol-naive controls ($*p = 0.01$) but not compared with nondependent animals [Taken with permission from Richardson, Lee, O'Dell, Koob, & Rivier, 2008]. (Right) In alcohol-dependent rats (n = 8), the levels of CRF mRNA, normalized to cyclophilin A, were significantly increased in punches of the central nucleus of the amygdala ($*p < 0.05$) compared with naive (n = 11) controls, measured by quantitative real-time polymerase chain reaction [Taken with permission from Roberto et al., 2010]

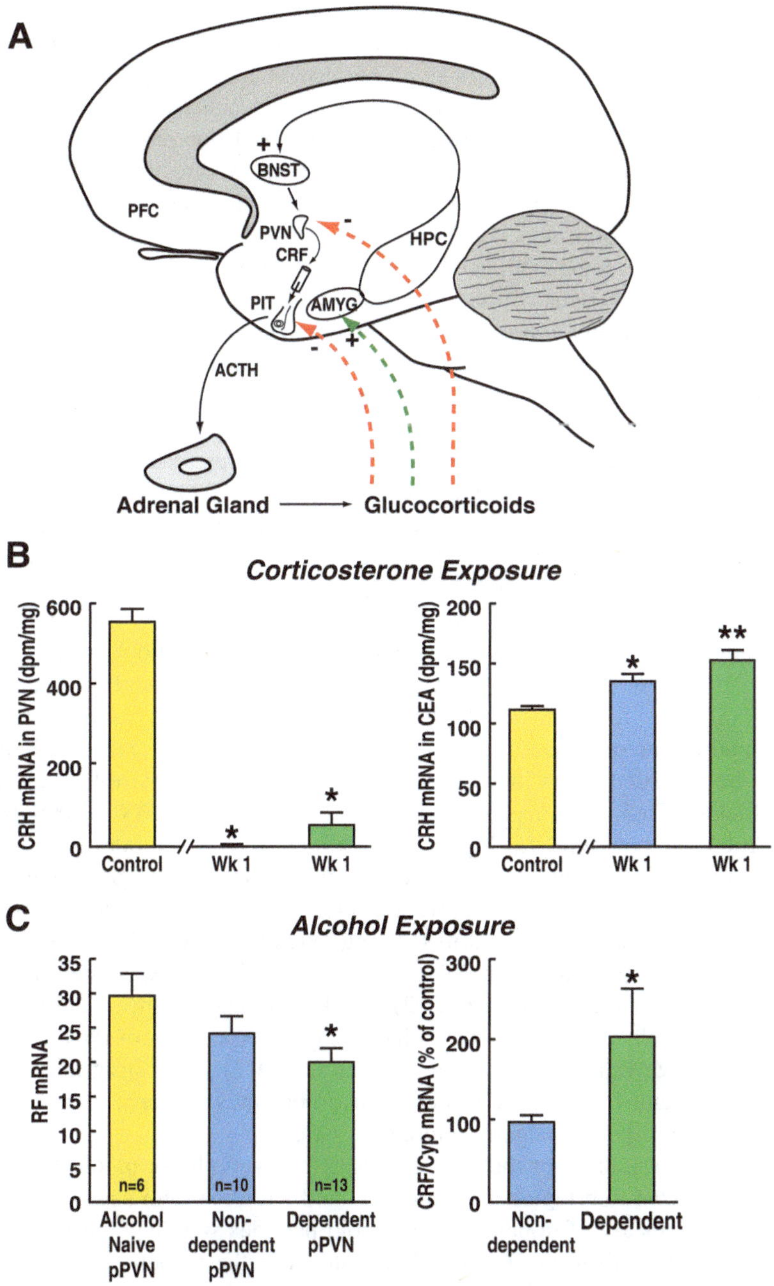

Fig. 1.10 (**a**) The central role of corticotropin-releasing factor in the hypothalamic–pituitary–adrenal stress axis. The functional interactions between glucocorticoids, CRF, and stress represent an exquisitely balanced hormonal stress response system and an allostatically sensitive brain stress system (see text). Hypothalamic–pituitary–adrenal stress system: Stressful stimuli increase CRF,

the increase in intravenous drug self-administration associated with extended access to cocaine (Specio et al., 2008), nicotine (George et al., 2007), and heroin (Greenwell et al., 2009). Systemic injections of small-molecule CRF_1 antagonists also blocked the escalated increase in alcohol intake associated with acute withdrawal following induction of dependence (Funk, Zorrilla, Lee, Rice, & Koob, 2007) and protracted abstinence (Gehlert et al., 2007). When administered directly into the central nucleus of the amygdala, a CRF_1/CRF_2 antagonist blocked alcohol self-administration in alcohol-dependent rats (Funk, O'Dell, Crawford, & Koob, 2006). These effects appear to be mediated by the actions of CRF on GABAergic interneurons in the central nucleus of the amygdala. A CRF receptor antagonist that was administered chronically during the development of dependence blocked the development of compulsive-like responding for alcohol (Roberto et al., 2010) and the escalation of heroin intake (Park et al., 2015). Altogether, these results suggest that CRF in the basal forebrain may also play an important role in the development of the negative emotional effects that drive the increase in drug seeking associated with cocaine, heroin, nicotine, and alcohol dependence (Fig. 1.11).

In contrast to the well-documented encephalin/endorphin-μ opioid receptor system that mediates positive hedonic effects, the dynorphin-κ opioid system has long been hypothesized to play a role in negative emotional states. κ opioid receptor agonists (dynorphins) produce aversive dysphoric-like effects in animals and humans and have been hypothesized to mediate negative emotional states (Mucha & Herz, 1985; Pfeiffer, Brantl, Herz, & Emrich, 1986; Shippenberg, Zapata, & Chefer, 2007; Wee & Koob, 2010). The depression-like aversive responses to stress and dysphoric-like responses during withdrawal from drugs of abuse are hypothesized to be mediated by an increase in dynorphin's actions (Chartoff et al., 2012; Knoll, Meloni, Thomas, Carroll, & Carlezon, 2007; Land et al., 2008, 2009; Mague et al., 2003; McLaughlin, Li, Valdez, Chavkin, & Chavkin, 2006; McLaughlin, Marton-Popovici, & Chavkin, 2003; Redila & Chavkin, 2008; Schindler, Li, & Chavkin, 2010). Dynorphin/κ opioid receptor antagonists can also block the compulsive-like responding for drugs during extended access (Schlosburg et al., 2013; Walker, Zorrilla, & Koob, 2010; Wee, Orio, Ghirmai, Cashman, & Koob, 2009; Whitfield et al., 2015; Fig. 1.12). A likely target for these actions is the extended amygdala, particularly the shell of the nucleus accumbens (Nealey, Smith, Davis, Smith, & Walker, 2011; Schlosburg et al., 2013), suggesting that multiple distributed systems from the brainstem and hypothalamus converge in the extended amygdala to contribute to negative emotional states.

Even more intriguing for the present thesis, the dynorphin-κ opioid system has been hypothesized to bridge between-system and within-system neuroadaptations. The excessive release of dopamine and opioid peptides was hypothesized to produce subsequent activation of dynorphin systems in the nucleus accumbens and then feedback to decrease dopamine release and contribute to the dysphoric syndrome that is associated with cocaine dependence (Carlezon, Nestler, & Neve, 2000; Nestler, 2001).

Other pro-stress, pro-dysphoria-inducing brain neurotransmitter systems that converge on the extended amygdala include norepinephrine, vasopressin, substance

Addiction / Corticotropin-Releasing Factor Interactions

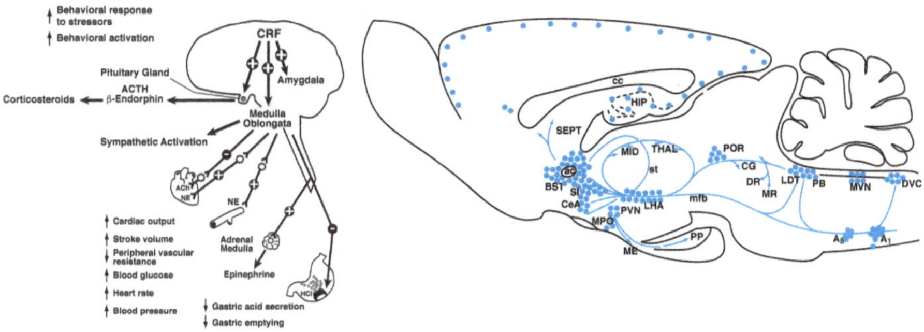

	CRF Antagonist Effects			
Withdrawal-induced changes in extracellular CRF in CeA	Withdrawal-induced anxiety-like or aversive responses	Baseline self-administration or place preference	Dependence-induced increases in self-administration	Stress-induced reinstatement
↑	↓	—	↓	↓

Fig. 1.11 (Top left) The multiple actions of CRF in mediating stress responses in the body. CRF drives the hypothalamic–pituitary–adrenal axis by acting to release adrenocorticotropic hormone (ACTH) in the portal system of the pituitary. CRF activates the sympathetic system by actions in the brainstem and mediates arousal and behavioral responses to stressors by actions in the amygdala, other basal forebrain regions, and the ventral midbrain, such as the ventral tegmental area. *Ach* acetylcholine, *NE* norepinephrine [Taken with permission from Koob, 2010]. (Top right) Localizations and projections of brain stress systems—CRF. The major CRF-stained cell groups (dots) and fiber systems in the rat brain. Most of the immunoreactive cells and fibers appear to be associated with systems that regulate the output of the pituitary and the autonomic nervous system and with cortical interneurons. Most of the longer central fibers course either ventrally through the medial forebrain bundle and its caudal extension in the reticular formation or dorsally through a periventricular system in the thalamus and brainstem central gray. The direction of fibers in these systems is unclear because they appear to interconnect regions that contain CRF-stained cell bodies. Three adjacent CRF-stained cell groups—laterodorsal tegmental nucleus, locus coeruleus, and parabrachial nucleus—lie in the dorsal pons. Uncertain is which of these cell groups contribute to each of the pathways shown and which of them receives inputs from the same pathways [Modified with permission from Swanson, Sawchenko, Rivier, & Vale, 1983]. *ac* anterior commissure, *BST* bed nucleus of the stria terminalis, *cc* corpus callosum, *CeA* central nucleus of the amygdala, *CG* central gray, *DR* dorsal raphe, *DVC* dorsal vagal complex, *HIP* hippocampus, *LDT* laterodorsal tegmental nucleus, *LHA* lateral hypothalamic area, *ME* median eminence, *mfb* medial forebrain bundle, *MID THAL* midline thalamic nuclei, *MPO* medial preoptic area, *MR* median raphe, *MVN* medial vestibular nucleus, *PB* parabrachial nucleus, *POR* perioculomotor nucleus, *PP* peripeduncular nucleus, *PVN* paraventricular nucleus, *SEPT* septal region, *SI* substantia innominata, *st* stria terminalis [Modified with permission from Swanson et al., 1983]. (Bottom) The role of CRF in drug dependence (see text for details)

P, hypocretin (orexin), and dynorphin, which may all contribute to negative emotional states associated with drug withdrawal or protracted abstinence (Koob, 2008). Using a compulsive-like alcohol seeking model of excessive drinking in dependent rats during withdrawal, a β-adrenergic receptor antagonist, α_1 adrenergic receptor antagonist, κ opioid receptor antagonist, vasopressin 1b receptor antagonist, glucocorticoid receptor antagonist, and neuroimmune system antagonist all blocked

Summary of Drugs of Abuse Interactions with κ-Opiod / Dynorphin Systems

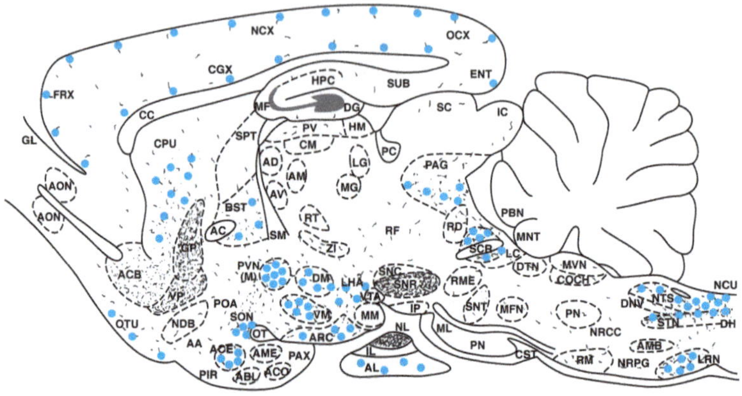

	κ-Opioid Antagonist Effects			
Withdrawal-induced changes in dynorphin peptide and prodynorphin mRNA in NAc	**Withdrawal-induced anxiety-like or aversive responses**	**Baseline self-administration or place preference**	**Dependence-induced increases in self-administration**	**Stress-induced reinstatement**
↑	↓	↑	↓	↓

Fig. 1.12 Localizations and projections of brain stress systems. Dynorphin. Schematic representation of the distribution of prodynorphin-derived peptides in the rat central nervous system determined by immunohistochemistry. Prodynorphin codes for several active opioid peptides that contain the sequence of [Leu]enkephalin, including dynorphin A, dynorphin B, and α-neoendorphin. This precursor is distributed in neuronal systems that are found at all levels of the neuraxis. Like their proenkephalin counterparts, the prodynorphin neurons form both short- and long-tract projections that are often found in parallel with the proenkephalin systems. Neuronal perikarya are shown as solid circles, and fibers-terminals are shown as short curved lines and dots [Modified with permission from Khachaturian, Lewis, Schafer, & Watson, 1985]. *AA* anterior amygdala, *ABL* basolateral nucleus of amygdala, *AC* anterior commissure, *ACB* nucleus accumbens, *ACE* central nucleus of the amygdala, *ACO* cortical nucleus of amygdala, *AD* anterodorsal nucleus of thalamus, *AL* anterior lobe of pituitary, *AM* anteromedial nucleus of thalamus, *AMB* nucleus ambiguus, *AME* medial nucleus of the amygdala, *AON* anterior olfactory nucleus, *ARC* arcuate nucleus, *AV* anteroventral nucleus of thalamus, *BST* bed nucleus of the stria terminalis, *CC* corpus callosum, *CGX* cingulate cortex, *CM* central-medial nucleus of thalamus, *COCH* cochlear nuclear complex, *CPU* caudate-putamen, *CST* corticospinal tract, *DH* dorsal horn of spinal cord, *DG* dentate gyrus, *DM* dorsomedial nucleus of hypothalamus, *DNV* dorsal motor nucleus of vagus, *DTN* dorsal tegmental nucleus, *ENT* entorhinal cortex, *FN* fastigial nucleus of cerebellum, *FRX* frontal cortex, *GL* glomerular layer of olfactory bulb, *GP* globus pallidus, *HM* medial habenular nucleus, *HPC* hippocampus, *IC* inferior colliculus, *IL* intermediate lobe of pituitary, *IP* interpeduncular nuclear complex, *LC* nucleus locus coeruleus, *LG* lateral geniculate nucleus, *LHA* lateral hypothalamic area, *LRN* lateral reticular nucleus, *MF* mossy fibers of hippocampus, *MFN* motor facial nucleus, *MG* medial geniculate nucleus, *ML* medial lemniscus, *MM* medial mammillary nucleus, *MNT* mesencephalic nucleus of trigeminal, *MVN* medial vestibular nucleus, *NCU* nucleus cuneatus, *NCX* neocortex, *NDB* nucleus of diagonal band, *NL* neural lobe of pituitary, *NRGC* nucleus reticularis gigantocellularis, *NRPG* nucleus reticularis paragigantocellularis, *NTS* nucleus tractus solitarius, *OCX* occipital cortex, *OT* optic tract, *OTU* olfactory tubercle, *PAG* periaqueductal gray, *PAX* periamygdaloid cortex, *PBN* parabrachial nucleus, *PC* posterior commissure, *PIR* piriform cortex, *PN* pons, *POA* preoptic area, *PP* perforant path, *PV* periventricular nucleus of thalamus, *PVN(M)*

excessive drinking (Edwards, Guerrero, Ghoneim, Roberts, & Koob, 2011; Gilpin & Koob, 2010; June et al., 2015; Vendruscolo et al., 2012; Walker & Koob, 2008; Walker, Rasmussen, Raskind, & Koob, 2008). Using the extended-access self-administration model of compulsive-like drug seeking, a substance P antagonist and hypocretin-2 antagonist blocked heroin intake (Barbier et al., 2013; Schmeichel et al., 2015). Thus, the activation of pro-stress, pro-negative emotional states that set up negative reinforcement is multi-determined and comprises the neurochemical bases for the hedonic opponent processes that are described above.

However, a neurotransmitter buffer system, also multi-determined, in the extended amygdala may be activated by the brain stress systems and is hypothesized to help return the organism to motivational homeostasis. Neurotransmitter systems that are implicated in such anti-stress actions include neuropeptide Y, nociceptin, and endocannabinoids (Koob, 2017). For example, neuropeptide Y has been hypothesized to act in opposition to the actions of increases in CRF (Heilig & Koob, 2007). Substantial evidence suggests that the activation of neuropeptide Y in the central nucleus of the amygdala can block the motivational aspects of dependence associated with chronic alcohol administration (Gilpin, Misra, & Koob, 2008; Gilpin, Stewart, Murphy, Li, & Badia-Elder, 2003; Thorsell et al., 2007; Thorsell, Slawecki, & Ehlers, 2005a, 2005b). The role of neuropeptide Y in the actions of other drugs of abuse is limited, particularly with regard to dependence and compulsive drug seeking, but the hypothesis here would be that neuropeptide Y is a buffer or homeostatic response to between-system neuroadaptations that can return the brain emotional systems to a homeostatic state (Heilig & Koob, 2007; Valdez & Koob, 2004). Similar hypotheses have been generated for nociceptin (also known as orphanin FQ), which generally attenuates stress-like responses and has a broad anxiolytic-like profile in animals (Ciccocioppo, Economidou, Fedeli, & Massi, 2003; Martin-Fardon, Zorrilla, Ciccocioppo, & Weiss, 2010), and endocannabinoids, in which the elevation of interstitial endocannabinoid levels through the inhibition of endocannabinoid clearance mechanisms in the amygdala is hypothesized to produce anxiolytic-like effects in various animal models of anxiety, particularly under stressful or aversive conditions (Serrano & Parsons, 2011). Thus, one could hypothesize that in parallel with activated brain stress systems, the decreased function of stress buffer systems (e.g., neuropeptide Y, nociceptin, and endocannabinoids) may also contribute to the negative affective disturbances that are associated with drug dependence and protracted withdrawal (Fig. 1.13).

Fig. 1.12 (continued) paraventricular nucleus (pars magnocellularis), *PVN(P)* paraventricular nucleus (pars parvocellularis), *RD* nucleus raphe dorsalis, *RE* nucleus reuniens of thalamus, *RF* reticular formation, *RM* nucleus raphe magnus, *RME* nucleus raphe medianus, *SC* superior colliculus, *SCP* superior cerebellar peduncle, *SM* stria medullaris thalami, *SNC* substantia nigra (pars compacta), *SNR* substantia nigra (pars reticulata), *SNT* sensory nucleus of trigeminal (main), *SON* supraoptic nucleus, *SPT* septal nuclei, *STN* spinal nucleus of trigeminal, *SUB* subiculum, *VM* ventromedial nucleus of hypothalamus, *VP* ventral pallidum, *ZI* zona incerta [Modified with permission from Khachaturian et al., 1985]. (Bottom) The role of dynorphin in drug dependence (see text for details)

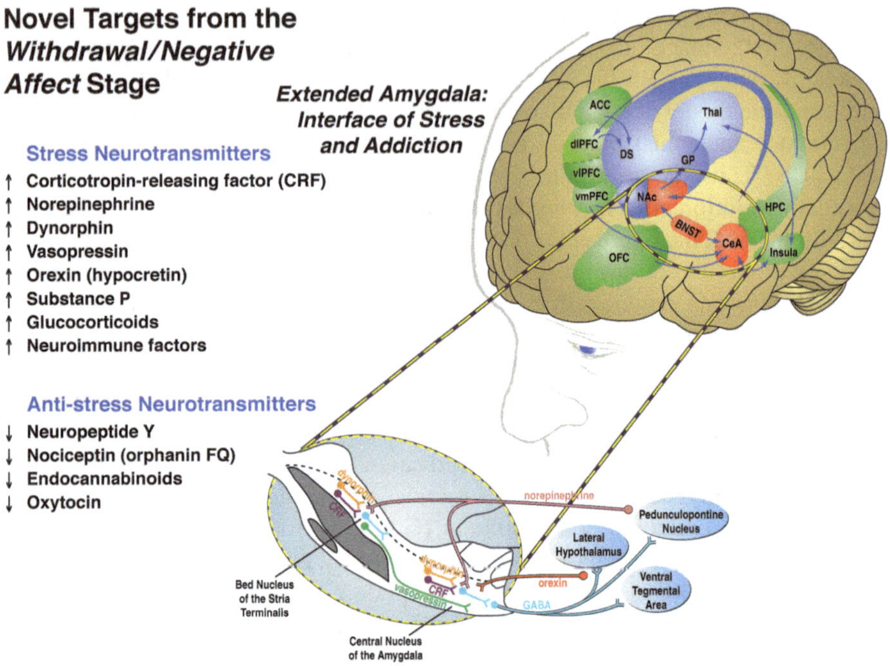

Fig. 1.13 Neurochemical players and neuroanatomical connections hypothesized to contribute to the negative emotional states that drive negative reinforcement. The neurotransmitters/neuromodulators with an up-arrow indicate activation associated with the induction of negative emotional states. The neurotransmitters/neuromodulators with a down-arrow indicate hypoactivation associated with the induction or prolongation of negative emotional states. *CeA* central nucleus of the amygdala, *DS* dorsal striatum, *GP* globus pallidus, *HPC* hippocampus, *NAC* nucleus accumbens, *Thal* thalamus [Taken with permission from George & Koob, 2013]. The enlargement shows the hypothesized interaction of the brain stress systems and the extended amygdala. Note that dynorphin may activate CRF neurons or be activated by CRF neurons, that norepinephrine and CRF are hypothesized to be involved in a feed-forward circuit, and that vasopressin for the central nucleus of the amygdala is hypothesized to derive from the bed nucleus of the stria terminalis. Neuropeptide Y and nociceptin are not depicted in this figure but may act either via modulation of the CRF system or independently, directly on the output of the central nucleus of the amygdala (to be determined) [Taken with permission from Koob, 2008]

Compulsivity in Addiction: A Dark Side View

Compulsivity is a term that has multiple meanings and certainly multiple etiologies. Compulsivity has been defined as elements of behavior that result in repetitive, perseverative behaviors in the face of adverse consequences and repetitive behaviors that are inappropriate to a particular situation. From a psychiatric perspective, individuals who suffer from compulsions often recognize that the behaviors are harmful, but they nonetheless feel emotionally compelled to perform them.

Doing so reduces tension, stress, or anxiety (Berlin & Hollander, 2014; Robbins, Gillan, Smith, de Wit, & Ersche, 2012). A similar argument has been made for addiction (see above), where the development of the negative emotional state of motivational withdrawal serves as an unconditioned reinforcer to drive the negative reinforcement associated with addiction (Koob & Le Moal, 2005, 2008).

Thus, the overall conceptual hypothesis here is that drug addiction represents a break with homeostatic emotional regulatory mechanisms. Such a break begins with initial excessive drug use and subsequent acute motivational withdrawal, followed by chronic excessive drug self-administration and the sensitization of motivational withdrawal. However, even with the cessation of excessive drug taking and prolonged abstinence, the perturbations to the brain reward and stress systems are hypothesized to leave a residual neuroadaptive trace that allows rapid "re-addiction" even months and years after detoxification and abstinence. Indeed, environmental cues and contexts are well known in addiction to trigger craving for the drug because of pairing with the positive hedonic effects of the drug and to trigger craving for the drug via conditioned withdrawal (O'Brien, Testa, O'Brien, Brady, & Wells, 1977). This phenomenon was replicated in an experimental setting where the subjective and physiological manifestations of the narcotic withdrawal syndrome were produced as a conditioned response. Here, the withdrawal reactions that were precipitated by the opioid antagonist naloxone in methadone-dependent volunteers were the unconditioned response, and a peppermint smell was the conditioned stimulus. After numerous pairings of the peppermint smell with the precipitated withdrawal produced by naloxone, the smell alone precipitated withdrawal (O'Brien et al., 1977). Conditioned withdrawal has also been observed in animal models using the conditioned place aversion paradigm (Schulteis et al., 1994) and operant responding for opioids (Kenny et al., 2006). In a study of rats that were allowed unlimited access to heroin via intravenous self-administration over a 23 h period, heroin intake escalated across sessions and was associated with a gradual decrease in reward sensitivity, reflected in progressively elevated ICSS thresholds. Additionally, stimuli that were repeatedly paired with naloxone-precipitated withdrawal provoked heroin consumption and elevated ICSS thresholds in rats that were allowed 23 h access. The observation that conditioned stimuli predict the onset of heroin withdrawal and the reward deficits that couple with this state suggest that motivational withdrawal may play a critical role in provoking craving and relapse (Kenny et al., 2006). Neurobiological studies using Fos measures paralleled with conditioned place aversion suggest activation of the extended amygdala (Gracy, Dankiewicz, & Koob, 2001), and functional studies suggest a key role for the basolateral amygdala, one of the major inputs to the extended amygdala (Schulteis, Ahmed, Morse, Koob, & Everitt, 2000). Thus, the emotional dysregulation of drug addiction represents the acute dysregulation of hedonic function (opponent process) and a residual dysregulation or break with hedonic homeostasis that has been termed allostasis (Koob & Le Moal, 1997).

Allostatic View of the Dark Side of Addiction

Allostasis was originally conceptualized to explain persistent morbidity of arousal and autonomic function associated with chronic stress to physiological function and can be defined as "stability through change" (Sterling & Eyer, 1988). Allostasis involves a feed-forward mechanism rather than the negative feedback mechanisms of homeostasis, with continuous re-evaluation of need and continuous readjustment of all parameters toward new set points. In the context of addiction, allostatic mechanisms have been hypothesized to be involved in maintaining a functioning brain reward system in the face of the growing motivational pathology of addiction (Koob & Le Moal, 2001). Two components are hypothesized to adjust to challenges to the brain that are produced by drugs of abuse: underactivation of brain reward transmitters and circuits and recruitment of the brain stress systems. The combination of a deficit in the reward system (negative hedonic valence) and recruitment of the brain stress systems, also termed anti-reward system (negative hedonic valence), provides a powerful motivational state that drives negative reinforcement (Koob & Le Moal, 2005). Anti-reward is a construct that is based on the hypothesis that brain systems (between-system brain stress systems) are in place to limit reward (Koob & Le Moal, 2005, 2008). Repeated challenges to reward function by drugs of abuse leads to attempts of the brain via molecular, cellular, and neurocircuitry changes to maintain stability but at a cost. This residual deviation from normal brain reward threshold regulation is termed an allostatic state. This state represents a combination of chronic elevation of the reward set point that is fueled by a decrease in the function of reward circuits and recruitment of anti-reward systems, both of which lead to the compulsivity of drug seeking and drug taking (Fig. 1.14).

Elucidation of the neurocircuitry of the negative emotional system outlined here (where the elements of the extended amygdala project to convey emotional valence), the ways in which the brain cognitive executive function systems control the dysregulation of brain emotional systems, and the ways in which individuals differ at the molecular-genetic level to convey loading on these circuits remain challenges for future research.

In summary, the present chapter has elaborated the seminal discoveries that formed the foundation of my negative emotional state—negative reinforcement—allostasis model of compulsive drug seeking. Aversive stimuli can suppress behavior but also generate negative emotional states that take on an insidious motivational significance via negative reinforcement. In addition, the interaction between reward and stress represents the "two faces of Janus," in that low amounts of stress can be rewarding but excessive reward can drive stress systems. The negative emotional state that comprises the *withdrawal/negative affect* stage consists of key motivational elements, such as chronic irritability, emotional pain, malaise, dysphoria, alexithymia, and the loss of motivation for natural rewards. Such a negative emotional state has been termed hyperkatifeia. Two processes are hypothesized to form the neurobiological basis for the negative emotional state of withdrawal or in the terms of Dr. Richard Solomon, the *b-process*: the loss of function in the reward systems (within-system neuroadaptation) and recruitment of the brain stress or

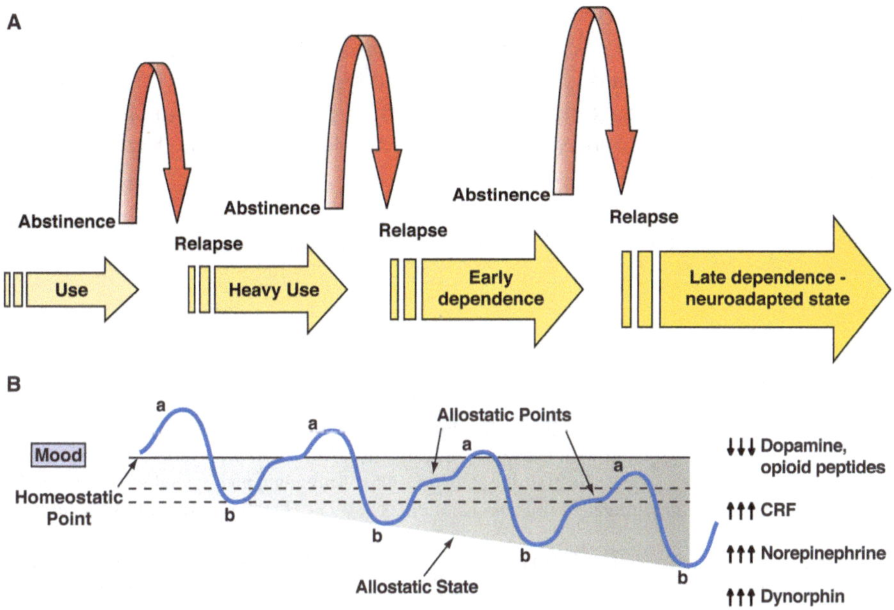

Fig. 1.14 (**a**) Schematic of the progression of drug dependence over time, illustrating the shift in underlying motivational mechanisms. From initial, positive reinforcing, pleasurable drug effects, the addictive process progresses over time to a point at which it is maintained by negative reinforcing relief from a negative emotional state. Neuroadaptations that encompass the recruitment of extrahypothalamic CRF systems are key to this shift [Taken with permission from Heilig & Koob, 2007]. (**b**) The *a-process* represents a positive hedonic or positive mood state, and the *b-process* represents the negative hedonic or negative mood state. The affective stimulus (state) has been argued to be the sum of both the *a-process* and *b-process*. An individual who experiences a positive hedonic mood state from a drug of abuse with sufficient time between re-administering the drug is hypothesized to retain the *a-process*. An appropriate counteradaptive opponent process (*b-process*) that balances the activational process (*a-process*) does not lead to an allostatic state. The changes in the affective stimulus (state) in an individual with repeated frequent drug use may represent a transition to an allostatic state in the brain reward systems and, by extrapolation, a transition to addiction. Notice that the apparent *b-process* never returns to the original homeostatic level before drug taking begins again, thus creating a progressively greater allostatic state in the brain reward system. The counteradaptive opponent process (*b-process*) does not balance the activational process (*a-process*) but in fact shows residual hysteresis. Although these changes that are illustrated in the figure are exaggerated and condensed over time, the hypothesis is that even during post-detoxification (a period of protracted abstinence), the reward system still bears allostatic changes. The following definitions apply: *allostasis*, the process of achieving stability through change; *allostatic state*, a state of chronic deviation of the regulatory system from its normal (homeostatic) operating level; *allostatic load*, the cost to the brain and body of the deviation, accumulating over time, and reflecting in many cases pathological states and accumulation of damage [Modified with permission from Koob & Le Moal, 2001]

anti-reward systems (between-system neuroadaptation; Koob & Bloom, 1988; Koob & Le Moal, 1997). During the development of withdrawal and dependence, the brain reward systems are compromised, and the brain stress systems (e.g., CRF, norepinephrine, and dynorphin) are recruited, producing aversive or stress-like states. The combination of decreases in reward neurotransmitter function and recruitment of anti-reward systems provides a powerful source of negative reinforcement that contributes to compulsive drug-seeking behavior and addiction. The source of motivational drive that is produced by negative reinforcement and its neurobiological components provides a foundation for our efforts to better understand, prevent, and treat addiction and other pathologies associated with motivational dysregulation.

Acknowledgements The author thanks Michael Arends for assistance with manuscript preparation.

References

Ahmed, S. H., Kenny, P. J., Koob, G. F., & Markou, A. (2002). Neurobiological evidence for hedonic allostasis associated with escalating cocaine use. *Nature Neuroscience, 5*, 625–626.

Alheid, G. F., De Olmos, J. S., & Beltramino, C. A. (1995). Amygdala and extended amygdala. In G. Paxinos (Ed.), *The rat nervous system* (2nd ed., pp. 495–578). San Diego, CA: Academic Press.

Ashok, A. H., Mizuno, Y., Volkow, N. D., & Howes, O. D. (2017). Association of stimulant use with dopaminergic alterations in users of cocaine, amphetamine, or methamphetamine: A systematic review and meta-analysis. *JAMA Psychiatry, 74*, 511–519.

Barbier, E., Vendruscolo, L. F., Schlosburg, J. E., Edwards, S., Juergens, N., Park, P. E., ... Heilig, M. (2013). The NK1 receptor antagonist L822429 reduces heroin reinforcement. *Neuropsychopharmacology, 38*, 976–984.

Berlin, G. S., & Hollander, E. (2014). Compulsivity, impulsivity, and the DSM-5 process. *CNS Spectrums, 19*, 62–68.

Brady, J. V. (1956). Assessment of drug effects on emotional behavior. *Science, 123*(3206), 1033–1034.

Brady, J. V. (1975). Toward a behavioral biology of emotion. In L. Levi (Ed.), *Emotions: Their Parameters and Measurement* (pp. 17–45). New York: Raven Press.

Brady, J. V., & Emurian, H. H. (1978). Behavioral analysis of motivational and emotional interactions in a programmed environment. In R. A. Dienstbier (Ed.), *Human Emotion* (series title: Nebraska Symposium on Motivation, vol. 26, pp. 81–122). Lincoln: University of Nebraska Press.

Breiter, H. C., Gollub, R. L., Weisskoff, R. M., Kennedy, D. N., Makris, N., Berke, J. D., ... Hyman, S. E. (1997). Acute effects of cocaine on human brain activity and emotion. *Neuron, 19*, 591–611.

Bruijnzeel, A. W., Bishnoi, M., van Tuijl, I. A., Keijzers, K. F., Yavarovich, K. R., Pasek, T. M., ... Yamada, H. (2010). Effects of prazosin, clonidine, and propranolol on the elevations in brain reward thresholds and somatic signs associated with nicotine withdrawal in rats. *Psychopharmacology, 212*, 485–499.

Bruijnzeel, A. W., Ford, J., Rogers, J. A., Scheick, S., Ji, Y., Bishnoi, M., & Alexander, J. C. (2012). Blockade of CRF1 receptors in the central nucleus of the amygdala attenuates the dysphoria associated with nicotine withdrawal in rats. *Pharmacology, Biochemistry, and Behavior, 101*, 62–68.

Bruijnzeel, A. W., Prado, M., & Isaac, S. (2009). Corticotropin-releasing factor-1 receptor activation mediates nicotine withdrawal-induced deficit in brain reward function and stress-induced relapse. *Biological Psychiatry, 66*, 110–117.

Bruijnzeel, A. W., Zislis, G., Wilson, C., & Gold, M. S. (2007). Antagonism of CRF receptors prevents the deficit in brain reward function associated with precipitated nicotine withdrawal in rats. *Neuropsychopharmacology, 32*, 955–963.

Burchfield, S. (1979). The stress response: A new perspective. *Psychosomatic Medicine, 41*, 661–672.

Carlezon, W. A., Jr., Nestler, E. J., & Neve, R. L. (2000). Herpes simplex virus-mediated gene transfer as a tool for neuropsychiatric research. *Critical Reviews in Neurobiology, 14*, 47–67.

Chartoff, E., Sawyer, A., Rachlin, A., Potter, D., Pliakas, A., & Carlezon, W. A. (2012). Blockade of kappa opioid receptors attenuates the development of depressive-like behaviors induced by cocaine withdrawal in rats. *Neuropharmacology, 62*, 1167–1176.

Ciccocioppo, R., Economidou, D., Fedeli, A., & Massi, M. (2003). The nociceptin/orphanin FQ/NOP receptor system as a target for treatment of alcohol abuse: A review of recent work in alcohol-preferring rats. *Physiology & Behavior, 79*, 121–128.

Cohen, A., Koob, G. F., & George, O. (2012). Robust escalation of nicotine intake with extended access to nicotine self-administration and intermittent periods of abstinence. *Neuropsychopharmacology, 37*, 2153–2160.

Collins, A. C., Bhat, R. V., Pauly, J. R., & Marks, M. J. (1990). Modulation of nicotine receptors by chronic exposure to nicotinic agonists and antagonists. In G. Bock & J. Marsh (Eds.), *The biology of nicotine dependence, Ciba foundation symposium* (Vol. 152, pp. 87–105). New York, NY: John Wiley.

Dani, J. A., & Heinemann, S. (1996). Molecular and cellular aspects of nicotine abuse. *Neuron, 16*, 905–908.

Davidson, M., Shanley, B., & Wilce, P. (1995). Increased NMDA-induced excitability during ethanol withdrawal: A behavioural and histological study. *Brain Research, 674*, 91–96.

Delfs, J. M., Zhu, Y., Druhan, J. P., & Aston-Jones, G. (2000). Noradrenaline in the ventral forebrain is critical for opiate withdrawal-induced aversion. *Nature, 403*, 430–434.

Deroche-Gamonet, V., Belin, D., & Piazza, P. V. (2004). Evidence for addiction-like behavior in the rat. *Science, 305*, 1014–1017.

Diana, M., Pistis, M., Carboni, S., Gessa, G. L., & Rossetti, Z. L. (1993). Profound decrement of mesolimbic dopaminergic neuronal activity during ethanol withdrawal syndrome in rats: Electrophysiological and biochemical evidence. *Proceedings of the National Academy of Sciences of the United States of America, 90*, 7966–7969.

Diana, M., Pistis, M., Muntoni, A., & Gessa, G. (1995). Profound decrease of mesolimbic dopaminergic neuronal activity in morphine withdrawn rats. *The Journal of Pharmacology and Experimental Therapeutics, 272*, 781–785.

Edwards, S., Guerrero, M., Ghoneim, O. M., Roberts, E., & Koob, G. F. (2011). Evidence that vasopressin V1b receptors mediate the transition to excessive drinking in ethanol-dependent rats. *Addiction Biology, 17*, 76–85.

Edwards, S., & Koob, G. F. (2010). Neurobiology of dysregulated motivational systems in drug addiction. *Future Neurology, 5*, 393–410.

Epping-Jordan, M. P., Watkins, S. S., Koob, G. F., & Markou, A. (1998). Dramatic decreases in brain reward function during nicotine withdrawal. *Nature, 393*, 76–79.

Estes, W. K., & Skinner, B. F. (1941). Some quantitative properties of anxiety. *Journal of Experimental Psychology, 29*, 390–400.

Everitt, B. J., & Robbins, T. W. (2005). Neural systems of reinforcement for drug addiction: From actions to habits to compulsion. *Nature Neuroscience, 8*, 1481–1489 [erratum: 9(7):979].

Funk, C. K., O'Dell, L. E., Crawford, E. F., & Koob, G. F. (2006). Corticotropin-releasing factor within the central nucleus of the amygdala mediates enhanced ethanol self-administration in withdrawn, ethanol-dependent rats. *The Journal of Neuroscience, 26*, 11324–11332.

Funk, C. K., Zorrilla, E. P., Lee, M. J., Rice, K. C., & Koob, G. F. (2007). Corticotropin-releasing factor 1 antagonists selectively reduce ethanol self-administration in ethanol-dependent rats. *Biological Psychiatry, 61*, 78–86.

Gantt, W. H. (1942). The origin and development of nervous disturbances experimentally produced. *The American Journal of Psychiatry, 98*, 475–481.

Gardner, E. L., & Vorel, S. R. (1998). Cannabinoid transmission and reward-related events. *Neurobiology of Disease, 5*, 502–533.

Gawin, F. H., & Kleber, H. D. (1986). Abstinence symptomatology and psychiatric diagnosis in cocaine abusers: Clinical observations. *Archives of General Psychiatry, 43*, 107–113.

Gehlert, D. R., Cippitelli, A., Thorsell, A., Le, A. D., Hipskind, P. A., Hamdouchi, C., … Heilig, M. (2007). 3-(4-Chloro-2-morpholin-4-yl-thiazol-5-yl)-8-(1-ethylpropyl)-2,6-dimethyl-imidazo[1,2-b]pyridazine: A novel brain-penetrant, orally available corticotropin-releasing factor receptor 1 antagonist with efficacy in animal models of alcoholism. *The Journal of Neuroscience, 27*, 2718–2726.

George, O., Ghozland, S., Azar, M. R., Cottone, P., Zorrilla, E. P., Parsons, L. H., … Koob, G. F. (2007). CRF-CRF_1 system activation mediates withdrawal-induced increases in nicotine self-administration in nicotine-dependent rats. *Proceedings of the National Academy of Sciences of the United States of America, 104*, 17198–17203.

George, O., & Koob, G. F. (2013). Control of craving by the prefrontal cortex. *Proceedings of the National Academy of Sciences of the United States of America, 110*, 4165–4166.

Gilpin, N. W., & Koob, G. F. (2010). Effects of β-adrenoceptor antagonists on alcohol drinking by alcohol-dependent rats. *Psychopharmacology, 212*, 431–439.

Gilpin, N. W., Misra, K., & Koob, G. F. (2008). Neuropeptide Y in the central nucleus of the amygdala suppresses dependence-induced increases in alcohol drinking. *Pharmacology Biochemistry and Behavior, 90*, 475–480.

Gilpin, N. W., Stewart, R. B., Murphy, J. M., Li, T. K., & Badia-Elder, N. E. (2003). Neuropeptide Y reduces oral ethanol intake in alcohol-preferring (P) rats following a period of imposed ethanol abstinence. *Alcoholism, Clinical and Experimental Research, 27*, 787–794.

Gracy, K. N., Dankiewicz, L. A., & Koob, G. F. (2001). Opiate withdrawal-induced Fos immunoreactivity in the rat extended amygdala parallels the development of conditioned place aversion. *Neuropsychopharmacology, 24*, 152–160.

Greenwell, T. N., Funk, C. K., Cottone, P., Richardson, H. N., Chen, S. A., Rice, K., … Koob, G. F. (2009). Corticotropin-releasing factor-1 receptor antagonists decrease heroin self-administration in long-, but not short-access rats. *Addiction Biology, 14*, 130–143.

Grieder, T. E., George, O., Tan, H., George, S. R., Le Foll, B., Laviolette, S. R., & van der Kooy, D. (2012). Phasic D1 and tonic D2 dopamine receptor signaling double dissociate the motivational effects of acute nicotine and chronic nicotine withdrawal. *Proceedings of the National Academy of Sciences of the United States of America, 109*, 3101–3106.

Haber, S. N., Fudge, J. L., & McFarland, N. R. (2000). Striatonigrostriatal pathways in primates form an ascending spiral from the shell to the dorsolateral striatum. *The Journal of Neuroscience, 20*, 2369–2382.

Heilig, M., & Koob, G. F. (2007). A key role for corticotropin-releasing factor in alcohol dependence. *Trends in Neurosciences, 30*, 399–406.

Himmelsbach, C. K. (1943). Can the euphoric, analgetic, and physical dependence effects of drugs be separated? IV. With reference to physical dependence. *Federation Proceedings, 2*, 201–203.

Jang, C. G., Whitfield, T., Schulteis, G., Koob, G. F., & Wee, S. (2013). A dysphoric-like state during early withdrawal from extended access to methamphetamine self-administration in rats. *Psychopharmacology, 225*, 753–763.

June, H. L., Liu, J., Warnock, K. T., Bell, K. A., Balan, I., Bollino, D., … Aurelian, L. (2015). CRF-amplified neuronal TLR4/MCP-1 signaling regulates alcohol self-administration. *Neuropsychopharmacology, 40*, 1549–1559.

Kenny, P. J., Chen, S. A., Kitamura, O., Markou, A., & Koob, G. F. (2006). Conditioned withdrawal drives heroin consumption and decreases reward sensitivity. *The Journal of Neuroscience, 26*, 5894–5900.

Kenny, P. J., Gasparini, F., & Markou, A. (2003). Group II metabotropic and α-amino-3-hydroxy-5-methyl-4-isoxazole propionate (AMPA)/kainate glutamate receptors regulate the deficit in brain reward function associated with nicotine withdrawal in rats. *The Journal of Pharmacology and Experimental Therapeutics, 306*, 1068–1076.

Khachaturian, H., Lewis, M. E., Schafer, M. K. H., & Watson, S. J. (1985). Anatomy of the CNS opioid systems. *Trends in Neurosciences, 8*, 111–119.

Knoll, A. T., Meloni, E. G., Thomas, J. B., Carroll, F. I., & Carlezon, W. A., Jr. (2007). Anxiolytic-like effects of κ-opioid receptor antagonists in models of unlearned and learned fear in rats. *The Journal of Pharmacology and Experimental Therapeutics, 323*, 838–845.

Koob, G. F. (2008). A role for brain stress systems in addiction. *Neuron, 59*, 11–34.

Koob, G. F. (2009). Brain stress systems in the amygdala and addiction. *Brain Research, 1293*, 61–75.

Koob, G. F. (2010). The role of CRF and CRF-related peptides in the dark side of addiction. *Brain Research, 1314*, 3–14.

Koob, G. F. (2015). The dark side of emotion: The addiction perspective. *European Journal of Pharmacology, 753*, 73–87.

Koob, G. F. (2017). The dark side of addiction: The Horsley Gantt to Joseph Brady connection. *Journal of Nervous and Mental Disease, 205*, 270–272.

Koob, G. F., & Annau, Z. (1973). Effect of hypoxia on hypothalamic mechanisms. *American Journal of Physiology, 224*, 1403–1408.

Koob, G. F., & Bloom, F. E. (1988). Cellular and molecular mechanisms of drug dependence. *Science, 242*, 715–723.

Koob, G. F., Heinrichs, S. C., Menzaghi, F., Pich, E. M., & Britton, K. T. (1994). Corticotropin releasing factor, stress and behavior. *Seminars in Neuroscience, 6*, 221–229.

Koob, G. F., & Kreek, M. J. (2007). Stress, dysregulation of drug reward pathways, and the transition to drug dependence. *The American Journal of Psychiatry, 164*, 1149–1159.

Koob, G. F., & Le Moal, M. (1997). Drug abuse: Hedonic homeostatic dysregulation. *Science, 278*, 52–58.

Koob, G. F., & Le Moal, M. (2001). Drug addiction, dysregulation of reward, and allostasis. *Neuropsychopharmacology, 24*, 97–129.

Koob, G. F., & Le Moal, M. (2005). Plasticity of reward neurocircuitry and the "dark side" of drug addiction. *Nature Neuroscience, 8*, 1442–1444.

Koob, G. F., & Le Moal, M. (2008). Addiction and the brain antireward system. *Annual Review of Psychology, 59*, 29–53.

Koob, G. F., & Volkow, N. D. (2010). Neurocircuitry of addiction. *Neuropsychopharmacology Reviews, 35*, 217–238 [erratum: 35: 1051].

Kornetsky, C., & Esposito, R. U. (1981). Reward and detection thresholds for brain stimulation: Dissociative effects of cocaine. *Brain Research, 209*, 496–500.

Kreek, M. J., & Koob, G. F. (1998). Drug dependence: Stress and dysregulation of brain reward pathways. *Drug and Alcohol Dependence, 51*, 23–47.

Land, B. B., Bruchas, M. R., Lemos, J. C., Xu, M., Melief, E. J., & Chavkin, C. (2008). The dysphoric component of stress is encoded by activation of the dynorphin κ-opioid system. *The Journal of Neuroscience, 28*, 407–414.

Land, B. B., Bruchas, M. R., Schattauer, S., Giardino, W. J., Aita, M., Messinger, D., … Chavkin, C. (2009). Activation of the kappa opioid receptor in the dorsal raphe nucleus mediates the aversive effects of stress and reinstates drug seeking. *Proceedings of the National Academy of Sciences of the United States of America, 106*, 19168–19173.

Liu, J., & Schulteis, G. (2004). Brain reward deficits accompany naloxone-precipitated withdrawal from acute opioid dependence. *Pharmacology, Biochemistry, and Behavior, 79*, 101–108.

Mague, S. D., Pliakas, A. M., Todtenkopf, M. S., Tomasiewicz, H. C., Zhang, Y., Stevens, W. C., Jr., … Carlezon, W. A., Jr. (2003). Antidepressant-like effects of κ-opioid receptor antagonists in the forced swim test in rats. *The Journal of Pharmacology and Experimental Therapeutics, 305*, 323–330.

Makino, S., Gold, P. W., & Schulkin, J. (1994). Effects of corticosterone on CRH mRNA and content in the bed nucleus of the stria terminalis: Comparison with the effects in the central nucleus of the amygdala and the paraventricular nucleus of the hypothalamus. *Brain Research, 657*, 141–149.

Markou, A., & Koob, G. F. (1991). Post-cocaine anhedonia: An animal model of cocaine withdrawal. *Neuropsychopharmacology, 4*, 17–26.

Martin-Fardon, R., Zorrilla, E. P., Ciccocioppo, R., & Weiss, F. (2010). Role of innate and drug-induced dysregulation of brain stress and arousal systems in addiction: Focus on corticotropin-releasing factor, nociceptin/orphanin FQ, and orexin/hypocretin. *Brain Research, 1314*, 145–161.

McLaughlin, J. P., Li, S., Valdez, J., Chavkin, T. A., & Chavkin, C. (2006). Social defeat stress-induced behavioral responses are mediated by the endogenous kappa opioid system. *Neuropsychopharmacology, 31*, 1241–1248.

McLaughlin, J. P., Marton-Popovici, M., & Chavkin, C. (2003). κ Opioid receptor antagonism and prodynorphin gene disruption block stress-induced behavioral responses. *The Journal of Neuroscience, 23*, 5674–5683.

Merlo-Pich, E., Lorang, M., Yeganeh, M., Rodriguez de Fonseca, F., Raber, J., Koob, G. F., & Weiss, F. (1995). Increase of extracellular corticotropin-releasing factor-like immunoreactivity levels in the amygdala of awake rats during restraint stress and ethanol withdrawal as measured by microdialysis. *The Journal of Neuroscience, 15*, 5439–5447.

Morrisett, R. A. (1994). Potentiation of N-methyl-D-aspartate receptor-dependent afterdischarges in rat dentate gyrus following in vitro ethanol withdrawal. *Neuroscience Letters, 167*, 175–178.

Mucha, R. F., & Herz, A. (1985). Motivational properties of kappa and mu opioid receptor agonists studied with place and taste preference conditioning. *Psychopharmacology, 86*, 274–280.

Nealey, K. A., Smith, A. W., Davis, S. M., Smith, D. G., & Walker, B. M. (2011). κ-Opioid receptors are implicated in the increased potency of intra-accumbens nalmefene in ethanol-dependent rats. *Neuropharmacology, 61*, 35–42.

Nestler, E. J. (2001). Molecular basis of long-term plasticity underlying addiction. *Nature Reviews. Neuroscience, 2*, 119–128.

Nestler, E. J. (2005). Is there a common molecular pathway for addiction? *Nature Neuroscience, 8*, 1445–1449.

O'Brien, C. P., Testa, J., O'Brien, T. J., Brady, J. P., & Wells, B. (1977). Conditioned narcotic withdrawal in humans. *Science, 195*, 1000–1002.

Olive, M. F., Koenig, H. N., Nannini, M. A., & Hodge, C. W. (2002). Elevated extracellular CRF levels in the bed nucleus of the stria terminalis during ethanol withdrawal and reduction by subsequent ethanol intake. *Pharmacology, Biochemistry, and Behavior, 72*, 213–220.

Park, P. E., Schlosburg, J. E., Vendruscolo, L. F., Schulteis, G., Edwards, S., & Koob, G. F. (2015). Chronic CRF_1 receptor blockade reduces heroin intake escalation and dependence-induced hyperalgesia. *Addiction Biology, 20*, 275–284.

Parsons, L. H., & Justice, J. B., Jr. (1993). Perfusate serotonin increases extracellular dopamine in the nucleus accumbens as measured by in vivo microdialysis. *Brain Research, 606*, 195–199.

Paterson, N. E., & Markou, A. (2003). Increased motivation for self-administered cocaine after escalated cocaine intake. *Neuroreport, 14*, 2229–2232.

Paterson, N. E., Myers, C., & Markou, A. (2000). Effects of repeated withdrawal from continuous amphetamine administration on brain reward function in rats. *Psychopharmacology, 152*, 440–446.

Pavlov, I. P. (1927). *Conditioned reflexes: An investigation of the physiological activity of the cerebral cortex*. London, England: Oxford University Press.

Pavlov, I. P., & Gantt, W. A. H. (1941). *Lectures on conditioned reflexes: Vol. 2. Conditioned reflexes and psychiatry*. London, England: Lawrence and Wishart.

Pfeiffer, A., Brantl, V., Herz, A., & Emrich, H. M. (1986). Psychotomimesis mediated by κ opiate receptors. *Science, 233*, 774–776.

Piazza, P. V., & Le Moal, M. (1997). Glucocorticoids as a biological substrate of reward: Physiological and pathophysiological implications. *Brain Research Reviews, 25*, 359–372.

Poulos, C. X., & Cappell, H. (1991). Homeostatic theory of drug tolerance: A general model of physiological adaptation. *Psychological Review, 98*, 390–408.

Rasmussen, D. D., Boldt, B. M., Bryant, C. A., Mitton, D. R., Larsen, S. A., & Wilkinson, C. W. (2000). Chronic daily ethanol and withdrawal: 1. Long-term changes in the hypothalamo-pituitary-adrenal axis. *Alcoholism, Clinical and Experimental Research, 24*, 1836–1849.

Redila, V. A., & Chavkin, C. (2008). Stress-induced reinstatement of cocaine seeking is mediated by the kappa opioid system. *Psychopharmacology, 200*, 59–70.

Richardson, H. N., Lee, S. Y., O'Dell, L. E., Koob, G. F., & Rivier, C. L. (2008). Alcohol self-administration acutely stimulates the hypothalamic-pituitary-adrenal axis, but alcohol dependence leads to a dampened neuroendocrine state. *European Journal of Neuroscience, 28*, 1641–1653.

Rivier, C., Bruhn, T., & Vale, W. (1984). Effect of ethanol on the hypothalamic-pituitary-adrenal axis in the rat: Role of corticotropin-releasing factor (CRF). *The Journal of Pharmacology and Experimental Therapeutics, 229*, 127–131.

Robbins, T. W., Gillan, C. M., Smith, D. G., de Wit, S., & Ersche, K. D. (2012). Neurocognitive endophenotypes of impulsivity and compulsivity: Towards dimensional psychiatry. *Trends in Cognitive Sciences, 16*, 81–91.

Roberto, M., Cruz, M. T., Gilpin, N. W., Sabino, V., Schweitzer, P., Bajo, M., … Parsons, L. H. (2010). Corticotropin releasing factor-induced amygdala gamma-aminobutyric acid release plays a key role in alcohol dependence. *Biological Psychiatry, 67*, 831–839.

Roberts, A. J., Cole, M., & Koob, G. F. (1996). Intra-amygdala muscimol decreases operant ethanol self-administration in dependent rats. *Alcoholism, Clinical and Experimental Research, 20*, 1289–1298.

Russell, M. A. H. (1976). What is dependence? In G. Edwards (Ed.), *Drugs and drug dependence* (pp. 182–187). Lexington, MA: Lexington Books.

Russo, S. J., Dietz, D. M., Dumitriu, D., Morrison, J. H., Malenka, R. C., & Nestler, E. J. (2010). The addicted synapse: Mechanisms of synaptic and structural plasticity in nucleus accumbens. *Trends in Neurosciences, 33*, 267–276.

Schindler, A. G., Li, S., & Chavkin, C. (2010). Behavioral stress may increase the rewarding valence of cocaine-associated cues through a dynorphin/-opioid receptor-mediated mechanism without affecting associative learning or memory retrieval mechanisms. *Neuropsychopharmacology, 35*, 1932–1942.

Schlosburg, J. E., Whitfield, T. W., Jr., Park, P. E., Crawford, E. F., George, O., Vendruscolo, L. F., & Koob, G. F. (2013). Long-term antagonism of κ opioid receptors prevents escalation of and increased motivation for heroin intake. *The Journal of Neuroscience, 33*, 19384–19392.

Schmeichel, B. E., Barbier, E., Misra, K. K., Contet, C., Schlosburg, J. E., Grigoriadis, D., … Vendruscolo, L. F. (2015). Hypocretin receptor 2 antagonism dose-dependently reduces escalated heroin self-administration in rats. *Neuropsychopharmacology, 40*, 1123–1129.

Schulteis, G., Ahmed, S. H., Morse, A. C., Koob, G. F., & Everitt, B. J. (2000). Conditioning and opiate withdrawal: The amygdala links neutral stimuli with the agony of overcoming drug addiction. *Nature, 405*, 1013–1014.

Schulteis, G., & Koob, G. (1994). Dark side of drug dependence. *Nature, 371*, 108–109.

Schulteis, G., & Liu, J. (2006). Brain reward deficits accompany withdrawal (hangover) from acute ethanol in rats. *Alcohol, 39*, 21–28.

Schulteis, G., Markou, A., Cole, M., & Koob, G. (1995). Decreased brain reward produced by ethanol withdrawal. *Proceedings of the National Academy of Sciences of the United States of America, 92*, 5880–5884.

Schulteis, G., Markou, A., Gold, L. H., Stinus, L., & Koob, G. F. (1994). Relative sensitivity to naloxone of multiple indices of opiate withdrawal: A quantitative dose-response analysis. *The Journal of Pharmacology and Experimental Therapeutics, 271*, 1391–1398.

Serrano, A., & Parsons, L. H. (2011). Endocannabinoid influence in drug reinforcement, dependence and addiction-related behaviors. *Pharmacology & Therapeutics, 132*, 215–241.

Shippenberg, T. S., Zapata, A., & Chefer, V. I. (2007). Dynorphin and the pathophysiology of drug addiction. *Pharmacology & Therapeutics, 116*, 306–321.

Shurman, J., Koob, G. F., & Gutstein, H. B. (2010). Opioids, pain, the brain, and hyperkatifeia: A framework for the rational use of opioids for pain. *Pain Medicine, 11*, 1092–1098.

Siegel, S. (1975). Evidence from rats that morphine tolerance is a learned response. *Journal of Comparative and Physiological Psychology, 89*, 498–506.

Solomon, R. L. (1980). The opponent-process theory of acquired motivation: The costs of pleasure and the benefits of pain. *The American Psychologist, 35*, 691–712.

Solomon, R. L., & Corbit, J. D. (1974). An opponent-process theory of motivation: 1. Temporal dynamics of affect. *Psychological Review, 81*, 119–145.
Specio, S. E., Wee, S., O'Dell, L. E., Boutrel, B., Zorrilla, E. P., & Koob, G. F. (2008). CRF1 receptor antagonists attenuate escalated cocaine self-administration in rats. *Psychopharmacology, 196*, 473–482.
Sterling, P., & Eyer, J. (1988). Allostasis: A new paradigm to explain arousal pathology. In S. Fisher & J. Reason (Eds.), *Handbook of life stress, cognition and health* (pp. 629–649). Chichester, England: John Wiley.
Stinus, L., Le Moal, M., & Koob, G. F. (1990). Nucleus accumbens and amygdala are possible substrates for the aversive stimulus effects of opiate withdrawal. *Neuroscience, 37*, 767–773.
Swanson, L. W., Sawchenko, P. E., Rivier, J., & Vale, W. (1983). The organization of ovine corticotropin-releasing factor immunoreactive cells and fibers in the rat brain: An immunohistochemical study. *Neuroendocrinology, 36*, 165–186.
Tan, H., Bishop, S. F., Lauzon, N. M., Sun, N., & Laviolette, S. R. (2009). Chronic nicotine exposure switches the functional role of mesolimbic dopamine transmission in the processing of nicotine's rewarding and aversive effects. *Neuropharmacology, 56*, 741–751.
Thorsell, A., Rapunte-Canonigo, V., O'Dell, L., Chen, S. A., King, A., Lekic, D., … Sanna, P. P. (2007). Viral vector-induced amygdala NPY overexpression reverses increased alcohol intake caused by repeated deprivations in Wistar rats. *Brain, 130*, 1330–1337.
Thorsell, A., Slawecki, C. J., & Ehlers, C. L. (2005a). Effects of neuropeptide Y and corticotropin-releasing factor on ethanol intake in Wistar rats: Interaction with chronic ethanol exposure. *Behavioural Brain Research, 161*, 133–140.
Thorsell, A., Slawecki, C. J., & Ehlers, C. L. (2005b). Effects of neuropeptide Y on appetitive and consummatory behaviors associated with alcohol drinking in Wistar rats with a history of ethanol exposure. *Alcoholism, Clinical and Experimental Research, 29*, 584–590.
Valdez, G. R., & Koob, G. F. (2004). Allostasis and dysregulation of corticotropin-releasing factor and neuropeptide Y systems: Implications for the development of alcoholism. *Pharmacology, Biochemistry, and Behavior, 79*, 671–689.
Van Dyke, C., & Byck, R. (1982). Cocaine. *Scientific American, 246*, 128–141.
Vanderschuren, L. J., & Everitt, B. J. (2004). Drug seeking becomes compulsive after prolonged cocaine self-administration. *Science, 305*, 1017–1019.
Vendruscolo, L. F., Barbier, E., Schlosburg, J. E., Misra, K. K., Whitfield, T., Jr., Logrip, M. L., … Koob, G. F. (2012). Corticosteroid-dependent plasticity mediates compulsive alcohol drinking in rats. *The Journal of Neuroscience, 32*, 7563–7571.
Volkow, N. D., Fowler, J. S., & Wang, G. J. (2003). The addicted human brain: Insights from imaging studies. *The Journal of Clinical Investigation, 111*, 1444–1451.
Walker, B. M., & Koob, G. F. (2007). The γ-aminobutyric acid-B receptor agonist baclofen attenuates responding for ethanol in ethanol-dependent rats. *Alcoholism, Clinical and Experimental Research, 31*, 11–18.
Walker, B. M., & Koob, G. F. (2008). Pharmacological evidence for a motivational role of κ-opioid systems in ethanol dependence. *Neuropsychopharmacology, 33*, 643–652.
Walker, B. M., Rasmussen, D. D., Raskind, M. A., & Koob, G. F. (2008). α1-Noradrenergic receptor antagonism blocks dependence-induced increases in responding for ethanol. *Alcohol, 42*, 91–97.
Walker, B. M., Zorrilla, E. P., & Koob, G. F. (2010). Systemic κ-opioid receptor antagonism by nor-binaltorphimine reduces dependence-induced excessive alcohol self-administration in rats. *Addiction Biology, 16*, 116–119.
Wee, S., & Koob, G. F. (2010). The role of the dynorphin-κ opioid system in the reinforcing effects of drugs of abuse. *Psychopharmacology, 210*, 121–135.
Wee, S., Mandyam, C. D., Lekic, D. M., & Koob, G. F. (2008). α1-Noradrenergic system role in increased motivation for cocaine intake in rats with prolonged access. *European Neuropsychopharmacology, 18*, 303–311.
Wee, S., Orio, L., Ghirmai, S., Cashman, J. R., & Koob, G. F. (2009). Inhibition of kappa opioid receptors attenuated increased cocaine intake in rats with extended access to cocaine. *Psychopharmacology, 205*, 565–575.

Wee, S., Wang, Z., Woolverton, W. L., Pulvirenti, L., & Koob, G. F. (2007). Effect of aripiprazole, a partial D2 receptor agonist, on increased rate of methamphetamine self-administration in rats with prolonged access. *Neuropsychopharmacology, 32*, 2238–2247.

Weiss, F., Markou, A., Lorang, M. T., & Koob, G. F. (1992). Basal extracellular dopamine levels in the nucleus accumbens are decreased during cocaine withdrawal after unlimited-access self-administration. *Brain Research, 593*, 314–318.

Weiss, F., Parsons, L. H., Schulteis, G., Hyytia, P., Lorang, M. T., Bloom, F. E., & Koob, G. F. (1996). Ethanol self-administration restores withdrawal-associated deficiencies in accumbal dopamine and 5-hydroxytryptamine release in dependent rats. *The Journal of Neuroscience, 16*, 3474–3485.

Whitfield, T. W., Jr., Schlosburg, J., Wee, S., Gould, A., George, O., Grant, Y., … Koob, G. F. (2015). κ Opioid receptors in the nucleus accumbens shell mediate escalation of methamphetamine intake. *The Journal of Neuroscience, 35*, 4296–4305.

Chapter 2
Changing Drug Use and Other Health-Related Behavior in Vulnerable Populations

Stephen T. Higgins, Allison N. Kurti, and Danielle R. Davis

Introduction

The focus of this report is on reducing drug use and promoting other health-related behavior change in vulnerable populations. However, it is important to understand this effort and target problems in a larger context. The US population health is quite poor relative to other industrialized nations. Among the 34 developed nations with membership in the Organization for Economic Cooperation and Development, for example, the USA ranks 25th in life expectancy, 29th in infant mortality, and 25th in maternal mortality (Higgins, 2015; Schroeder, 2016). These outcomes occur despite spending orders of magnitude more on healthcare than any other country (Woolf & Aron, 2013). When population health experts assess how to improve the relatively dismal status of the US population health, the domain of personal behavior is identified as the area that offers the greatest potential for improvements (Schroeder, 2007, 2016). Cigarette smoking, other substance abuse, physical inactivity, unhealthy food choices, and nonadherence with the recommended medical regimens are strikingly harmful to long-term health and longevity (Avendano & Kawachi, 2014; Higgins, 2015; Schroeder, 2016; Woolf & Aron, 2013). The current opioid addiction epidemic, which is having a devastating impact throughout the USA, is a striking example (Compton, Boyle, & Wargo, 2015; Sigmon et al., 2016; Volkow & Collins, 2017). Such unhealthy personal behavior patterns increase the risk for numerous chronic diseases, including coronary heart disease, stroke, site-specific cancers, and type-2 diabetes, and are estimated to be the largest contributor to premature deaths in the USA (~40%) (Avendano & Kawachi, 2014; Danaei et al., 2009; Higgins, 2015; Schroeder, 2016; U.S. Department of Health and Human

S. T. Higgins (✉) · A. N. Kurti · D. R. Davis
Vermont Center on Behavior and Health, Departments of Psychiatry and Psychological Science, University of Vermont, Burlington, VT, USA
e-mail: Stephen.Higgins@uvm.edu

D. A. Hope, R. A. Bevins (eds.), *Change and Maintaining Change*, Nebraska Symposium on Motivation 65, https://doi.org/10.1007/978-3-319-96920-6_2

Services, 2014; Woolf & Aron, 2013). Development of more effective strategies to promote and sustain smoking cessation and other health-related behavior change is critical to resolving this national problem.

Cigarette smoking is the biggest killer among the unhealthy behavior patterns above and is responsible for more than 480,000 premature deaths annually in the USA and 5,000,000 globally (U.S. Department of Health and Human Services, 2014). Cigarette smoking is also a substantial economic burden on the healthcare system. Direct medical costs associated with cigarette smoking in the USA, for example, exceed $170 billion annually (U.S. Department of Health and Human Services, 2014). Cigarette smoking is also a bit of a paradox in that it remains the biggest killer while also representing one of the most compelling examples that large-scale health-related behavior change is possible and can drive tremendous improvements in health. The US smoking prevalence dropped precipitously following the landmark US Surgeon General's report from approximately 42% in 1964 to 15% in 2015. That change is estimated to have prevented eight million premature deaths between 1964 and 2012 with a mean extended life span of 19–20 years (Holford et al., 2014), and also netted tremendous health care cost savings (U.S. Department of Health and Human Services, 2014). Unfortunately though, those gains were disproportionately realized among the more affluent. Smoking prevalence decreased substantially less or not at all among socioeconomically disadvantaged and other vulnerable populations (e.g., those with comorbid substance use disorders, those with mental illness, and sexual minorities), and even increased in some segments of the US population (e.g., socioeconomically disadvantaged women) (Chilcoat, 2009; Higgins & Chilcoat, 2009; Schroeder, 2016; U.S. Department of Health and Human Services, 2014). This overrepresentation of cigarette smoking in vulnerable populations is not unique. It also occurs across a wide range of other health-related behavior problems (e.g., other substance use disorders, nonadherence with recommended medical regimens, violence, and unplanned pregnancies) and is a major contributor, although not the sole contributor, to the problem of health disparities (Cutler & Lleras-Muney, 2010; Higgins & Chilcoat, 2009; Isaacs & Schroeder, 2004; Kumanyika, 2012). More effective strategies to promote smoking cessation and other health-related behavior change in vulnerable populations are especially needed and it is the focus of the research reviewed below.

Considerable scientific effort to understand what motivates cigarette smoking, other substance abuse, unhealthy food choices, and many of these other risk behaviors identifies a fundamental role of the reinforcement process. This process has been reviewed at length previously, including with regard to cigarette smoking and other substance use disorders in several volumes of the Nebraska Symposium on Motivation series (Bevins & Bardo, 2004; Bevins & Caggiula, 2009). Thus, it is discussed only briefly here. What is abundantly clear is that the nicotine in cigarettes, cocaine, opioids, and other abused drugs, fatty and sweet foods, and sexual activity all stimulate dopamine-based mesolimbic brain reward centers, which directly increases the likelihood that these same activities will be repeated in the future (Kelley & Berridge, 2002). Nicotine also enhances the efficacy of other reinforcers experienced while under the influence of its psychoactive effects

(Caggiula et al., 2009). Other abused drugs can have similar effects where, for example, they enhance the efficacy of social reinforcement (Higgins, Hughes, & Bickel, 1989; Higgins, Roll, & Bickel, 1996). These reward pathways evolved to assure that humans and other organisms would learn to: (a) consume the basic nutrients necessary to sustain themselves, (b) engage in reproductive behavior to sustain the species, and (c) engage in other similarly basic behavior patterns critical to survival. When considered in the context of reinforcement's connection to survival, the powerful control that abused drugs and other highly reinforcing substances can exert is somewhat less perplexing.

Also important to note is that there are several additional factors associated with the reinforcement process that are involved as well. First, humans and many other species evolved with certain biases in how they choose between different reinforcement options with a major one being a bias for more immediate over delayed reinforcement even when the more immediate option is smaller (Bickel, Moody, & Higgins, 2016). Indeed, there is a growing literature demonstrating a relatively greater bias for the present among individuals with various addictions, obesity, and low compliance with the disease prevention regimens relative to otherwise comparable individuals who are without those problems (e.g., Bickel et al., 2007; Bradford, 2010). Moreover, the degree of this bias is negatively associated with level of income or educational attainment, which likely also contributes to the overrepresentation of these risk behaviors and chronic health problems among disadvantaged populations (Green, Myerson, Lichtman, Rosen, & Fry, 1996; Jaroni, Wright, Lerman, & Epstein, 2004). Indeed, environmental conditions where reinforcement availability is scarce appear to accentuate this bias for the present (Mani, Mullainathan, Shafir, & Zhao, 2013; Shah, Mullainathan, & Shafir, 2012). Second, there is also considerable evidence from preclinical laboratory settings, clinical laboratory settings, treatment outcome research, and epidemiological studies supporting the position that impoverished environments where there are few competing sources of alternative reinforcement render responding that is maintained by drugs and other basic sources of reinforcement more resistant to change (e.g., Campbell & Carroll, 2000; Carroll, 1993; Higgins, 1997; Higgins, Heil, & Lussier, 2004). That appears to be another substantive factor underpinning the overrepresentation of these risk behaviors and associated problems among socioeconomically disadvantaged populations. Third, a factor relevant to humans and other social primates is that this same reinforcement pathway appears to be impacted by one's relative status in social hierarchies and has been shown to moderate the reinforcing effects of drugs in nonhuman primates (e.g., lower social status increases sensitivity to cocaine-produced reinforcement) (Nader, Czoty, Nader, & Morgan, 2012). Lastly, an additional characteristic of human decision-making that merits mention in this context is a greater sensitivity to discrete and salient behavioral consequences over those that are more diffuse or subtle (Loewenstein, Brennan, & Volpp, 2007). To grasp the potential impact of this characteristic, contrast the readily discernible onset and salient tastes associated with the consumption of fatty and salty foods that contribute to hypertension compared to the relatively diffuse and largely imperceptible benefits of exercise-related reductions in blood pressure (Loewenstein et al., 2007).

While the reinforcement process and associated features are highly adaptive, humans residing in contemporary industrialized societies are now confronted with pharmacological agents and associated drug administration regimens that are highly effective at stimulating these same reward pathways. We reside in environments where fatty and sweet foods are abundantly available and, for some, are available to the relative exclusion of healthier food options. We also reside in complex social environments with well-developed and sometimes inflexible social hierarchies. As such, many individuals experience levels of scarcity or impoverishment that can accentuate the tendency to prefer more immediate over delayed sources of reinforcement even under conditions where the magnitude or subjective value of the latter is larger. In short, there is overwhelming evidence that the reinforcement process plays a substantial role in the genesis and maintenance of cigarette smoking and other unhealthy behavior patterns and their overrepresentation and resilience in socioeconomically disadvantaged and otherwise vulnerable populations.

The overarching aim of the research reviewed below is to leverage that same reinforcement process to reduce drug use and promote other health-related behavior change in vulnerable populations. We review a body of research using financial incentives to promote changes in drug use among socioeconomically disadvantaged populations. That is, we offer financial incentives as an immediate reward for objective evidence of behavior change thereby leveraging the same reinforcement process and the tendency to prefer immediate reinforcement that drives drug use, abuse, and dependence to encourage cessation. To put that research in context, we begin by reviewing a body of research that successfully used that strategy in outpatient treatment of cocaine dependence, work that catalyzed interest in the use of financial incentives to reduce drug use and promote health-related behavior change more generally (Higgins, Heil, & Lussier, 2004). We next review the successful extension of that model to tackling a major public health challenge of smoking during pregnancy, which in the USA is largely although not exclusively constrained to socioeconomically disadvantaged women (Higgins et al., 2012; Higgins & Solomon, 2016). We also briefly review several studies where financial incentives were used to promote greater use of medically recommended contraceptives in women at risk for unplanned pregnancies (Heil et al., 2016), and to increase adherence with cardiac rehabilitation in socioeconomically disadvantaged cardiac patients (Gaalema et al., 2016), to illustrate the generality of this behavior-change approach to a wide range of health problems in vulnerable populations. Finally, consistent with the multipronged approach to health promotion in vulnerable populations that we believe is necessary for improving population health, we shift to reviewing research with vulnerable populations of cigarette smokers where again the reinforcement process is leveraged with the goal of reducing cigarette smoking in vulnerable populations. Rather than the overarching goal of devising more effective treatment interventions, this research is conducted to evaluate the potential feasibility and efficacy of a national policy that would reduce the maximal nicotine content in cigarettes below levels necessary to produce reinforcement thereby decreasing the likelihood that cigarette smoking would produce or sustain addiction (Benowitz & Henningfield, 1994; Benowitz & Henningfield, 2013; Donny et al., 2015; Higgins,

Heil, et al., 2017, Higgins, Redner, et al., 2017). In the parlance of the field of tobacco research, the former falls under the heading of tobacco control research while the latter is under the heading of tobacco regulatory science. Important to keep in mind is that most smokers, other substance abusers, and those with other behavioral health problems will never seek or otherwise receive formal treatment for those problems. Thus, additional behavior-change and health promotion strategies are needed to reach the majority of those who need to change health-related behavior patterns but will never receive formal treatment to do so. We conclude by reviewing overarching themes reflected in all of the research presented, as well as providing recommendations for future research focused on promoting and maintaining health-related behavior change particularly among vulnerable populations.

Intervention for Cocaine-Dependent Outpatients

The US cocaine epidemic in the 1980s and 1990s was comparable to the current opioid epidemic. Nationally representative surveys administered during this time indicated that cocaine use peaked around 1985 with approximately 5.8 million users, but persisted at epidemic levels well into the 1990s (Cornish & O'Brien, 1996). The clinical and scientific communities were strikingly unprepared to deal with the adverse consequences of such rampant cocaine use and with the resulting cocaine-related deaths and disabilities. Indeed, the program of research described below was conducted in a context in which behavioral and pharmacological treatments targeting cocaine use were failing miserably, and the pharmacology of cocaine (i.e., mechanisms of action-targeted brain dopamine systems) suggested substantial challenges in developing an efficacious medication that reduced cocaine use while leaving the dopamine systems sufficiently intact to support basic everyday functioning. It was in this context that the use of financial incentives gained a substantial toehold in the domain of health promotion when it was used as part of a multicomponent intervention for outpatient treatment of cocaine dependence (Higgins, Heil, & Lussier, 2004). The intervention offered financial incentives in the form of vouchers exchangeable for retail items contingent on objective evidence of recent abstinence from cocaine use. More details on the incentive program are outlined below. The voucher program was combined with an intensive behavior therapy program originally developed for alcohol use disorders known as the Community Reinforcement Approach (CRA) (Hunt & Azrin, 1973). The overarching aim of CRA is to assist patients with creating a community that will reinforce healthy, drug-free lifestyle choices in order to compete with the allure of obtaining reinforcement through the substance abusing lifestyle. CRA integrates several treatment components, including building motivation to abstain from drug use, reengaging with earlier source or identifying new sources of nondrug reinforcement, and developing new coping skills, all of which are designed to teach an individual how to recruit nondrug sources of reinforcement for healthy living in his or her surrounding community.

The content of the CRA plus Vouchers intervention is described in detail in a therapist manual (see Budney & Higgins, 1994) available on the National Institute on Drug Abuse webpage (https://archives.drugabuse.gov/TXManuals/CRA/CRA1.html). Briefly, cocaine-dependent individuals received a 24-week treatment intervention and a subsequent 24 weeks of aftercare. The initial 12 weeks consisted of twice-weekly counseling with thrice-weekly urine toxicology testing to detect any cocaine use during the initial 12 weeks. This schedule of counseling and urine toxicology testing was subsequently thinned to once-weekly counseling and twice-weekly urinalysis during weeks 13–24, and months 7–12 consisted of an aftercare program wherein participants completed once-monthly check-ins with a counselor and random urinalysis. During those initial 12 weeks, patients could earn vouchers for providing objective evidence of cocaine abstinence. The rationale for including the incentive program was that assisting patients with establishing naturalistic sources of reinforcement for a healthy lifestyle (e.g., establishing healthy social relationships, securing a meaningful job, and learning how to recreate without drugs involved) takes time, and during that period a lack of reinforcement relative to what patients were used to in the cocaine-abusing lifestyle could precipitate treatment dropout and relapse. Thus, these contrived sources of relatively immediate reinforcement in the form of vouchers exchangeable for retail items were provided to bridge that temporal gap between entering treatment and initiating cocaine abstinence and establishing natural sources of nondrug reinforcement in one's community that would be necessary to sustain longer-term abstinence.

In this voucher system, participants earned points (1 point = $0.25) for providing cocaine-negative urine specimens at their thrice-weekly visits. The first negative urine sample was worth 10 points (the equivalent of $2.50), and points earned per sample (i.e., magnitude of reinforcement) increased across consecutive negative samples to reinforce sustained cocaine abstinence. In addition, points equivalent to a $10.00 bonus were provided for every three consecutive negative tests with the goal of further reinforcing sustained abstinence. If participants tested positive for cocaine, they earned zero points for that sample and the value of the voucher available for the next cocaine-negative test result was reset back to the initial low 10 points ($2.50). However, to encourage patients to continue efforts to abstain from cocaine use following a reset, five consecutive negative urine toxicology tests following a reset restored voucher value back to where it was prior to the reset. Vouchers could be redeemed through study staff for retail items in the community, but had to be approved by their therapist as being aligned with the overarching CRA aim of recruiting natural sources of reinforcement for a cocaine-free lifestyle. Maximum total vouchers a patient could earn was $997.50 across the 12-week period. Of course, not all patients successfully abstained and thus the results below were achieved at a cost of approximately half of that maximum.

Efficacy Trials

The efficacy of the CRA plus Vouchers intervention was demonstrated in six randomized controlled clinical trials (Higgins et al., 1991, 1993, 2003, 2007; Higgins, Budney, et al., 1994; Higgins, Wong, Badger, Ogden, & Dantona, 2000). CRA plus Vouchers was compared to standard care for promoting cocaine abstinence in the initial two trials to assess whether the intervention was more effective than treatment that was already available in the community (Higgins et al., 1991, 1993). Next, three trials were completed, experimentally isolating the initial and longer-term effects of the voucher incentives on cocaine abstinence (Higgins et al., 2007; Higgins, Budney, et al., 1994; Higgins, Wong, et al., 2000). A sixth trial experimentally isolated the contributions of the CRA therapy component of the treatment on cocaine abstinence and other outcomes (Higgins et al., 2003).

Alongside these clinical trials, numerous complimentary clinical laboratory experimental studies were conducted as well, often substituting cigarette smoking for cocaine use as the target substance (e.g., Alessi, Badger, & Higgins, 2004; Higgins, Bickel, & Hughes, 1994; Roll & Higgins, 2000; Roll, Higgins, & Badger, 1996). These laboratory studies were used to experimentally examine questions in a more time-efficient manner than is feasible in clinical trials. For example, we demonstrated that including the reset contingency in the voucher delivery schedule increased the duration of continuous abstinence achieved compared to when the same value vouchers were available but without that contingency (Roll et al., 1996; Roll & Higgins, 2000). These studies also gave our research group the experience with using financial incentives to promote abstinence from cigarette smoking, which was the start of what eventually became the intervention we use in the research on smoking cessation among pregnant women described below.

CRA Plus Vouchers Versus Standard Care An initial pilot clinical trial (Higgins et al., 1991) and a subsequent fully randomized clinical trial (Higgins et al., 1993) were conducted examining the efficacy of this CRA plus Vouchers intervention versus standard care to see if this novel approach produced outcomes that were superior to what was already available in treatment seekers in the community. Results were highly consistent across those two studies and we report only those from the second trial. Participants were 38 cocaine-dependent adults who were randomly assigned to one of the two treatment conditions (19 participants per condition). Separate therapist teams trained in the respective treatment approaches delivered the interventions. Those assigned to the CRA plus Vouchers condition received the 24-week intervention outlined above. Those assigned to the Standard Care control condition received counseling based on the disease model of addiction and recovery often referred to as the "12-steps model."

Outcomes were strikingly different across the two conditions (Fig. 2.1). The two conditions were initially comparable in terms of cocaine use, but those assigned to Standard Care quickly resumed cocaine use or dropped out of treatment consistent

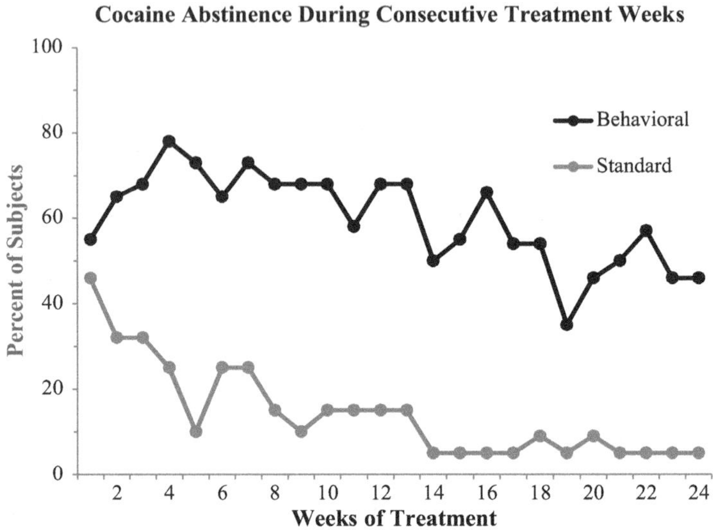

Fig. 2.1 Abstinence from cocaine among cocaine-dependent outpatients given behavioral treatment or standard drug abuse counseling. Behavioral treatment represented by closed circles and standard drug abuse counseling represented by open circles. Data originally reported in Higgins et al. (1993)

with the literature on outpatient treatment of cocaine dependence at that time. In contrast, those assigned the CRA plus Vouchers condition largely remained in treatment and sustained relatively high levels of cocaine abstinence throughout, which was an unprecedented observation in this clinical population. These promising results provided strong support for the efficacy of the multicomponent behavioral treatment for retaining patients in outpatient care and promoting cocaine abstinence.

Trials Isolating the Contribution of Financial Incentives In the initial trial isolating the effects of the incentives component of this treatment (Higgins, Budney, et al., 1994), 40 cocaine-dependent adults were randomly assigned to 24 weeks of either the CRA plus Vouchers intervention outlined above or to a CRA therapy only condition. Again, the results were quite clear: 75% of participants assigned to the CRA plus Vouchers group completed 24 weeks of treatment versus 40% of those assigned to the CRA alone condition. Further, average durations of continuous cocaine abstinence during weeks 1 through 24 of treatment were approximately doubled in the CRA plus Vouchers condition compared to the CRA alone condition (Fig. 2.2). These approximately twofold differences were also observed when duration of abstinence during weeks 1–12 and weeks 13–24 were examined separately.

In addition to increasing duration of continuous abstinence, participants assigned to the CRA plus Vouchers condition achieved greater improvements than those in the CRA alone condition on the Drug scale of the Addiction Severity Index (ASI) 24 weeks after treatment entry, and only participants receiving CRA plus Vouchers

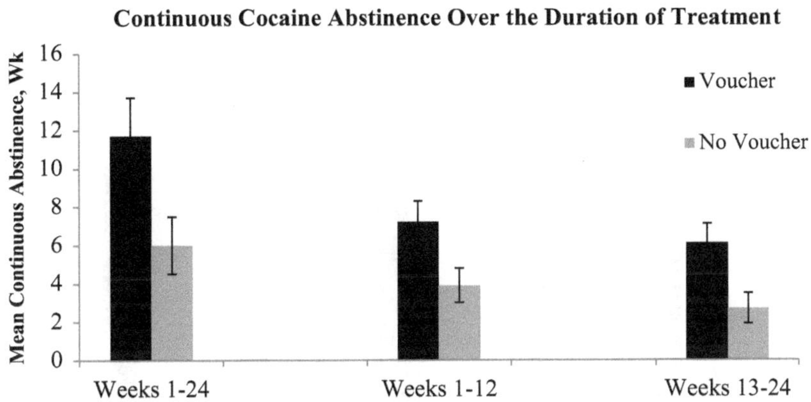

Fig. 2.2 Distributions of documented, continuous cocaine abstinence observed in each treatment group. The height of each bar represents the percentage of patients achieving a duration of abstinence greater than or equal to the number of weeks indicated. Mean durations of continuous abstinence achieved in the treatment group during weeks 1 through 24, 1 through 12, and 13 through 24. Solid bars indicate the voucher group; shaded bars, the no-voucher group. Data originally reported in Higgins, Budney, et al. (1994)

showed significant improvements on the ASI Psychiatric scale. Thus, the results of this study provided strong evidence that vouchers were an active component of this multicomponent intervention.

Examining Longer-term Outcomes While the above trials established the efficacy of incentives in promoting cocaine abstinence, longer-term effects were not reported. Consequently, this became a focus in subsequent trials. For example, participants in Higgins, Wong, et al. (2000) were 70 cocaine-dependent outpatients who were randomly assigned to one of two study conditions. All participants received 24 weeks of treatment and were followed for up to 1 year following treatment withdrawal. Participants in both treatment conditions also received CRA plus Vouchers. However, vouchers were provided contingent on cocaine-negative urine toxicology results in one condition, as they were in the earlier trials, while in the other condition they were provided independent of urine toxicology results (i.e., noncontingent incentives control condition). This noncontingent incentives control condition equates access to material resources across study conditions thereby permitting experimental isolation of the effect of the contingency requiring cocaine abstinence to obtain the incentives on treatment outcomes. Results were again clear: there were no differences in treatment retention as participants in both conditions had to come to the clinic to receive vouchers; the proportion of participants abstinent from cocaine use however was greater in the condition with contingencies on abstinence compared to the noncontingent condition during treatment and throughout 1 year of posttreatment follow-up assessments (Fig. 2.3). These results provided strong evidence that the effects of the voucher-based incentives were from the reinforcement contingency (i.e., had to abstain to obtain them), and that those effects

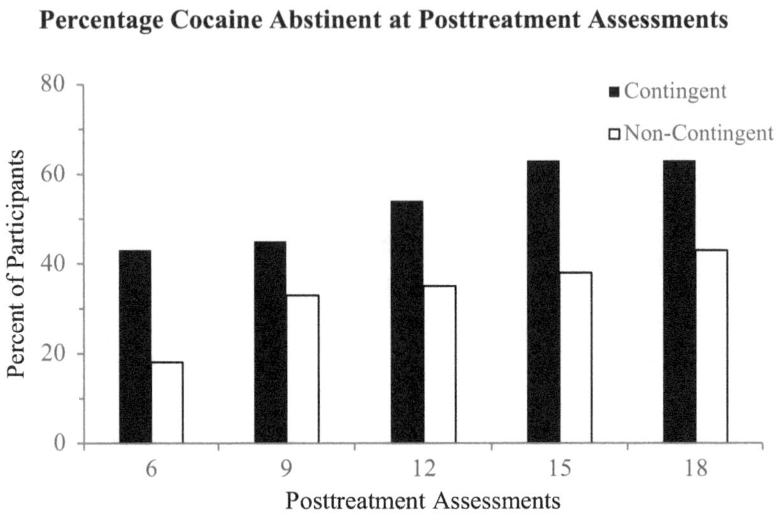

Fig. 2.3 Percentage of patients in two treatment conditions were cocaine abstinent at specific posttreatment assessments (i.e., point-prevalence abstinence). Patients were considered abstinent at an assessment period if they reported no cocaine use for the 30 days preceding the assessment and had the cocaine-negative urinalysis test results. Data originally reported in Higgins, Wong, et al. (2000)

remained discernible through 15 months after the incentive program was discontinued and 12 months after completion of the recommended 24-week course of treatment. Another important aspect of this study was that we investigated predictors of success in sustaining longer-term abstinence using multiple logistic regression modeling. The strongest predictor of longer-term abstinence was the duration of continuous abstinence achieved during the 24-week treatment period.

The observation about duration of continuous abstinence during treatment was followed up with a secondary study using 190 cocaine-dependent outpatients who participated in the earlier trials described above (Higgins, Badger, & Budney, 2000). Participants were divided into two groups: (a) those treated with CRA plus Contingent Vouchers ($n = 125$), and (b) those who received one of the control treatments ($n = 65$). In multiple logistic regression modeling, the duration of continuous cocaine abstinence during the 24-week treatment period was associated with significantly greater odds of sustaining abstinence following treatment, with no evidence of differences across treatment conditions in that regard. Where the treatment conditions differed was that those assigned to the CRA plus Contingent Vouchers condition were more likely to achieve a period of sustained abstinence during treatment. Results of this study underscored the importance of achieving early, sustained abstinence to longer-term success, an observation that was also concordant with the results reported with cigarette smokers (Kenford et al., 1994) and eventually with pregnant smokers described subsequently (Higgins et al., 2006).

Although retrospective data analysis provided strong evidence that early periods of sustained abstinence beget longer-term abstinence, retrospective results can be misleading. Thus, an important next step was to examine this relationship in a prospective experiment. A randomized controlled clinical trial was conducted in which 100 cocaine-dependent outpatients were randomly assigned to one of two CRA plus Contingent Voucher treatment conditions (Higgins et al., 2007). In one condition, vouchers were set at twice the usual monetary value (maximum of $1995 during the 12-week intervention) while in the other treatment condition they were set at half the usual value (maximum of $499 during the 12-week intervention). All else in the treatment conditions remained consistent with the usual CRA plus Vouchers treatment discussed above. As anticipated, increasing the value of the vouchers increased the duration of continuous cocaine abstinence achieved during the 24-week treatment period. Moreover, as hypothesized, point-prevalence cocaine abstinence was consistently greater among those treated in the high- compared to the low-magnitude voucher condition in assessments conducted every 3 months throughout an 18-month posttreatment follow-up period (Fig. 2.4). Considered together with the prior retrospective studies, these results provided compelling evidence that taking steps to assure success in abstaining from cocaine use during the recommended treatment period was key to achieving longer-term behavior change. The convergence of evidence from these studies on discontinuing cocaine use with evidence showing the same with quitting cigarette smoking (Kenford et al., 1994) further bolsters support for that conclusion. The results also demonstrated that the behavior change promoted with this multicomponent intervention was sustained well beyond treatment termination.

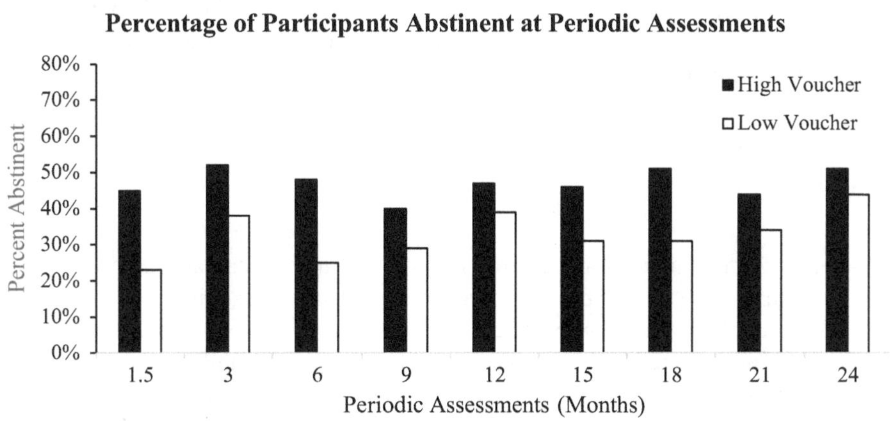

Fig. 2.4 Percentages of participants abstinent at each of the periodic assessments conducted with subjects retained in treatment as well as dropouts. Data points represent point-prevalence abstinence at the respective assessments. Abstinence was defined as a self-report of no cocaine use in the past 30 days and cocaine-negative urinalysis results. Data points for the high- and low-voucher conditions are represented by closed and open symbols, respectively. Brackets represent the categorization of periodic assessments and associated significance levels from the categorical modeling analysis. Data originally reported in Higgins et al. (2007)

The sixth randomized clinical trial in this series experimentally examined the effects of the Contingent Vouchers intervention delivered alone compared to the complete CRA plus Vouchers intervention (Higgins et al., 2003). One hundred cocaine-dependent adults were randomly assigned to one of two treatment conditions: CRA plus Vouchers or Vouchers Only. All patients earned vouchers exchangeable for retail items contingent on cocaine-free urinalysis results during treatment weeks 1–12. Incentives were combined with the 24-week course of CRA therapy in the CRA plus Vouchers condition as described above, while the voucher-based incentives represented the primary treatment in the Vouchers Only condition. Patient drug use and psychosocial functioning were assessed at intake and at least every 3 months for 2 years after treatment entry. Regarding outcomes, patients assigned to the CRA plus Vouchers condition were retained better in treatment and used cocaine at a lower frequency during the treatment period, but did not differ from those assigned to Vouchers Only on measures of continuous cocaine abstinence or cocaine abstinence at posttreatment follow-up. Those assigned to the full CRA plus Vouchers condition reported a lower frequency of drinking to intoxication during treatment and posttreatment follow-up compared with patients treated with Vouchers Only condition as well as a higher frequency of days of paid employment during treatment and the initial 6 months of follow-up, decreased depressive symptoms during the treatment period, and fewer hospitalizations and legal problems during posttreatment follow-up. Overall, the results demonstrated that the CRA component of this intervention produced a broad array of important therapeutic gains during treatment and posttreatment follow-up that should not be underestimated in terms of the overarching goal of improving health in this clinical population, the vast majority of whom have comorbid problems. That point notwithstanding, the results from this trial also indicated that the effects on posttreatment cocaine use observed in the earlier trials were likely attributable to the voucher component of the intervention which was shared across the two treatment conditions in this trial and did not differ between them.

Conclusions

This series of randomized clinical trials and supporting clinical laboratory and secondary studies provide robust empirical evidence that this reinforcement-based CRA plus Vouchers treatment produces meaningful and sustained behavior change among cocaine-dependent outpatients. The studies experimentally isolated the contribution of the voucher-based incentives program to increasing cocaine abstinence. Moreover, the studies demonstrated the importance of achieving a period of early and continuous abstinence to sustaining that behavior change longer-term. The CRA therapy was also an active component of this multicomponent intervention, decreasing drinking to intoxication, depressive symptoms, legal problems, and hospitalizations, and increasing employment—in short, increasing social stability and health.

One question initially raised about the findings early on was whether treatment effects achieved in a relatively homogeneous Caucasian, rural sample in Vermont could be achieved with more ethnically diverse, urban samples. That possibility was soon addressed through a collaborative study between the Vermont investigators and investigators located in Baltimore, MD. In that collaboration, the voucher program was demonstrated to produce substantial increases in cocaine abstinence in a sample of ethnic minority, intravenous drug users who were enrolled in methadone maintenance treatment for heroin dependence but were continuing to use cocaine (Silverman et al., 1996). Silverman and colleagues went on to develop a highly efficacious treatment model based on an adaptation of this vouchers model that is known as the Therapeutic Workplace (e.g., Silverman et al., 2002, 2007; Silverman, Svikis, Robles, Stitzer, & Bigelow, 2001). In this model, patients earn daily access to a supported work environment contingent on providing a cocaine-negative urine specimen. Upon entering the work environment, they are able to earn vouchers contingent on acquiring basic educational and vocational skills. Rather than discontinue the incentives program after 12 weeks as in the CRA plus Vouchers model, incentives in the Therapeutic Workplace Model may remain in place for as long as several years supporting abstinence from cocaine or other drug use while patients acquire vocational skills.

As noted above, because these studies were conducted in a context in which other behavioral and pharmacological approaches to treating cocaine dependence were failing miserably when examined in controlled clinical trials, this research garnered considerable attention. A literature of controlled studies examining the efficacy and effectiveness of vouchers and related financial incentives interventions across a wide range of different types of substance use disorders, populations, and settings grew rapidly. That literature has been reviewed in a three-report series that encompassed all controlled studies on treating substance use disorders using vouchers and related monetary incentives from 1991 when the first report on CRA plus Vouchers was reported through 2014 (Davis et al., 2016; Higgins, Sigmon, & Heil, 2011; Lussier, Heil, Mongeon, Badger, & Higgins, 2006). The first of these three reviews spanned the duration from January, 1991 through March, 2004 (13.25 years). The second review covered from April, 2004 through October, 2009 (5.5 years), and the most recent review covered from November, 2009 through December, 2014 (5.2 years). Across the 24 years encompassed by these three reviews, 176 controlled studies were reviewed with 151 (86%) reporting statistically significant treatment effects.

The larger literature supporting the efficacy of financial incentives for substance use disorders provided the evidence to support the adoption of financial incentives as (a) part of intensive outpatient treatment for substance use disorders within the US Veterans Administration hospital system (Petry, DePhilippis, Rash, Drapkin, & McKay, 2014), (b) a component of employee wellness programs that is now offered by the majority of major US employers (Mattke et al., 2013), and (c) a cornerstone of the empirical rationale for the World Bank's Conditional Cash Transfer program to combat chronic poverty in developing countries (Ranganathan & Lagarde, 2012). These efforts have been substantial, although the approach still has considerable unrealized potential in public-sector efforts to promote health and reduce disparities in vulnerable populations in the USA and other developed countries.

The CRA component of the CRA plus Vouchers intervention has garnered less attention, although it has been adapted into an efficacious intervention for treating (a) adolescent substance use disorders (e.g., Godley, Smith, Passetti, & Subramaniam, 2014), (b) alcohol use disorders, which is the disorder for which CRA was initially developed (Meyers, Roozen, & Smith, 2011), and (c) assisting family members with how to effectively encourage treatment entry among addicted adults who are reluctant to seek treatment (Kirby et al., 2017).

Intervention for Pregnant Cigarette Smokers

Cigarette smoking during pregnancy is a substantial public health problem in the USA and other developed countries. Smoking during pregnancy is the leading preventable cause of poor pregnancy outcomes, increasing risk for pregnancy complications, preterm birth, stillbirth, infant death, impaired lung development, childhood illness and developmental/behavioral problems, and later-in-life increased risk for cardiovascular disease, obesity, and metabolic syndrome (Barker, 2004; Dietz et al., 2010; Leslie, 2013). About 22% of women of childbearing age are regular cigarette smokers (Lopez et al., 2018), as are about 13% of pregnant women, a number that has remained stable over the past decade (Alshaarawy & Anthony, 2015; Kurti et al., 2017). Smoking prevalence is not distributed equally across subgroups of pregnant women, with rates being orders of magnitude higher among more socioeconomically disadvantaged women. For example, prevalence of smoking during pregnancy among women with less than a high school education has been estimated to be nine times higher than prevalence among those with a college degree (Kandel, Griesler, & Schaffran, 2009), and less educated women are also more likely to begin smoking at a younger age, to be heavy smokers, and to be nicotine dependent, all of which decrease the likelihood of quitting smoking during pregnancy (Higgins et al., 2009; Kandel et al., 2009). Although approximately 20% of pregnant smokers quit smoking soon after learning of pregnancy, the vast majority continue smoking through pregnancy in the absence of a formal intervention (Heil et al., 2014; Solomon & Quinn, 2004). Clearly, more effective interventions to promote smoking cessation in this vulnerable population are sorely needed.

Efficacy Trials

Seminal Trial The seminal controlled clinical trial examining smoking cessation for pregnant women was reported in the 1980s (Sexton & Hebel, 1984). Women enrolled in the intervention condition in this trial received a relatively intensive multicomponent treatment involving counseling, home visits, self-help materials, and follow-up phone calls, whereas women in the control condition received usual care for smoking cessation. Results were promising, with women in the intervention condition smoking significantly fewer cigarettes per day than those in the control condition at the final antepartum assessment (6.4 vs. 12.8), demonstrating significantly lower salivary thiocyanate levels (2094 vs. 2452 *u*mole/L), and delivering infants with higher average birth weights (3278 + 566 g vs. 3186 + 627 g, variance = SDs).

Although those results provided empirical support for the efficacy of this intensive approach to smoking cessation among pregnant women, subsequent interventions were almost exclusively developed to be brief (e.g., 5–15 min) and deliverable in the context of medical visits. Unfortunately, few of these brief interventions produced significant treatment effects on smoking abstinence (<10% of reported trials) and only one study reported statistically significant improvements in birth outcomes (decrease in infant growth-restricted births from 7.3 to 1.7%) (Lumley et al., 2009). Meta-analyses including over 70 controlled trials and 25,000 pregnant women indicated that, on average, these behavioral and psychosocial interventions increase late-pregnancy abstinence rates but only by an average of approximately 6% above control levels (Chamberlain et al., 2013; Lumley et al., 2009). The one exception to that pattern was financial incentives, which increased late-pregnancy abstinence by an average of 24% above control levels.

Financial Incentives The financial-incentive interventions studied with pregnant women are adaptations of the voucher-based program initially developed for cocaine dependence that was described above. A recent quantitative review (Cahill, Hartmann-Boyce, & Perera, 2015) examined effect sizes across eight of those trials (Donatelle et al., 2000a, as reported in Donatelle, Prows, Champeau, & Hudson, 2000; Donatelle et al., 2000b, as reported in Donatelle et al., 2004; Heil et al., 2008; Higgins, Heil, Solomon, et al., 2004; Higgins et al., 2014; Ondersma et al., 2012; Tappin et al., 2015; Tuten, Fitzsimons, Chisolm, Nuzzo, & Jones, 2012) involving 1297 women (675 treated with incentives and 622 without). Overall, those treated with incentives had 3.60 times greater odds (95% CI: 2–5.43) of being abstinent at the final assessment conducted, which typically ran out to 24 weeks postpartum (Table 2.1).

To illustrate the basic incentives treatment approach with pregnant smokers, below we describe the voucher-based incentives program used in trials conducted at the University of Vermont. Other adaptations are detailed in narrative reviews of this approach to promoting smoking cessation with pregnant women (Higgins et al., 2012; Higgins & Solomon, 2016). Trial participants in the Vermont trials were recruited from obstetric practices and WIC programs in the greater Burlington, VT community. The majority were Caucasian, <25 years old, unemployed, without health insurance, and have <12 years of education. After enrolling in the study, women were assigned to an abstinence-contingent vouchers condition or a noncontingent vouchers control condition. Women assigned to abstinence-contingent condition earned vouchers exchangeable for retail items contingent on biochemically verified smoking abstinence whereas women in the noncontingent condition earned vouchers independent of their smoking status. Vouchers were available in both conditions from study enrollment, which on average was approximately 11 weeks gestation, through 12 weeks postpartum. In the abstinence-contingent incentives

Table 2.1 Pregnancy trials at longest follow up

Study or subgroup	Log[odds ratio]	Incentives SE	Control Total	Total	Odds ratio Weight (%)	IV, fixed, 95% CI
Donatelle (2000a)	1.470176	0.48486864	103	102	18.8	4.35 [1.68, 11.25]
Donatelle (2000b)	0.598837	0.5086189	67	60	17.1	1.82 [0.67, 4.93]
Heil et al. (2008)	1.235471	1.17961923	37	40	3.2	3.44 [0.34, 34.73]
Higgins et al. (2004)	2.876949	1.48401171	30	23	2.0	17.76 [0.97, 325.56]
Higgins et al. (2014)	0.936093	0.72979458	40	39	8.3	2.55 [0.61, 10.66]
Ondersma et al. (2012)	1.324418966	1.10352688	48	23	3.6	3.76 [0.43, 32.70]
Tappin et al. (2015)	1.355835	0.31290118	306	303	45.1	3.88 [2.10, 7.16]
Tuten et al. (2012)	3.392829	1.4628312	42	32	2.1	29.75 [1.69, 523.18]
Total (95% CI)			673	622	100.0	3.60 [2.39, 5.43]

Data originally reported in Cahill et al. (2015)

condition, voucher value began at $6.25 for the first urine specimen indicating no smoking and escalated by $1.25 for each consecutive negative sample up to a maximum of $45.00. Women in the noncontingent incentives condition received vouchers for $11.50 per urine specimen submitted during pregnancy and $20.00 per specimen postpartum. Average earnings were similar across the two conditions with mean earnings in the abstinence-contingent incentives condition being an average of $461.00 + $456.00 versus $413.00 + $163.00 (variance = SDs) in the noncontingent incentives control condition. In addition to vouchers, women in both conditions received usual care from their providers plus pregnancy-specific smoking-cessation educational materials provided by research staff. Women in both conditions also received serial ultrasounds at 30 and 34 weeks gestation to examine fetal growth trajectories, and medical records were examined to evaluate birth outcomes.

Across trials, end of pregnancy point-prevalence abstinence rates have been almost fivefold greater in the abstinence-contingent incentives condition compared to controls (34.1% vs. 7.4%), and treatment effect has remained discernible out through 24 weeks postpartum (14.1% vs. 1.2%), 12 weeks after discontinuation of the incentives (Fig. 2.5).

In addition to effects on abstinence, infants born to mothers who received contingent incentives had greater mean birth weights (3295 + 63.8 g vs. 3093.6 + 67.0 g) (variance = SEMs) and a lower percentage of low birth weight (<2500 g) (5.9% vs. 18.5%) (Table 2.2) with trends in the same direction for gestational age at delivery among infants born to mothers who received contingent incentives (39.1 + 0.2 weeks vs. 38.5 + 0.3 weeks), (variance = SEMs) as well as a lower percentage of preterm

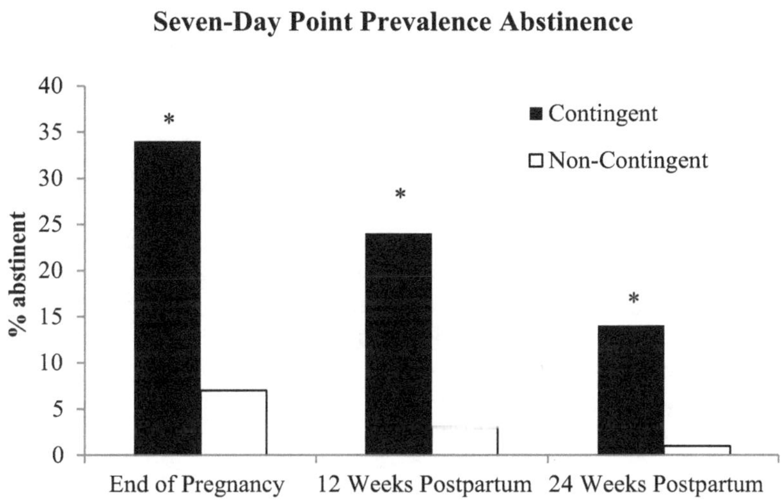

Fig. 2.5 Seven-day point-prevalence abstinence at the end-of-pregnancy, 12-, and 24-week postpartum assessments in the contingent ($n = 85$) and noncontingent ($n = 81$) treatment conditions. Treatment conditions are the same as described in Fig. 2.1. Asterisks indicate a significant difference between conditions ($p = 0.003$ or below across the three assessments). Data originally reported in Higgins et al. (2012)

Table 2.2 Infant outcomes at delivery by treatment group

Measure	Contingent ($n = 85$)	Non-contingent ($n = 81$)	*P* values
Birth weight (g)	3295.6 ± 63.8	3093 ± 67.0	0.03
% Low birth weight	5.9	18.5	0.02
Gestational age	39.1 ± 0.2	38.5 ± 0.3	0.06
% Preterm births	5.9	13.6	0.09
% NICU admissions	4.7	13.8	0.06

Data originally reported in Higgins et al. (2010). Values represent mean ± standard error, unless otherwise specified. Women in the contingent condition received vouchers exchangeable for retail items contingent on biochemically verified smoking abstinence while those in the non-contingent condition received vouchers of comparable value but independent of smoking status. *NICU* neonatal intensive care unit. Gestational age reported is in weeks. Based on results reported in Higgins et al. (2010)

births (5.9% vs. 13.6%, $p = 0.09$) among the contingent versus noncontingent conditions and a trend in the same direction for NICU admissions (4.7% vs. 13.8%). A higher proportion of women in the contingent condition also continued to breastfeed at 8 weeks (41% vs. 26%) and 12 weeks postpartum (35% vs. 17%), and postpartum depressive symptoms were reduced among depression-prone women treated with abstinence-contingent incentives (Lopez, Skelly, & Higgins, 2015; Zvorsky, Skelly, & Higgins, 2017).

Predictors of Treatment Response Other research questions examined by the University of Vermont investigators included which baseline participant characteristics predicted quit success. Nicotine-dependence indicators including cigarettes smoked per day and time to first cigarette (Kurti, Davis, Skelly, Redner, & Higgins, 2016), as well as educational attainment (Higgins et al., 2016) have been demonstrated to independently predict late-pregnancy smoking status. Also investigated was whether the relationships between early and longer-term abstinence occurred among pregnant smokers as it does for cocaine-dependent outpatients and smokers from the general population. Consistent with those prior results, a women's smoking status in the initial 2 weeks of a quit attempt was a remarkably strong predictor of late-pregnancy smoking status (Higgins et al., 2006). Among women who abstained during the first 2 weeks of the cessation effort, 88% were abstinent at their late-pregnancy assessment compared to only 15% among those who smoked even just a few puffs during the first 2 weeks.

Conclusions

There is robust evidence supporting the efficacy of financial incentives for promoting smoking-cessation among pregnant women that is evident at the level of individual trials and in three Cochrane meta-analyses (Cahill et al., 2015; Chamberlain et al., 2013; Lumley et al., 2009). Antepartum treatment effects are strikingly positive and important in light of accumulating evidence regarding the broad range of adverse effects from in utero smoke exposure across the life span of exposed offspring. Treatment effects of the incentives are not as strong postpartum as they are antepartum, but typically produce abstinence levels several fold above control levels (e.g., Heil et al., 2008 ; Higgins, Heil, Solomon, et al., 2004) and aggregated across trials (Cahill et al., 2015). Where there is more to be learned is regarding efficacy for sustaining longer-term maternal cessation rates after the incentives have been discontinued. There is evidence of significant sustained treatment effects for 3 months after discontinuation of the incentives in two trials conducted at the University of Vermont (Heil et al., 2008; Higgins, Heil, Solomon, et al., 2004), and a clear trend in that direction in a third trial (Higgins et al., 2014). Nonetheless, this is an area that merits further investigation and also further attention in terms of treatment efforts specifically designed to prepare women to sustain abstinence longer-term.

We know of no alternative strategy in this population with comparable support. For this reason, it should come as no surprise that there is strong and growing international interest in the use of financial incentives for pregnant smokers. To date, the UK has made the most progress in moving this model into routine care. Specifically, Ierfino et al. (2015) demonstrated the effectiveness of the incentives intervention when delivered by clinicians in a clinical rather than research setting in a large urban community hospital in Chesterfield, England, where incentives produced cessation rates of 20% above control levels, a difference that is consistent with Cahill et al. (2015) meta-analysis.

The cost-effectiveness of financial incentives targeting pregnant cigarette smokers has been examined in one trial comparing the incremental cost per late-pregnancy quitter in the incentives versus control treatment (Boyd, Briggs, Bauld, Sinclair, & Tappin, 2016). Comparing against standardized incremental cost-effectiveness ratio tables in the literature for smoking cessation in the general population, the model was deemed to be highly cost effective. Consideration of impacts on birth outcomes and infant health in future cost-effectiveness studies certainly would be expected to improve cost-effectiveness even further.

Interventions to Promote Adherence with Medical Regimens Among Vulnerable Populations

Although financial incentives have been most extensively researched with regard to treating substance use disorders, this behavioral economic approach to behavior change can be used across a wide range of health problems (Higgins et al., 2012). Below, we review two areas of research underway at the University of Vermont that illustrate the generality of this behavior-change approach.

Increasing the Use of Medically Recommended Contraception Among Opioid-Dependent Women One of the most unsettling aspects of the current US opioid dependence epidemic is the high rate of in utero drug exposure among infants born to opioid-dependent women. Most of those pregnancies are unplanned and result from low rates of effective contraceptive use in this population. In a seminal controlled study on this topic, 31 opioid-dependent women were randomly assigned to usual care or an experimental intervention (Heil et al., 2016). Usual care included receiving an informational booklet about birth control methods (Planned Parenthood's "Facts About Birth Control"), a list of nearby providers of contraceptive services, and an offer of free condoms and a dose of emergency contraception (i.e., Plan B or ella). The experimental intervention included receiving usual care plus (a) the World Health Organization's (WHO) contraception initiation protocol, including free contraceptives, and (b) financial incentives for attending 13 follow-up visits over 6 months to help manage side effects and other issues with maximal potential earnings of $390—note that incentives were earned for meeting with staff to discuss side effects, etc. and not for contraceptive use.

In terms of outcomes, more women assigned to the experimental vs. usual care control conditions initiated prescription contraceptive use (100% vs. 29%) and reported prescription contraceptive use at the 1-month (63% vs.13%), 3-month (88% vs. 20%), and 6-month (94% vs. 13%) assessments. None of the experimental condition participants became pregnant during the 6-month protocol versus three women (20%) in the control condition. In addition, 38% of women in the experimental condition chose the most effective prescription contraceptive methods versus 7% of women in the control condition.

These results provided the first experimental evidence supporting the efficacy of an intervention for increasing prescription contraceptive use among at-risk opioid-maintained women. We consider this model to have tremendous potential for promoting effective contraceptive use among other vulnerable populations. Preliminary research results from an ongoing trial examining the relative efficacy of the WHO and incentives components of this intervention suggest that both are active contributors to the positive results outlined above.

Increasing Adherence to Cardiac Rehabilitation among Socioeconomically Disadvantaged Patients Cardiac rehabilitation (CR) is a structured, progressive exercise program (often 36 sessions) with interventions for coronary risk factor reduction that is highly effective at reducing morbidity and mortality rates following a myocardial infarction (MI) or coronary revascularization (Lawler, Filion, & Eisenberg, 2011) producing an approximately one-third reduction in cardiac rehospitalizations over 12 months and one-quarter to one-third decrease in cardiac mortality over 2–3 years (Lawler et al., 2011). Unfortunately, lower socioeconomic status (SES) patients are substantially less likely to participate in or complete CR compared to more affluent patients. This initial study examined whether financial incentives may increase participation and adherence to CR among lower-SES patients (Gaalema et al., 2016).

Ten patients with Medicaid insurance coverage who were eligible to participate in CR were approached for inclusion. Patients received financial incentives contingent upon completion of each of the 36 CR sessions with a maximal potential earnings of $1368. CR participation was compared to a usual care group of 101 Medicaid patients eligible for CR in the 18 months prior to the study. Attendance (participating in ≥ one CR sessions) and adherence (sessions completed out of 36) were compared between conditions. All 10 (100%) patients who received incentives completed at least one session of CR compared to only 25/101 (25%) in the control condition. Of patients in both conditions who attended at least one session of CR, adherence was higher in the intervention conditions (average of 31.1 sessions completed vs. 13.6 in the control group). CR completion rates were also higher in the intervention with 8 of 10 (80%) patients completing all 36 sessions compared to only 2 of 25 (8%) control patients.

The results provided strong initial evidence that financial incentives appear to be a highly efficacious strategy for increasing CR participation among Medicaid patients. Preliminary results from a large randomized controlled trial being conducted to follow up these results appear to be replicating and extending the positive outcomes obtained with incentives in this initial proof-of-concept study.

Conclusions

The studies on the efficacy of financial incentives in promoting use of effective contraception and adherence to critical medical services like cardiac rehabilitation illustrate the breadth and potential of this behavior-change model for addressing medically important but often ignored challenges to improving health and reducing disparities in vulnerable populations. Financial incentives clearly have a potentially substantive contribution to make in efforts to promote health and reduce disparities in vulnerable populations. Cost-effectiveness is likely to be an important factor in determining the extent to which that potential is realized.

Another Component of a Multipronged Approach to Promoting Health-Related Behavior Change in Vulnerable Populations: Tobacco Regulatory Science Research

Tobacco Regulatory Science

Above, we focused on leveraging the reinforcement process in efforts to develop more effective treatment interventions for promoting health-related behavior change in vulnerable populations. However, because so many of those with substance use disorders and other behavioral health conditions never receive formal treatment for those problems, it is important that we also look for opportunities to leverage the reinforcement process in ways that can promote health outside of formal treatment settings. In the remaining section of this report, we focus on tobacco regulatory science as an exemplar of such an effort. After providing a brief introduction to the relatively new field of tobacco regulatory science, we review research that is examining the potential feasibility and efficacy of a national policy that would reduce the maximal nicotine content of commercial cigarettes in order to decrease their reinforcing effects and hence their potential to produce addiction. We specifically address the potential benefits of reduced-nicotine content cigarettes among those populations who are considered especially vulnerable to tobacco use, addiction, or experiencing greater adverse health effects from smoking relative to the general population.

Reduced-Nicotine Standards in Cigarettes

The 2009 US Family Smoking Prevention and Tobacco Control Act for the first time granted the Food and Drug Administration (FDA) authority to regulate the manufacture, marketing, and distribution of tobacco products in order to protect the public health. As part of this regulatory effort, the FDA in collaboration with the NIH's Office of Disease Prevention established a trans-NIH Tobacco Regulatory Science Program (Office of Disease Prevention, 2017). Important to note is that this act gives the FDA the authority to reduce, although not completely eliminate, the nicotine content in cigarettes and other tobacco and nicotine delivery products if doing so protects the public health. Interestingly, the notion that setting national standards for the maximum nicotine content allowable in cigarettes may benefit public health is not new. Indeed, a prescient essay by Benowitz and Henningfield (1994) first proposed reducing the nicotine content in cigarettes below a hypothesized threshold for developing addiction (0.7 mg/g) more than two decades ago. Since the passage of the Smoking Prevention and Tobacco Control Act in 2009, and the corresponding development of tobacco regulatory science research infrastructure, a growing body of research is accumulating in support of the potential feasibility and efficacy of a reduced-nicotine content policy among relatively stable and healthy smokers as well as in vulnerable populations. We review selected aspects of that research below, but first review some observational studies that bolster the rationale for considering such a policy.

Observational Studies on Use of Higher-Nicotine/Tar-Yield (Regular Full-Flavored) Cigarettes Among Vulnerable Populations

In this section, we review observational studies on whether use of machine-estimated high-nicotine and tar-yield (full-flavor, medium, light, and ultralight) commercial cigarettes increases risk for nicotine dependence. These studies provide an important context for considering the subsequent body of experimental research reviewed examining the effects of reducing the nicotine content of cigarettes to very low levels.

Commercial cigarettes come in a variety of types, including ultralight, light, medium, and full-flavor corresponding to machine-estimated levels nicotine/tar yield. Although there are now regulations that prevent manufacturers from using those particular labels, these different cigarette types are still marketed but are now designated by colors (e.g., Marlboro "silvers" indicate ultralight cigarettes whereas Marlboro "reds" indicate regular full-flavor cigarettes). Importantly, the nicotine content of the cigarette is equivalent across these four cigarette types, but the cigarettes are engineered to include differing levels of ventilation to dilute the smoke and corresponding different levels of machine-estimated nicotine yields, with ultralights estimated to have the lowest yield and full-flavor cigarettes the highest (Benowitz et al., 1986; Gori & Lynch, 1983; Kozlowski, Frecker, & Lei, 1982; Zacny, Stitzer, Brown, Yingling, & Griffiths, 1987). There is broad scientific consensus that users of lower-yield cigarettes commonly engage in compensatory smoking by blocking the ventilation holes or altering their smoking topography in order to achieve desired nicotine blood levels thereby undermining the goal of reducing health impacts by lowering exposure levels (Kozlowski & Pillitteri, 2001). However, less well recognized is that compensatory smoking is typically partial with regard to nicotine exposure (approximately 75%; Scherer & Lee, 2014). An important question is whether that 25% difference in nicotine exposure levels between lower and higher yield cigarettes might be sufficient to result in differences in nicotine-dependence risk, which is concerning as nicotine dependence is considered to be a major contributor to the emergence and persistence of chronic smoking and difficulties quitting (Shiffman, Dunbar, & Benowitz, 2014; U.S. Department of Health and Human Services, 1988, 2014). Below, we review three observational studies conducted by University of Vermont investigators examining whether use of higher-nicotine yield cigarettes is

(a) associated with increased risk for nicotine dependence, (b) overrepresented among socioeconomically disadvantaged and other populations known to be vulnerable to nicotine dependence, and (c) whether use of full-flavor cigarettes may be associated with the problem of women continuing to smoke despite being pregnant and aware of the harmful effects that smoking can have on the fetus.

The first of these three studies examined whether use of higher-nicotine/tar-yield cigarettes is associated with greater nicotine dependence after controlling for important potential confounding variables (e.g., sociodemographics, and cigarettes per day) in the US nationally representative samples of adults and adolescents (Redner, White, Bunn, & Higgins, 2016). The research was conducted using 3 years (2012, 2013, and 2014) of the National Survey on Drug Use and Health (NSDUH), with adults and adolescents examined separately. Nicotine dependence was measured using the Nicotine Dependence Syndrome Scale (NDSS) and the single item Fagerstrom Test of Nicotine Dependence question on the latency to first cigarette upon waking. Associations between cigarette type and these dependence indices were examined using multiple logistic regression modeling. Table 2.3 shows prevalence of nicotine dependence (NDSS and Time-to-first-Cigarette) by cigarette type among both adults and adolescents. The proportion of respondents meeting criteria for nicotine dependence was greatest among those using full-flavor cigarettes in adults and adolescents. This relationship was demonstrated across both measures of nicotine dependence, both study populations, and consecutive years of the survey. Even after controlling for sociodemographics and smoking characteristics known to influence dependence risk, the odds of being nicotine dependent were significantly higher among users of full-flavor cigarettes relative to users of medium, light, and ultralight cigarettes.

The second study collapsed data across 3 consecutive years of the NSDUH to have sufficient statistical power to examine whether use of full-flavor cigarettes among smokers was overrepresented among those with lower socioeconomic status and other characteristics associated with vulnerability to tobacco use and addiction

Table 2.3 Prevalence of nicotine dependence (NDSS and time-to-first-cigarette) by cigarette type among adults and adolescents (2011–2013 National Survey of Drug Use and Health [NSDUH])

	Adults, 2013 NSDUH (n = 10,361)		Adults, 2012 NSDUH (n = 11,092)		Adolescents, 2011–2013 NSDUH (n = 3682)	
	NDSS (%)	Time-to-first-cigarette (<30) (%)	NDSS (%)	Time-to-first-cigarette (<30) (%)	NDSS (%)	Time-to-first-cigarette (<30) (%)
Cigarette type						
Full-flavor	46.4	58.8	47.7	59.0	32.2	41.8
Medium	31.1	40.8	40.1	45.9	18.5	18.4
Light	31.1	38.9	32.2	38.3	8.7	18.0
Ultra-light	32.8	43.7	37.5	40.4	4.7	10.8

Data originally reported in Redner et al. (2016)
NDSS Nicotine Dependence Syndrome Scale

(Higgins et al., 2016). Indeed, use of full-flavor cigarettes was independently associated with six of the seven markers of vulnerability examined. Low educational attainment was the strongest predictor of using full-flavor cigarettes among current cigarette smokers followed by having an annual income below the federal poverty level, male sex, younger age, racial/ethnic minority status, past-year mental illness, and past-year drug abuse/dependence. Past-year alcohol abuse/dependence was the only vulnerable population in whom use of full-flavor cigarettes was not overrepresented. Use of full-flavor cigarettes was associated with greater odds of nicotine dependence within each of the six subpopulations associated with using that cigarette type.

The study examining the use of full-flavor cigarettes among pregnant women collapsed data across 10 years of the NSDUH (2005–2014) to assure a sufficient number of pregnant women. The study examined cigarette type preferences of non-pregnant women of reproductive age (ages 15–44 years) and women pregnant at the time of survey completion, comparing prevalence of smoking and use of full-flavor versus lower-yield cigarettes (Higgins, Redner, et al., 2017). The logic underpinning this study was that smoking prevalence is well known to be higher among nonpregnant than pregnant women as a subset of smokers quit upon learning of a pregnancy (e.g., Alshaarawy & Anthony, 2015; Kurti et al., 2017; Redner et al., in press). Thus, if prevalence of using full-flavor cigarettes is greater among pregnant compared to nonpregnant female smokers of reproductive age, it suggests that women using full-flavor cigarettes are less likely to quit smoking upon learning of a pregnancy. Similarly, overall smoking prevalence is known to decrease during the course of pregnancy with the lowest prevalence seen in the third trimester (Alshaarawy & Anthony, 2015). Thus, if prevalence of using full-flavor cigarettes increases among smokers in the third trimester compared to earlier in the course of pregnancy that too would suggest that women using full-flavor cigarettes are less likely to quit smoking during pregnancy. Among nonpregnant women, 39% of current cigarette smokers used full-flavor cigarettes compared to 55% among pregnant women (Fig. 2.6). Similarly, 53% of women in their first trimester of pregnancy used full-flavor cigarettes compared to 64% among those in their third trimester. Across nonpregnant and pregnant women, those using full-flavor cigarettes had greater odds of nicotine dependence than those using lower-yield cigarettes across both measures used in these studies.

Experimental Studies on Reduced-Nicotine Content Cigarettes

Rather than decrease nicotine exposure through ventilation, an alternative approach to reducing nicotine exposure levels from cigarette smoking is to reduce the nicotine content of the cigarette. A series of studies in relatively healthy smokers conducted since the FDA gained regulatory authority over tobacco products support a position that reducing nicotine content in cigarettes to very low levels significantly reduces the addiction potential of smoking (Benowitz et al., 2012; Donny et al., 2015; Hatsukami et al., 2010, 2013). Moreover, reduced-nicotine content cigarettes

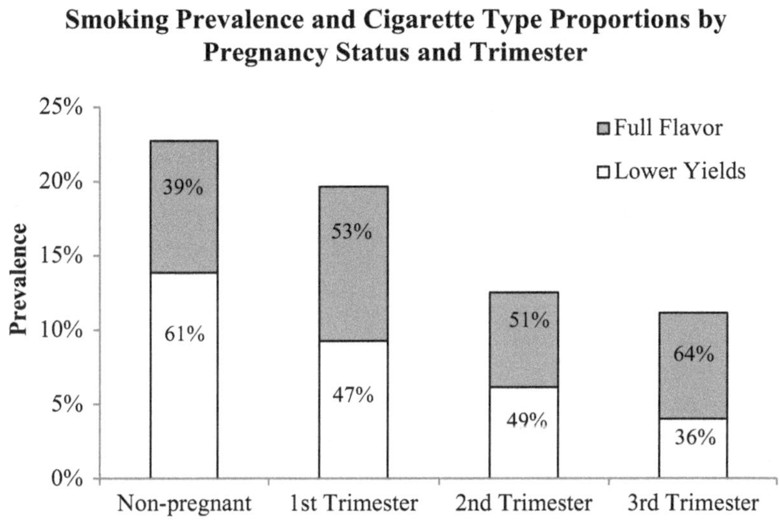

Fig. 2.6 Bar graph showing prevalence of smoking among nonpregnant and pregnant women of reproductive age (15–44 years), with results from the pregnant women displayed by trimester. Shown within each bar are the proportions of smokers whose usual brand of cigarette was full-flavor (gray) versus a lower yield (white). The data source in the National Survey on Drug Use and Health (2005–2014). Data originally reported in Higgins, Redner, et al. (2017)

appear to produce minimal compensatory smoking. To illustrate this approach, we describe results from a large randomized clinical trial reported by Donny and colleagues (Donny et al., 2015).

Donny et al. (2015) conducted a double-blind, parallel groups, randomized clinical trial with 840 adults (aged >18 years) across 10 sites who reported smoking five or more cigarettes per day and had no immediate plans to quit smoking. Participants were randomly assigned to study conditions involving 6 weeks of smoking either their usual brand of cigarettes, or one of six research cigarettes differing in nicotine content ranging from 15.8 mg/g of tobacco (comparable to commercial brand cigarettes) to 0.4 mg/g, with this lower-nicotine content cigarette being well below the 0.7 mg hypothetical threshold for addiction. The primary outcome was the number of cigarettes smoked per day during week 6.

Participants assigned to smoke their usual brand or the 15.8 mg/g content cigarette smoked a greater mean number of total cigarettes per day at week 6 than those assigned to the 2.4, 1.3, and 0.4 mg/g conditions (Fig. 2.7, upper panel). Smoking rates did not differ between those assigned to the 15 and 5.2 mg/g content conditions. Similar results were also observed when the analysis was restricted to the mean number of study cigarettes smoked per day across the varying nicotine content conditions (Fig. 2.7, lower panel).

In addition to promoting reductions in smoking, using lower-nicotine content cigarettes also reduced nicotine-dependence levels (Fig. 2.8). More specifically, participants' total scores on the Wisconsin Inventory of Smoking Dependence

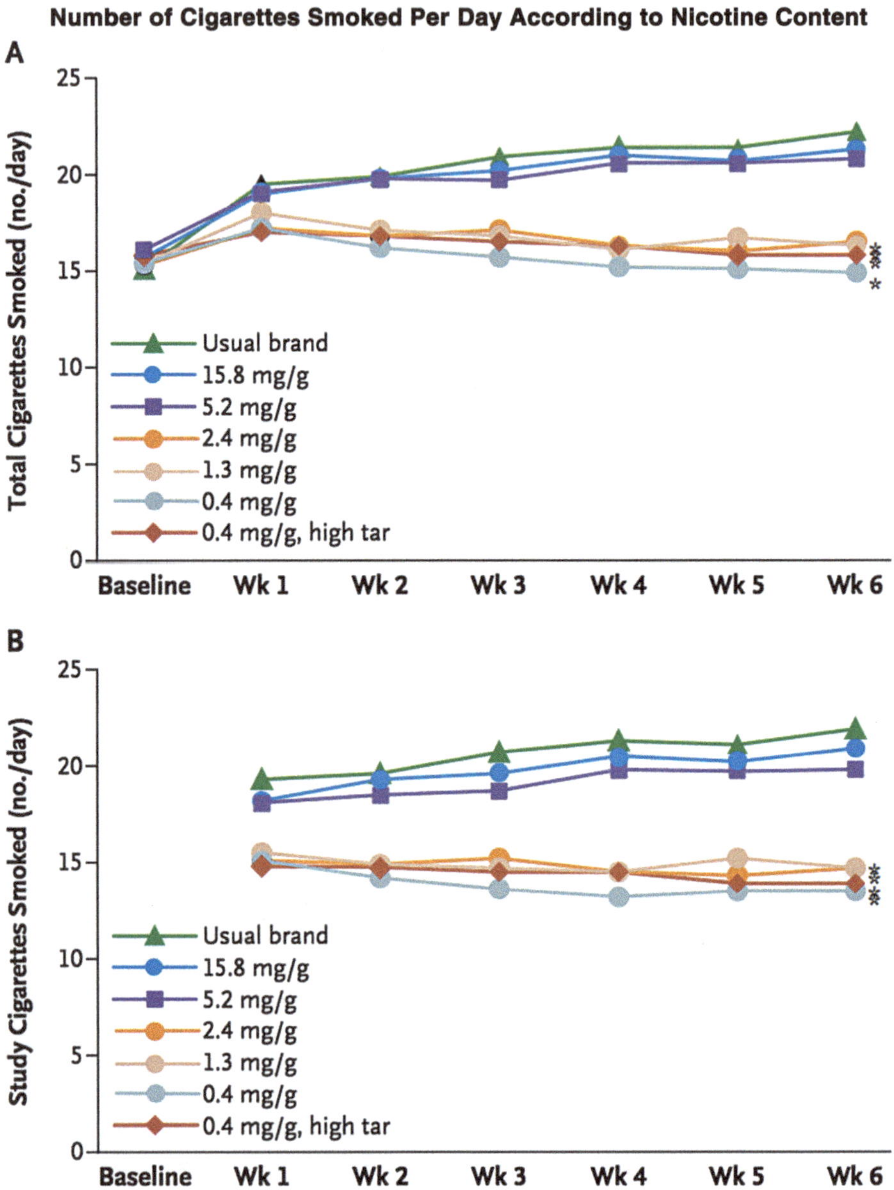

Fig. 2.7 Mean total number of cigarettes smoked per day, including both study cigarettes only (Panel **b**) and total cigarettes (Panel **a**). An asterisk indicated $p < 0.001$ for the comparison at week 6 with the primary control cigarettes (15.8 mg of nicotine per gram of tobacco). Figure reprinted with permission from Donny et al. (2015)

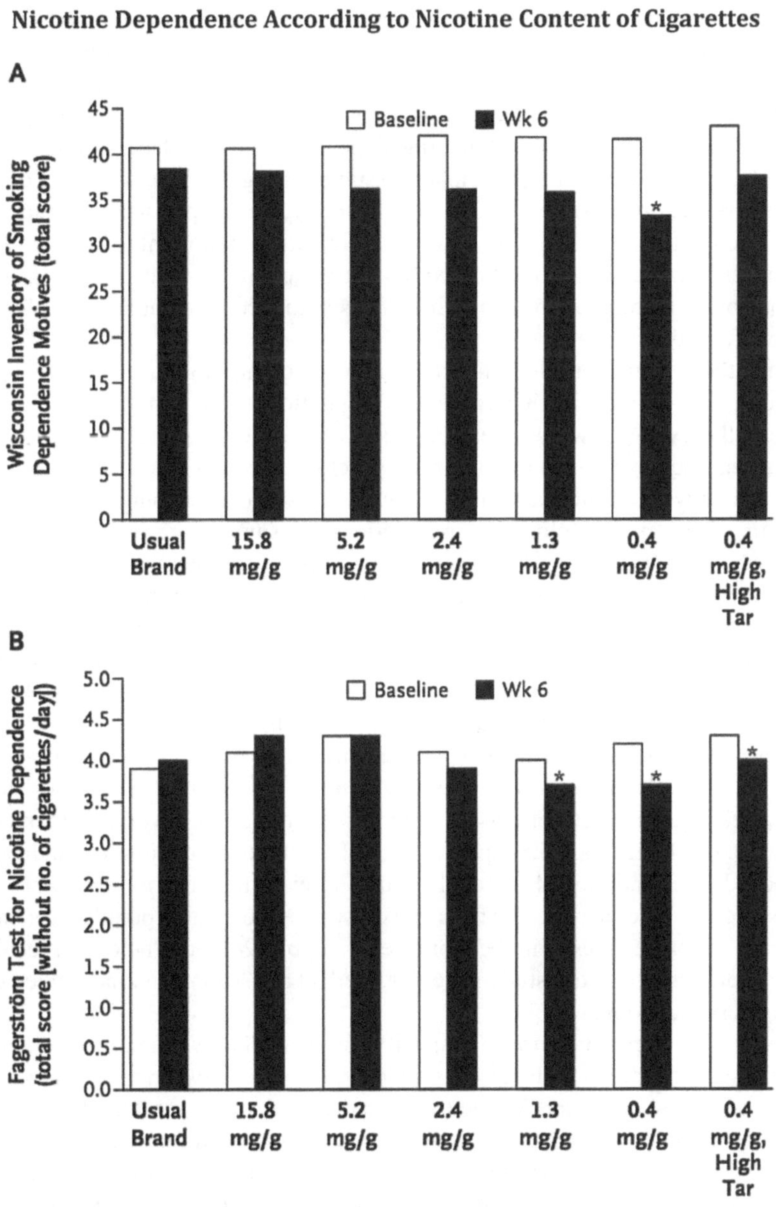

Fig. 2.8 Panel (**a**) shows total scores on the Wisconsin Inventory of Smoking Dependence Motives (score range, 11–77, with higher values indicating greater dependence), which is a multifactorial scale of nicotine dependence. Panel (**b**) shows total scores on the Fagerstrom Test for Nicotine Dependence, with the item concerning number of cigarettes smoked per day excluded (score range after exclusion of that item, 0–7, with higher values indicating greater dependence). All analyses were adjusted for the baseline score. An asterisk indicates $p \leq 0.002$ for the comparison at week 6 with cigarettes containing 15.8 mg of nicotine per gram. Figure reprinted with permission from Donny et al. (2015)

Motives (upper panel) was significantly lower at week 6 among participants assigned to the 0.4 mg/g compared to the 15.8 mg/g nicotine content conditions. Similar results were observed using the Fagerstrom Test for Nicotine Dependence (lower panel). Considered together, these results indicate that reduced-nicotine cigarettes decrease smoking frequency and nicotine dependence among the US general population of adult smokers, with participants assigned to cigarettes with 2.4 mg of nicotine or less per gram smoking 23–30% fewer cigarettes per week versus those randomized to the condition with 15.8 mg/g cigarettes. Important to note is that the differences in tar levels across the two 0.4 mg/g nicotine content cigarettes did not alter outcomes thereby eliminating differences in that constituent as an explanation for the effects observed.

While these results provide important information highlighting the potential for a policy reducing the nicotine content of cigarettes in the general population of smokers, the extent to which these results can be generalized to more vulnerable populations such as those with comorbid psychiatric conditions or socioeconomic disadvantage was left unclear in this study. University of Vermont investigators are examining how more vulnerable populations of smokers respond to reduced-nicotine content cigarettes. Those studies focus on three vulnerable populations: (a) economically disadvantaged women of reproductive age, (b) opioid-dependent individuals, and (c) individuals with affective disorders. These groups have higher rates of smoking relative to the general population (40%, 89%, 45%, respectively, versus 16.8%) and are less likely to quit than the general population of smokers (Higgins & Chilcoat, 2009; Hser, Hoffman, Grella, & Anglin, 2001; Lasser et al., 2000; Lawrence, Mitrou, & Zubrick, 2009). These investigators are conducting two multisite studies on the topic. The first is a within-subjects clinical laboratory experiment assessing the acute effects of four research cigarettes varying in nicotine content (0.4, 2.4, 5.2, and 15.8 mg/g) in each of the three populations of interest, and the second is a randomized, parallel groups, clinical trial examining response to these same cigarettes across 12 weeks of exposure in those same populations largely following the protocol used in the Donny et al. report. We focus below on results of the acute effects laboratory study (Higgins, Heil, et al., 2017); the randomized clinical trial is still ongoing.

Participants were 53 socioeconomically disadvantaged women of reproductive age, 60 men and women with current opioid dependence between the ages of 18 and 70 years, and 56 men and women with current or past-year affective disorder between the ages of 18 and 70 years. Participants completed fourteen 2–4 h experimental sessions in a within-subjects research design with a minimum of 48 h between sessions. Sessions were conducted following brief smoking abstinence (i.e., >50% reduction in expired breath carbon monoxide (CO) levels). Sessions were organized into three phases. In Phase 1 (Sessions 1–5), participants sampled the research cigarettes under double-blind conditions. Participants were oriented to the research protocol in Session 1 using their usual-brand cigarette. In Sessions 2–5, participants smoked one research cigarette per session, which were identical in appearance but varied in nicotine content (15.8, 5.2, 2.4, 0.4 mg/g) as in the Donny et al. study. The highest dose served as a control for nicotine levels typical of commercial cigarettes while the lowest dose represents a dose below the hypothesized 0.7 mg/g threshold dose for addiction. Participants were instructed to smoke the research cigarettes as usual, but used a plastic cigarette holder connected to a device that recorded smoking topography. After smoking the assigned cigarette each session, participants completed the Cigarette Purchase Task (CPT), which is a behavioral economic simulation task that models smoking under varying levels of hypothetical prices along with validated questionnaires assessing subjective effects and nicotine withdrawal. Phase 2 (Sessions 6–11) directly tested the relative reinforcing effects of the different dose cigarettes by allowing participants to choose which cigarette they preferred to smoke. Each of the six possible cigarette dose-pair combinations was tested once in separate sessions. In these 3-h sessions, a participant sat alone in a comfortable, ventilated room with reading materials. When they wished to smoke, they used a computer mouse to click on one of two icons on a screen representing the two cigarettes available in that session. After ten clicks on the icon, they could take two puffs of the associated cigarette. Participants were free to choose either option as often as they wished or to abstain. Lastly, Phase 3 (Sessions 12–14) used the same arrangement as in Phase 2, but compared only the lowest and highest doses (0.4 and 15.8 g/mg). This phase assessed whether preference could be reliably shifted away from the high dose. Puffs from the low dose were always available by clicking that option ten times, but the number of clicks necessary to earn puffs from the high dose started at 10 and increased each time it was chosen to 160, 320, 640, 1280, 2400, 3600, 4800, 6000, 7200, and 8400 clicks. Participants were informed of the different response requirements in advance. Lastly, participants completed the CPT for both the 0.4 and 15.8 g/mg doses following the concurrent choice sessions in Phase 3 to assess relative demand for the two cigarettes outside of the concurrent choice test arrangement.

There were minimal between-population differences in this study, and results overall were very consistent with reduced-nicotine content cigarettes having a lower addiction potential in these three vulnerable populations. In tests of subjective effects, positive ratings of smoking decreased as a function of reducing nicotine content consistent with reduced addiction potential. Each of the doses significantly reduced nicotine withdrawal symptoms and craving across time and no changes indicative of compensatory smoking were noted across doses in smoking topography or breath CO exposure levels. Turning to direct measures of the relative reinforcing effects of the varying nicotine content cigarettes in the concurrent choice testing of each of the six possible dose pairs, participants reliably chose to smoke the higher-nicotine content option across all dose pairs (Fig. 2.9). It is worth emphasizing again that these cigarettes were administered under double-blind conditions, thus the finding that participants reliably preferred the higher-nicotine content cigarettes indicates that they were acutely sensitive to drug effects associated with smoking the varying nicotine content cigarettes.

Importantly, this pronounced preference for the higher-nicotine content cigarette was malleable. That is, participants preferred the 15 mg/g over the 0.4 mg/g content cigarettes when the number of mouse clicks required to obtain them was equal in Phase 2 (Fig. 2.10, left panel), but that preference was reversed in Phase 3 sessions

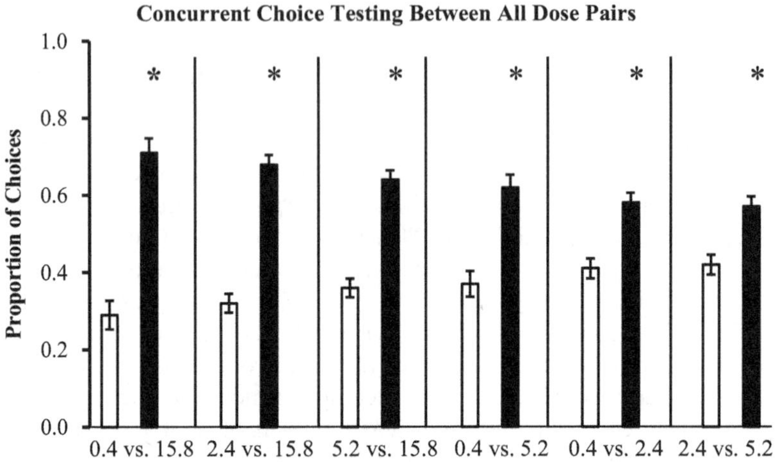

Fig. 2.9 Mean proportion of choices allocated to the different nicotine dose cigarettes across six 3-h two-dose concurrent choice sessions. Data points are means across participants and populations and error bars represent ±SEM. All possible two-dose comparisons across the four nicotine dose cigarettes (0.4, 2.4, 5.2, and 15.8 mg/g tobacco) were examined. The varying two-dose comparisons are shown on the *x*-axis with mean proportion of choice allocated to each shown on the *y*-axis. Dose pairs are ordered to show those with largest to least preference differences going left to right. Asterisks indicate that the higher dose was chosen at significantly greater than chance level after Bonferroni correction. Data originally reported in Higgins, Heil, et al. (2017)

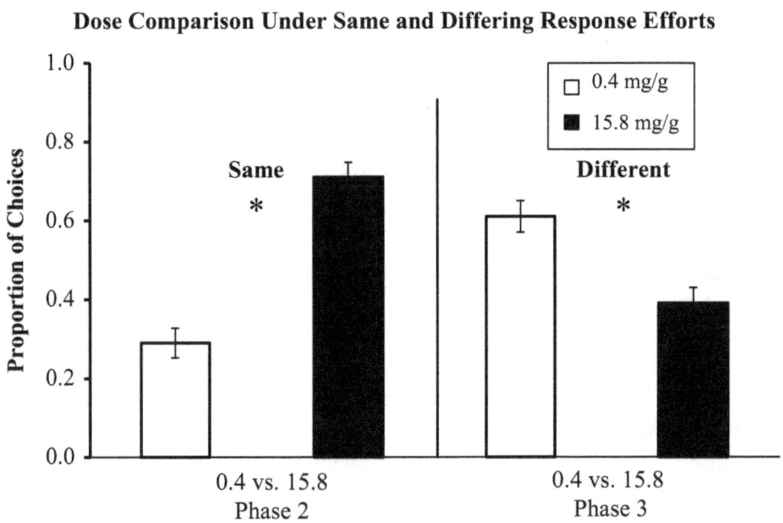

Fig. 2.10 Mean proportion of choices allocated to the 15.8 mg/g dose when it was available at the *same* (left-most plot) response effort as the 0.4 mg/g dose (fixed ratio of 10 responses) as shown in closed bars and when it was available at *different* (right-most plot) response effort (progressive ratio starting at 10 responses that incremented upwards to a maximum of 8400 responses) than the 4 mg/g dose (fixed ratio 10) as shown in open bars. Data points are means across participants and sessions (Phase 3) and error bars represent ±SEM. Asterisks indicate significant differences in dose preferences (p's < 0.001). Data originally reported in Higgins, Redner, et al. (2017)

where access to the 15 mg/g nicotine content cigarette was increased according to a progressive ratio schedule of reinforcement.

Conclusions

Results of the observational studies indicate that use of full-flavor nicotine/tar-yield cigarettes is associated with greater risk of nicotine dependence in both adults and adolescents, is overrepresented in subpopulations known to be most vulnerable to tobacco use and addiction, and is associated with the unsettling public health problem of women continuing to smoke during pregnancy. Of course, these observational studies cannot support causal inferences meaning that we cannot know if the greater potential nicotine yield of full-flavor cigarettes is causing greater nicotine dependence or continuing to smoke during pregnancy. Nevertheless, it seems clear that the greater nicotine yield associated with full-flavor cigarettes is either contributing directly to these problems or is supporting an unhealthy practice that is driven by other factors. Either way, having relatively high-nicotine yield cigarettes available commercially is associated with practices that adversely impact the US public health.

At first blush, recommending lower machine-estimated yield cigarettes may appear to represent a viable alternative in terms of being associated with a lower likelihood of dependence and greater likelihood of quitting should a women become pregnant, but the empirically based concern is that use of commercially available lower-yield cigarettes promotes compensatory smoking involving greater puff volume, deeper inhalation, or increased smoking rates that can produce greater toxin exposure and unique adverse health risks. So, there is no obviously safer combusted substitute commercially available at this time. Thus, the results from those observational studies provide additional reasons for the FDA to consider a national policy that lowers the maximal nicotine content of cigarettes to very low levels.

Results from the experimental studies in the general population of smokers on reduced-nicotine content cigarettes suggest that such a policy has the potential to reduce nicotine exposure and dependence levels with minimal evidence of compensatory smoking. The more recent evidence from more vulnerable populations are encouraging and suggest that such effects will extend to population subgroups that are especially vulnerable to tobacco use, addiction, and adverse health impacts. Effects from extended exposure in those vulnerable populations will be necessary to further confirm that, and those studies are ongoing at the University of Vermont and elsewhere. The results from Phase 3 of the acute exposure study in vulnerable populations are important in that they illustrate the potential malleability of tobacco-product preferences depending on the conditions under which they are available. For example, allowing very low nicotine content cigarette to be sold in common retail outlets while restricting sale of higher content cigarettes to less plentiful or more regulated stores would be predicted to shift preference towards the former. This same concept may also extend to regulatory efforts to shift preference from combusted to less harmful non-combusted tobacco products. This observation is consistent with unit-price models of drug abuse wherein reinforcing value corresponds to the ratio of drug dose and cost (Bickel, DeGrandpre, Hughes, & Higgins, 1991; Smith, Sved, Hatsukami, & Donny, 2014).

Important to clarify is that chronic use of any nicotine content cigarette is highly toxic as is use of any combusted tobacco product. Nicotine causes relatively few of the adverse health effects of cigarette smoking. Those adverse effects are caused by the many other constituents in tobacco smoke. What nicotine does is reinforce the behavior of smoking and eventual addiction. The goal behind reducing the nicotine content of cigarettes is to decrease the reinforcing effects of smoking thereby making it easier for those who are already smoking to quit, and to keep those who may sample cigarette smoking for the first time from coming into contact with a sufficiently potent reinforcing effect to drive repeated use and eventual addiction. A recent announcement from the FDA Commissioner Scott Gottlieb, MD, indicates that the agency is moving forward with consideration of a national policy that would reduce the nicotine of cigarettes and other combusted tobacco products to achieve this goal and thereby better protect the US public health from the adverse health effects of cigarette smoking (U.S. Food and Drug Administration, 2017). That is an encouraging development on many fronts and certainly an example of policy makers recognizing the potential of leveraging the reinforcement process to improve the US population health.

Summary and Conclusions

We have reviewed how the US population health is relatively poor compared to that of other developed countries despite spending more on health care than any other nation. There is broad agreement that unhealthy behavior patterns in the form of substance abuse, physical inactivity, poor food choices, and nonadherence to recommended medical regimens represent the single biggest contributor to this problem, underscoring the need for more effective behavior-change strategies to promote health. We have reviewed more than 30 years of research illustrating how the same reinforcement process and associated biases in decision-making that underpin vulnerability to these unhealthy behavior patterns can be leveraged to promote and sustain behavior change. The greatest amount of research has been conducted around the strategy of using financial incentives to promote behavior change. We also illustrated how the reinforcement process can be leveraged in intensive behavior therapy interventions like CRA therapy. Lastly, we reviewed how that same process can be leveraged in population-based interventions such as the reduced-nicotine standards policy currently under consideration by the FDA. The research covered was by no means comprehensive but instead was meant to be illustrative of the potential of this approach to promote and sustain behavior change. Several areas where we see need for more research are (a) explicitly planning for sustaining treatment effects longer-term from the beginning of implementing incentives and other reinforcement-based interventions, (b) identifying additional vulnerable populations and health problems where these interventions might be efficacious and a positive step in the direction of reducing health disparities, and (c) examining the cost-effectiveness of this treatment approach. Finally, it merits underscoring that the behavioral economic conceptual framework taken in this report posits that the reinforcement process underpins parts or all of the unhealthy behavior patterns that are having such an adverse impact on the US population health (i.e., a trans-disease process—Bickel et al., 2017). As such, it should not be surprising that interventions leveraging that process would have the potential to contribute in a substantive manner across such a wide array of behavior health problems. We believe that the approach is still underutilized and has a great deal more to contribute going forward.

References

Alessi, S. M., Badger, G. J., & Higgins, S. T. (2004). An experimental examination of the initial weeks of abstinence in cigarette smokers. *Experimental and Clinical Psychopharmacology, 12*, 276–287.

Alshaarawy, O., & Anthony, J. C. (2015). Month-wise estimates of tobacco smoking during pregnancy for the United States, 2002-2009. *Maternal and Child Health Journal, 19*(5), 1010–1015. https://doi.org/10.1007/s10995-014-1599-4

Avendano, M., & Kawachi, I. (2014). Why do Americans have shorter life expectancy and worse health than do people in other high-income countries? *Annual Review of Public Health, 35*, 307–325.

Barker, D. J. (2004). The developmental origins of adult disease. *Journal of the American College of Nutrition, 23*(6 Suppl), 588S–595S.

Benowitz, N. L., Dains, K. M., Hall, S. M., Stewart, S., Wilson, M., Dempsey, D., & Jacob, P., 3rd. (2012). Smoking behavior and exposure to tobacco toxicants during 6 months of smoking progressively reduced nicotine content cigarettes. *Cancer Epidemiology, Biomarkers & Prevention, 21*(5), 761–769. https://doi.org/10.1158/1055-9965.EPI-11-0644

Benowitz, N. L., & Henningfield, J. E. (1994). Establishing a nicotine threshold for addiction. The implications for tobacco regulation. *The New England Journal of Medicine, 331*(2), 123–125. https://doi.org/10.1056/NEJM199407143310212

Benowitz, N. L., & Henningfield, J. E. (2013). Reducing the nicotine content to make cigarettes less addictive. *Tobacco Control, 22*(Suppl 1), i14–i17. https://doi.org/10.1136/tobaccocontrol-2012-0508

Benowitz, N. L., Jacob, P., 3rd, Yu, L., Talcott, R., Hall, S., & Jones, R. T. (1986). Reduced tar, nicotine, and carbon monoxide exposure while smoking ultralow- but not low-yield cigarettes. *JAMA, 256*(2), 241–246.

Bevins, R. A., & Bardo, M. T. (2004). Introduction: Motivation, drug abuse, and 50 years of theoretical and empirical inquiry. *Nebraska Symposium on Motivation, 50*, ix–xv.

Bevins, R. A., & Caggiula, A. R. (2009). Nicotine, tobacco use, and the 55th Nebraska symposium on motivation. *Nebraska Symposium on Motivation, 55*, 1–3.

Bickel, W. K., DeGrandpre, R. J., Hughes, J. R., & Higgins, S. T. (1991). Behavioral economics of drug self-administration. II. A unit-price analysis of cigarette smoking. *Journal of the Experimental Analysis of Behavior, 55*(2), 145–154. https://doi.org/10.1901/jeab.1991.55-145

Bickel, W. K., Mellis, A. M., Snider, S. E., Athamneh, L. N., Stein, J. S., & Pope, D. A. (2017). 21st century neurobehavioral theories of decision making in addiction: Review and evaluation. *Pharmacology, Biochemistry, and Behavior*. https://doi.org/10.1016/j.pbb.2017.09.009

Bickel, W. K., Miller, M. L., Yi, R., Kowal, B. P., Lindquist, D. M., & Pitcock, J. A. (2007). Behavioral and neuroeconomics of drug addiction: Competing neural systems and temporal

discounting processes. *Drug and Alcohol Dependence, 90*(Suppl 1), S85–S91. https://doi.org/10.1016/j.drugalcdep.2006.09.016
Bickel, W. K., Moody, L., & Higgins, S. T. (2016). Some current dimensions of the behavioral economics of health-related behavior change. *Preventive Medicine, 92*, 16–23. https://doi.org/10.1016/j.ypmed.2016.06.002
Boyd, K. A., Briggs, A. H., Bauld, L., Sinclair, L., & Tappin, D. (2016). Are financial incentives cost-effective to support smoking cessation during pregnancy? *Addiction, 111*(2), 360–370. https://doi.org/10.1111/add.13160
Bradford, W. D. (2010). The association between individual time preferences and health maintenance habits. *Medical Decision Making, 30*(1), 99–112. https://doi.org/10.1177/0272989X09342276
Budney, A., & Higgins, S. T. (1994). *A community reinforcement plus vouchers approach: Treating cocaine addiction* (NIDA Publication No. 98–4309 ed.). Rockville, MD: National Institute on Drug Abuse.
Caggiula, A. R., Donny, E. C., Palmatier, M. I., Liu, X., Chaudhri, N., & Sved, A. F. (2009). The role of nicotine in smoking: A dual-reinforcement model. *Nebraska Symposium on Motivation, 55*, 91–109.
Cahill, K., Hartmann-Boyce, J., & Perera, R. (2015). Incentives for smoking cessation. *Cochrane Database of Systematic Reviews, 5*, CD004307. https://doi.org/10.1002/14651858.CD004307.pub5
Campbell, U. C., & Carroll, M. E. (2000). Reduction of drug self-administration by an alternative non-drug reinforcer in rhesus monkeys: Magnitude and temporal effects. *Psychopharmacology (Berl), 147*, 418–425.
Carroll, M. E. (1993). The economic context of drug and non-drug reinforcers affects acquisition and maintenance of drug-reinforced behavior and withdrawal effects. *Drug and Alcohol Dependence, 33*(2), 201–210.
Chamberlain, C., O'Mara-Eves, A., Oliver, S., Caird, J. R., Perlen, S. M., Eades, S. J., & Thomas, J. (2013). Psychosocial interventions for supporting women to stop smoking in pregnancy. *Cochrane Database of Systematic Reviews, 10*, CD001055. https://doi.org/10.1002/14651858.CD001055.pub4
Chilcoat, H. D. (2009). An overview of the emergence of disparities in smoking prevalence, cessation, and adverse consequences among women. *Drug and Alcohol Dependence, 104*(Suppl 1), S17–S23. https://doi.org/10.1016/j.drugalcdep.2009.06.002
Compton, W. M., Boyle, M., & Wargo, E. (2015). Prescription opioid abuse: Problems and responses. *Preventive Medicine, 80*, 5–9. https://doi.org/10.1016/j.ypmed.2015.04.003
Cornish, J. W., & O'Brien, C. P. (1996). Crack cocaine abuse: An epidemic with many public health consequences. *Annual Reviews of Public Health, 17*, 259–273.
Cutler, D. M., & Lleras-Muney, A. (2010). Understanding differences in health behaviors by education. *Journal of Health Economics, 29*(1), 1–28. https://doi.org/10.1016/j.jhealeco.2009.10.003
Danaei, G., Ding, E. L., Mozaffarian, D., Taylor, B., Rehm, J., Murray, C. J., & Ezzati, M. (2009). The preventable causes of death in the United States: Comparative risk assessment of dietary, lifestyle, and metabolic risk factors. *PLoS Medicine, 6*(4), e1000058. https://doi.org/10.1371/journal.pmed.1000058
Davis, D. R., Kurti, A. N., Skelly, J. M., Redner, R., White, T. J., & Higgins, S. T. (2016). A review of the literature on contingency management in the treatment of substance use disorders, 2009-2014. *Preventive Medicine, 92*, 36–46. https://doi.org/10.1016/j.ypmed.2016.08.008
Dietz, P. M., England, L. J., Shapiro-Mendoza, C. K., Tong, V. T., Farr, S. L., & Callaghan, W. M. (2010). Infant morbidity and mortality attributable to prenatal smoking in the U.S. *American Journal of Preventive Medicine, 39*(1), 45–52. https://doi.org/10.1016/j.amepre.2010.03.009
Donatelle, R.J., Prows, S.L., Champeau, D., & Hudson, D. (2000a). Randomized controlled trial using social support and financial incentives for high risk pregnant smokers: significant other support (SOS) program. Tobacco Control, 9, Suppl 3:11167-9. PMID: 10982912

Donatelle, R.J., Prows, S.L., Champeau, D., et al. (2000b). Using social support, biochemical feedback, and incentives to motivate smoking cessation during pregnancy: comparison of three intervention trials. Poster presented at the annual meeting of the American Public Health Association; Boston, MA. Reported in Donatelle et al. (2004)

Donatelle, R., Hudson, D., Dobie, S., Goodall, A., Hunsberger, M., & Oswald, K. (2004). Incentives in smoking cessation: Status of the field and implications for research and practice with pregnant smokers. *Nicotine & Tobacco Research, 6*(Suppl 2), S163–S179. https://doi.org/10.1080/14622200410001669196

Donatelle, R. J., Prows, S. L., Champeau, D., & Hudson, D. (2000). Randomised controlled trial using social support and financial incentives for high risk pregnant smokers: Significant other supporter (SOS) program. *Tobacco Control, 9*(Suppl 3), III67–III69.

Donny, E. C., Denlinger, R. L., Tidey, J. W., Koopmeiners, J. S., Benowitz, N. L., Vandrey, R. G., … Hatsukami, D. K. (2015). Randomized trial of reduced-nicotine standards for cigarettes. *The New England Journal of Medicine, 373*(14), 1340–1349. https://doi.org/10.1056/NEJMsa1502403

Gaalema, D. E., Savage, P. D., Rengo, J. L., Cutler, A. Y., Higgins, S. T., & Ades, P. A. (2016). Financial incentives to promote cardiac rehabilitation participation and adherence among Medicaid patients. *Preventive Medicine, 92*, 47–50. https://doi.org/10.1016/j.ypmed.2015.11.032

Godley, S. H., Smith, J. E., Passetti, L. L., & Subramaniam, G. (2014). The adolescent community reinforcement approach (A-CRA) as a model paradigm for the management of adolescents with substance use disorders and co-occurring psychiatric disorders. *Substance Abuse, 35*(4), 352–363. https://doi.org/10.1080/08897077.2014.936993

Gori, G. B., & Lynch, C. J. (1983). Smoker intake from cigarettes in the 1-mg Federal Trade Commission tar class. *Regulatory Toxicology and Pharmacology, 3*(2), 110–120.

Green, L., Myerson, J., Lichtman, D., Rosen, S., & Fry, A. (1996). Temporal discounting in choice between delayed rewards: The role of age and income. *Psychology and Aging, 11*(1), 79–84.

Hatsukami, D. K., Heishman, S. J., Vogel, R. I., Denlinger, R. L., Roper-Batker, A. N., Mackowick, K. M., … Donny, E. (2013). Dose-response effects of spectrum research cigarettes. *Nicotine & Tobacco Research, 15*(6), 1113–1121. https://doi.org/10.1093/ntr/nts247

Hatsukami, D. K., Kotlyar, M., Hertsgaard, L. A., Zhang, Y., Carmella, S. G., Jensen, J. A., … Hecht, S. S. (2010). Reduced nicotine content cigarettes: Effects on toxicant exposure, dependence and cessation. *Addiction, 105*(2), 343–355. https://doi.org/10.1111/j.1360-0443.2009.02780.x

Heil, S. H., Hand, D. J., Sigmon, S. C., Badger, G. J., Meyer, M. C., & Higgins, S. T. (2016). Using behavioral economic theory to increase use of effective contraceptives among opioid-maintained women at risk of unintended pregnancy. *Preventive Medicine, 92*, 62–67. https://doi.org/10.1016/j.ypmed.2016.06.023

Heil, S. H., Herrmann, E. S., Badger, G. J., Solomon, L. J., Bernstein, I. M., & Higgins, S. T. (2014). Examining the timing of changes in cigarette smoking upon learning of pregnancy. *Preventive Medicine, 68*, 58–61. https://doi.org/10.1016/j.ypmed.2014.06.034

Heil, S. H., Higgins, S. T., Bernstein, I. M., Solomon, L. J., Rogers, R. E., Thomas, C. S., … Lynch, M. E. (2008). Effects of voucher-based incentives on abstinence from cigarette smoking and fetal growth among pregnant women. *Addiction, 103*(6), 1009–1018. https://doi.org/10.1111/j.1360-0443.2008.02237.x

Higgins, S. T. (1997). The influence of alternative reinforcers on cocaine use and abuse: A brief review. *Pharmacology, Biochemistry, and Behavior, 57*(3), 419–427.

Higgins, S.T., Bernstein, I.M., Washio, Y., Heil, S.H., Badger, G.J., Skelly, J.M., Higgins, T.M., & Solomon, L..J. (2010). Effects of smoking cessation with voucher-based contingency management on birth outcomes. Addiction, 105, 2023–30. https://doi.org/10.1111/j.1360-0443.2010.03073.x. Epub 2010 Sep 15. PMID: 20840188

Higgins, S. T. (2015). Editorial: 2nd special issue on behavior change, health, and health disparities. *Preventive Medicine, 80*, 1–4. https://doi.org/10.1016/j.ypmed.2015.07.020

Higgins, S. T., Badger, G. J., & Budney, A. J. (2000). Initial abstinence and success in achieving longer term cocaine abstinence. *Experimental and Clinical Psychopharmacology, 8*(3), 377–386.

Higgins, S. T., Bickel, W. K., & Hughes, J. R. (1994). Influence of an alternative reinforcer on human cocaine self-administration. *Life Sciences, 55*(3), 179–187.

Higgins, S. T., Budney, A. J., Bickel, W. K., Badger, G. J., Foerg, F. E., & Ogden, D. (1995). Outpatient behavioral treatment for cocaine dependence: One-year outcome. *Experimental and Clinical Psychopharmacology, 3*(2), 205–212.

Higgins, S. T., Budney, A. J., Bickel, W. K., Foerg, F. E., Donham, R., & Badger, G. J. (1994). Incentives improve outcome in outpatient behavioral treatment of cocaine dependence. *Archives of General Psychiatry, 51*, 568–576.

Higgins, S. T., Budney, A. J., Bickel, W. K., Hughes, J. R., Foerg, F., & Badger, G. (1993). Achieving cocaine abstinence with a behavioral approach. *The American Journal of Psychiatry, 150*(5), 763–769. https://doi.org/10.1176/ajp.150.5.763

Higgins, S. T., & Chilcoat, H. D. (2009). Women and smoking: An interdisciplinary examination of socioeconomic influences. *Drug and Alcohol Dependence, 104*(Suppl 1), S1–S5. https://doi.org/10.1016/j.drugalcdep.2009.06.006

Higgins, S. T., Delaney, D. D., Budney, A. J., Bickel, W. K., Hughes, J. R., Foerg, F., & Fenwick, J. W. (1991). A behavioral approach to achieving initial cocaine abstinence. *The American Journal of Psychiatry, 148*(9), 1218–1224. https://doi.org/10.1176/ajp.148.9.1218

Higgins, S. T., Heil, S. H., Badger, G. J., Skelly, J. M., Solomon, L. J., & Bernstein, I. M. (2009). Educational disadvantage and cigarette smoking during pregnancy. *Drug and Alcohol Dependence, 104*(Suppl 1), S100–S105. https://doi.org/10.1016/j.drugalcdep.2009.03.013

Higgins, S. T., Heil, S. H., Dantona, R., Donham, R., Matthews, M., & Badger, G. J. (2007). Effects of varying the monetary value of voucher-based incentives on abstinence achieved during and following treatment among cocaine-dependent outpatients. *Addiction, 102*, 271–281.

Higgins, S. T., Heil, S. H., Dumeer, A. M., Thomas, C. S., Solomon, L. J., & Bernstein, I. M. (2006). Smoking status in the initial weeks of quitting as a predictor of smoking-cessation outcomes in pregnant women. *Drug and Alcohol Dependence, 85*(2), 138–141. https://doi.org/10.1016/j.drugalcdep.2006.04.005

Higgins, S. T., Heil, S. H., & Lussier, J. P. (2004). Clinical implications of reinforcement as a determinant of substance use disorders. *Annual Review of Psychology, 55*, 431–461. https://doi.org/10.1146/annurev.psych.55.090902.142033

Higgins, S. T., Heil, S. H., Sigmon, S. C., Tidey, J. W., Gaalema, D. E., Hughes, J. R., … Tursi, L. (2017). Addiction potential of cigarettes with reduced nicotine content in populations with psychiatric disorders and other vulnerabilities to tobacco addiction. *JAMA Psychiatry, 74*(10), 1–9. https://doi.org/10.1001/jamapsychiatry.2017.2355

Higgins, S. T., Heil, S. H., Solomon, L. J., Bernstein, I. M., Lussier, J. P., Abel, R. L., … Badger, G. J. (2004). A pilot study on voucher-based incentives to promote abstinence from cigarette smoking during pregnancy and postpartum. *Nicotine & Tobacco Research, 6*(6), 1015–1020.

Higgins, S. T., Hughes, J. R., & Bickel, W. K. (1989). Human psychopharmacology of intranasal cocaine. *NIDA Research Monograph, 95*, 357–358.

Higgins, S. T., Kurti, A. N., Redner, R., White, T. J., Keith, D. R., Gaalema, D. E., … Priest, J. S. (2016). Co-occurring risk factors for current cigarette smoking in a U.S. nationally representative sample. *Preventive Medicine, 92*, 110–117. https://doi.org/10.1016/j.ypmed.2016.02.025

Higgins, S. T., Redner, R., Arger, C. A., Kurti, A. N., Priest, J. S., & Bunn, J. Y. (2017). Use of higher-nicotine/tar-yield (regular full-flavor) cigarettes is associated with nicotine dependence and smoking during pregnancy among U.S. women. *Preventive Medicine*. https://doi.org/10.1016/j.ypmed.2017.07.029

Higgins, S. T., Roll, J. M., & Bickel, W. K. (1996). Alcohol pretreatment increases preference for cocaine over monetary reinforcement. *Psychopharmacology, 123*(1), 1–8.

Higgins, S. T., Sigmon, S. C., & Heil, S. H. (2011). Contingency management in the treatment of substance use disorders. Trends in the literature. In P. Ruiz & E. Strain (Eds.), *Lowinson and*

Ruiz's substance abuse: A comprehensive textbook (pp. 603–621). Philadelphia, PA: Lippincott Williams & Wilkins.

Higgins, S. T., Sigmon, S. C., Wong, C. J., Heil, S. H., Badger, G. J., Donham, R., ... Anthony, S. (2003). Community reinforcement therapy for cocaine dependent outpatients. *Archives of General Psychiatry, 60*(10), 1043–1052. https://doi.org/10.1001/archpsyc.60.9.1043

Higgins, S. T., & Solomon, L. J. (2016). Some recent developments on financial incentives for smoking cessation among pregnant and newly postpartum women. *Current Addiction Reports, 3*(1), 9–18. https://doi.org/10.1007/s40429-016-0092-0

Higgins, S. T., Washio, Y., Heil, S. H., Solomon, L. J., Gaalema, D. E., Higgins, T. M., & Bernstein, I. M. (2012). Financial incentives for smoking cessation among pregnant and newly postpartum women. *Preventive Medicine, 55*(Suppl), S33–S40. https://doi.org/10.1016/j.ypmed.2011.12.016

Higgins, S. T., Washio, Y., Lopez, A. A., Heil, S. H., Solomon, L. J., Lynch, M. E., ... Bernstein, I. M. (2014). Examining two different schedules of financial incentives for smoking cessation among pregnant women. *Preventive Medicine, 68*, 51–57. https://doi.org/10.1016/j.ypmed.2014.03.024

Higgins, S. T., Wong, C. J., Badger, G. J., Ogden, D. E., & Dantona, R. L. (2000). Contingent reinforcement increases cocaine abstinence during outpatient treatment and 1 year of follow-up. *Journal of Consulting and Clinical Psychology, 68*, 64–72.

Holford, T. R., Meza, R., Warner, K. E., Meernik, C., Jeon, J., Moolgavkar, S. H., & Levy, D. T. (2014). Tobacco control and the reduction in smoking-related premature deaths in the United States, 1964-2012. *JAMA, 311*(2), 164–171. https://doi.org/10.1001/jama.2013.285112

Hser, Y. I., Hoffman, V., Grella, C. E., & Anglin, M. D. (2001). A 33-year follow-up of narcotics addicts. *Archives of General Psychiatry, 58*(5), 503–508.

Hunt, G. M., & Azrin, N. H. (1973). A community-reinforcement approach to alcoholism. *Behaviour Research and Therapy, 11*(1), 91–104.

Ierfino, D., Mantzari, E., Hirst, J., Jones, T., Aveyard, P., & Marteau, T. M. (2015). Financial incentives for smoking cessation in pregnancy: A single-arm intervention study assessing cessation and gaming. *Addiction, 110*(4), 680–688. https://doi.org/10.1111/add.12817

Isaacs, S. L., & Schroeder, S. A. (2004). Class—the ignored determinant of the nation's health. *The New England Journal of Medicine, 351*(11), 1137–1142. https://doi.org/10.1056/NEJMsb040329

Jaroni, J. L., Wright, S. M., Lerman, C., & Epstein, L. H. (2004). Relationship between education and delay discounting in smokers. *Addictive Behaviors, 29*(6), 1171–1175. https://doi.org/10.1016/j.addbeh.2004.03.014

Kandel, D. B., Griesler, P. C., & Schaffran, C. (2009). Educational attainment and smoking among women: Risk factors and consequences for offspring. *Drug and Alcohol Dependence, 104*(Suppl 1), S24–S33. https://doi.org/10.1016/j.drugalcdep.2008.12.005

Kelley, A. E., & Berridge, K. C. (2002). The neuroscience of natural rewards: Relevance to addictive drugs. *The Journal of Neuroscience, 22*(9), 3306–3311.

Kenford, S. L., Fiore, M. C., Jorenby, D. E., Smith, S. S., Wetter, D., & Baker, T. B. (1994). Predicting smoking cessation. Who will quit with and without the nicotine patch. *JAMA, 271*(8), 589–594.

Kirby, K.C., Benishek, L.A., Kerwin, M.E., Dugosh, K.L., Carpendo, C.M., Bresani, E., Haugh, J.A., Washio, Y., & Meyers, R.J. (2017). Analyzing components of Community Reinforcement and Family Training (CRAFT): Is treatment entry training sufficient? Psychology of Addictive Behavior, 31, 818-827. https://doi.org/10.1037/adb0000306. Epub 2017 Aug 24. PMID: 28836796

Kozlowski, L. T., Frecker, R. C., & Lei, H. (1982). Nicotine yields of cigarettes, plasma nicotine in smokers, and public health. *Preventive Medicine, 11*(2), 240–244.

Kozlowski, L. T., & Pillitteri, J. L. (2001). Beliefs about "light" and "ultra light" cigarettes and efforts to change those beliefs: An overview of early efforts and published research. *Tobacco Control, 10*(Suppl 1), i12–i16.

Kumanyika, S. (2012). Health disparities research in global perspective: New insights and new directions. *Annual Review of Public Health, 33*, 1–5. https://doi.org/10.1146/annurev-publhealth-112911-155504

Kurti, A. N., Davis, D. R., Skelly, J. M., Redner, R., & Higgins, S. T. (2016). Comparison of nicotine dependence indicators in predicting quitting among pregnant smokers. *Experimental and Clinical Psychopharmacology, 24*(1), 12–17. https://doi.org/10.1037/pha0000056

Kurti, A. N., Redner, R., Lopez, A. A., Keith, D. R., Villanti, A. C., Stanton, C. A., … Higgins, S. T. (2017). Tobacco and nicotine delivery product use in a national sample of pregnant women. *Preventive Medicine*. https://doi.org/10.1016/j.ypmed.2017.07.030

Lasser, K., Boyd, J., Woolhandler, S., Himmelstein, D. U., McCormick, D., & Bor, D. H. (2000). Smoking and mental illness: A population-based prevalence study. *JAMA, 284*(20), 2606–2610. https://doi.org/10.1001/jama.284.20.2606

Lawler, P. R., Filion, K. B., & Eisenberg, M. J. (2011). Efficacy of exercise-based cardiac rehabilitation post-myocardial infarction: A systematic review and meta-analysis of randomized controlled trials. *American Heart Journal, 162*(4), 571–584.e572. https://doi.org/10.1016/j.ahj.2011.07.017

Lawrence, D., Mitrou, F., & Zubrick, S. R. (2009). Smoking and mental illness: Results from population surveys in Australia and the United States. *BMC Public Health, 9*, 285. https://doi.org/10.1186/1471-2458-9-285

Leslie, F. M. (2013). Multigenerational epigenetic effects of nicotine on lung function. *BMC Medicine, 11*, 27. https://doi.org/10.1186/1741-7015-11-27

Loewenstein, G., Brennan, T., & Volpp, K. G. (2007). Asymmetric paternalism to improve health behaviors. *JAMA, 298*(20), 2415–2417. https://doi.org/10.1001/jama.298.20.2415

Lopez, A. A., Skelly, J. M., & Higgins, S. T. (2015). Financial incentives for smoking cessation among depression-prone pregnant and newly postpartum women: Effects on smoking abstinence and depression ratings. *Nicotine & Tobacco Research, 17*(4), 455–462. https://doi.org/10.1093/ntr/ntu193

Lopez, A.A., Redner, R., Kurti, A.N., Keith, D.R., Villanti, A.C., Stanton, C.A., Gaalema, D.E., Bunn, J.Y., Doogan, N.J., Cepeda-Benito, A., Roberts, M.E., & Higgins, S.T. (2018). Tobacco and nicotine delivery product use in a U.S. national sample of women of reproductive age. Preventive Medicine, pii: S0091-7435(18)30090-2. https://doi.org/10.1016/j.ypmed.2018.03.001. [Epub ahead of print] PMID:29559222

Lumley, J., Chamberlain, C., Dowswell, T., Oliver, S., Oakley, L., & Watson, L. (2009). Interventions for promoting smoking cessation during pregnancy. *Cochrane Database of Systematic Reviews, 3*, CD001055. https://doi.org/10.1002/14651858.CD001055.pub3

Lussier, J. P., Heil, S. H., Mongeon, J. A., Badger, G. J., & Higgins, S. T. (2006). A meta-analysis of voucher-based reinforcement therapy for substance use disorders. *Addiction, 101*, 192–203.

Mani, A., Mullainathan, S., Shafir, E., & Zhao, J. (2013). Poverty impedes cognitive function. *Science, 341*(6149), 976–980. https://doi.org/10.1126/science.1238041

Mattke, S., Liu, H., Caloyeras, J., Huang, C. Y., Van Busum, K. R., Khodyakov, D., & Shier, V. (2013). Workplace wellness programs study: Final report. *Rand Health Quarterly, 3*(2), 7.

Meyers, R. J., Roozen, H. G., & Smith, J. E. (2011). The community reinforcement approach: An update of the evidence. *Alcohol Research & Health, 33*(4), 380–388.

Nader, M. A., Czoty, P. W., Nader, S. H., & Morgan, D. (2012). Nonhuman primate models of social behavior and cocaine abuse. *Psychopharmacology, 224*(1), 57–67. https://doi.org/10.1007/s00213-012-2843-5

Office of Disease Prevention. (2017). National Institutes of Health. Retrieved September 30, 2017, from https://prevention.nih.gov/tobacco-regulatory-science-program

Ondersma, S. J., Svikis, D. S., Lam, P. K., Connors-Burge, V. S., Ledgerwood, D. M., & Hopper, J. A. (2012). A randomized trial of computer-delivered brief intervention and low-intensity contingency management for smoking during pregnancy. *Nicotine & Tobacco Research, 14*(3), 351–360. https://doi.org/10.1093/ntr/ntr221

Petry, N. M., DePhilippis, D., Rash, C. J., Drapkin, M., & McKay, J. R. (2014). Nationwide dissemination of contingency management: The Veterans Administration initiative. *The American Journal on Addictions, 23*(3), 205–210. https://doi.org/10.1111/j.1521-0391.2014.12092.x

Ranganathan, M., & Lagarde, M. (2012). Promoting healthy behaviours and improving health outcomes in low and middle income countries: A review of the impact of conditional cash transfer programmes. *Preventive Medicine, 55*(Suppl), S95–S105. https://doi.org/10.1016/j.ypmed.2011.11.015

Redner R., Lopez, A. A., Kurti, A. N., Keith, D. R., Villanti, A. C., Stanton, C. A., Gaalema, D. E., Bunn, J. Y., Doogan, N. J., Cepeda-Benito, A., Roberts, M. E., & Higgins, S. T. (in press). Tobacco and nicotine delivery product use in a U.S. national sample of women of reproductive age. *Preventive Medicine.*

Redner, R., White, T. J., Bunn, J. Y., & Higgins, S. T. (2016). Use of high-nicotine/tar-yield (full-flavor) cigarettes and risk for nicotine dependence in nationally representative samples of US smokers. *Nicotine & Tobacco Research, 18*(6), 1424–1430. https://doi.org/10.1093/ntr/ntv252

Roll, J. M., & Higgins, S. T. (2000). A within-subject comparison of three different schedules of reinforcement of drug abstinence using cigarette smoking as an exemplar. *Drug and Alcohol Dependence, 58*, 103–109.

Roll, J. M., Higgins, S. T., & Badger, G. J. (1996). An experimental comparison of three different schedules of reinforcement of drug abstinence using cigarette smoking as an exemplar. *Journal of Applied Behavior Analysis, 29*, 495–505.

Scherer, G., & Lee, P. N. (2014). Smoking behaviour and compensation: A review of the literature with meta-analysis. *Regulatory Toxicology and Pharmacology, 70*(3), 615–628. https://doi.org/10.1016/j.yrtph.2014.09.008

Schroeder, S. A. (2007). Shattuck lecture. We can do better—improving the health of the American people. *The New England Journal of Medicine, 357*(12), 1221–1228. https://doi.org/10.1056/NEJMsa073350

Schroeder, S. A. (2016). American health improvement depends upon addressing class disparities. *Preventive Medicine, 92*, 6–15. https://doi.org/10.1016/j.ypmed.2016.02.024

Sexton, M., & Hebel, J. R. (1984). A clinical trial of change in maternal smoking and its effect on birth weight. *JAMA, 251*(7), 911–915.

Shah, A. K., Mullainathan, S., & Shafir, E. (2012). Some consequences of having too little. *Science, 338*(6107), 682–685. https://doi.org/10.1126/science.1222426

Shiffman, S., Dunbar, M. S., & Benowitz, N. L. (2014). A comparison of nicotine biomarkers and smoking patterns in daily and nondaily smokers. *Cancer Epidemiology, Biomarkers & Prevention, 23*(7), 1264–1272. https://doi.org/10.1158/1055-9965.epi-13-1014

Sigmon, S. C., Ochalek, T. A., Meyer, A. C., Hruska, B., Heil, S. H., Badger, G. J., … Higgins, S. T. (2016). Interim buprenorphine vs. waiting list for opioid dependence. *The New England Journal of Medicine, 375*(25), 2504–2505. https://doi.org/10.1056/NEJMc1610047

Silverman, K., Higgins, S. T., Brooner, R. K., Montoya, I. D., Cone, E. J., Schuster, C. R., & Preston, K. L. (1996). Sustained cocaine abstinence in methadone maintenance patients through voucher-based reinforcement therapy. *Archives of General Psychiatry, 53*(5), 409–415.

Silverman, K., Svikis, D., Robles, E., Stitzer, M. L., & Bigelow, G. E. (2001). A reinforcement-based therapeutic workplace for the treatment of drug abuse: Six-month abstinence outcomes. *Experimental and Clinical Psychopharmacology, 9*(1), 14–23.

Silverman, K., Svikis, D., Wong, C. J., Hampton, J., Stitzer, M. L., & Bigelow, G. E. (2002). A reinforcement-based therapeutic workplace for the treatment of drug abuse: Three-year abstinence outcomes. *Experimental and Clinical Psychopharmacology, 10*(3), 228–240.

Silverman, K., Wong, C. J., Needham, M., Diemer, K. N., Knealing, T., Crone-Todd, D., … Kolodner, K. (2007). A randomized trial of employment-based reinforcement of cocaine abstinence in injection drug users. *Journal of Applied Behavior Analysis, 40*(3), 387–410.

Smith, T. T., Sved, A. F., Hatsukami, D. K., & Donny, E. C. (2014). Nicotine reduction as an increase in the unit price of cigarettes: A behavioral economics approach. *Preventive Medicine, 68*, 23–28. https://doi.org/10.1016/j.ypmed.2014.07.005

Solomon, L., & Quinn, V. (2004). Spontaneous quitting: Self-initiated smoking cessation in early pregnancy. *Nicotine & Tobacco Research, 6*(Suppl 2), S203–S216. https://doi.org/10.1080/14622200410001669132

Tappin, D., Bauld, L., Purves, D., Boyd, K., Sinclair, L., MacAskill, S., … Cessation in Pregnancy Incentives Trial. (2015). Financial incentives for smoking cessation in pregnancy: Randomised controlled trial. *BMJ, 350*, h134. https://doi.org/10.1136/bmj.h134

Tuten, M., Fitzsimons, H., Chisolm, M. S., Nuzzo, P. A., & Jones, H. E. (2012). Contingent incentives reduce cigarette smoking among pregnant, methadone-maintained women: Results of an initial feasibility and efficacy randomized clinical trial. *Addiction, 107*(10), 1868–1877. https://doi.org/10.1111/j.1360-0443.2012.03923.x

U.S. Department of Health and Human Services. (1988). *The health consequences of smoking: Nicotine addiction a report of the surgeon general*. Atlanta, GA: U.S. Department of Health and Human Services.

U.S. Department of Health and Human Services. (2014). *The health consequences of smoking—50 years of progress: A report of the surgeon general*. Atlanta, GA: U.S. Department of Health and Human Services.

U.S. Food and Drug Administration. (2017). *FDA news release: FDA announces comprehensive regulatory plan to shift trajectory of tobacco-related disease, death*. Retrieved October 1, 2017 from https://www.fda.gov/newsevents/newsroom/pressannouncements/ucm568923.htm

Volkow, N. D., & Collins, F. S. (2017). The role of science in addressing the opioid crisis. *The New England Journal of Medicine, 377*(4), 391–394. https://doi.org/10.1056/NEJMsr1706626

Woolf, S. H., & Aron, L. Y. (2013). The US health disadvantage relative to other high-income countries: Findings from a National Research Council/Institute of Medicine report. *JAMA, 309*(8), 771–772. https://doi.org/10.1001/jama.2013.91

Zacny, J. P., Stitzer, M. L., Brown, F. J., Yingling, J. E., & Griffiths, R. R. (1987). Human cigarette smoking: Effects of puff and inhalation parameters on smoke exposure. *The Journal of Pharmacology and Experimental Therapeutics, 240*(2), 554–564.

Zvorsky, I., Skelly, J. M., & Higgins, S. T. (2017). Effects of financial incentives for smoking cessation on mood and anxiety symptoms among pregnant and newly postpartum women. *Nicotine & Tobacco Research*. https://doi.org/10.1093/ntr/ntx111

Chapter 3
Action, Inaction, and Actionability: Definitions and Implications for Communications and Interventions to Change Behaviors

Dolores Albarracín, Aashna Sunderrajan, and Wenhao Dai

Persuasive communications are designed with different objectives. For example, religious ministers try to strengthen their audiences' beliefs in the afterlife, and presidents defend the veracity of their statements. Marketing firms try to promote liking for a brand, and political campaign managers try to foster positive attitudes towards a candidate. Yet, other communications and programs try to change behavior, as when religious ministers solicit financial contributions, campaign managers strive to obtain votes for a candidate, or marketers seek to increase purchase. These communications to change behaviors bring up a number of important questions, including what contents maximize behavioral impact and the degree to which communications are successful in trying to induce actions or inactions. We begin this chapter with a discussion of action and inaction judgments that may affect one's disposition towards behaviors, such as those recommended in persuasive communications. We then follow with the notion of actionability, or the degree to which a communication or intervention is likely to influence behavior.

D. Albarracín (✉)
Department of Psychology and Department of Business Administration, Gies College of Business, University of Illinois at Urbana–Champaign, Champaign, IL, USA
e-mail: dalbarra@illinois.edu

A. Sunderrajan · W. Dai
Department of Psychology, University of Illinois at Urbana–Champaign, Champaign, IL, USA
e-mail: sunderr2@illinois.edu; wdai7@illinois.edu

D. A. Hope, R. A. Bevins (eds.), *Change and Maintaining Change*, Nebraska Symposium on Motivation 65, https://doi.org/10.1007/978-3-319-96920-6_3

Action and Inaction

An important consideration when assessing the likely impact of communications intended to change behavior is the construal of the recommendation as an action or an inaction. We define behavior as something that involves either motor or cognitive processes, such as sleeping, walking, or solving an intellectual problem. Behavior can be objectively conceptualized as active or inactive depending on the effort or energy expenditure involved in the process (Albarracín et al., 2008). For example, behaviorally, running is more active than sleeping. As such, the ends of an action/inaction continuum may be represented by a sprint on the action end and non-REM sleep on the inaction end. As analyzed presently, however, a person may arrive to a state of inaction in a restful or effortful manner, which leads to the distinction between restful and inhibitory inaction.

Factors Influencing Judgments of Action and Inaction

Although one may classify behavior objectively, whether a behavior is an action or an inaction is primarily a judgment, which has implications for other judgments, goals, and behaviors. For example, the contents of a communication may convey actions or inactions as goals and our judgments of each may influence adherence to the recommended behavior. These judgments are represented in Fig. 3.1 and concern evaluative valence (whether a behavior is positive or negative), intentionality (whether a behavior can be initiated willfully), control (whether a behavior can be stopped willfully), and effort (whether a behavior demands energy). Interventions may recommend actions and inactions, and their potential at achieving each is

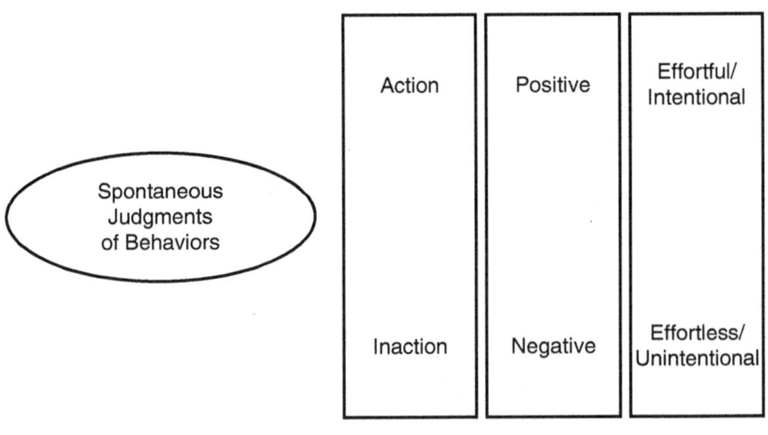

Fig. 3.1 Judgments of action and inaction

hereafter termed "actionability," which is the degree to which the program is successful at eliciting the recommended behaviors, be those actions or inactions.

Actions Are Seen as More Positive than Inactions Past evidence suggests that naïve definitions of action and inaction likely diverge in terms of valence, with evaluations of action being more positive than those of inaction. For example, work by McCulloch, Li, Hong, and Albarracín (2012) has found that people tend to rate words like "active," "run," and "jump" more positively than words like "inactive," "stationary," and "still." Similarly, cultural research has revealed that the general concept of action (e.g., "action is good") is rated subjectively more favorably than the general concept of inaction (e.g., "inaction is good"), especially in Western cultures (Ireland, Hepler, Li, & Albarracín, 2015; Zell et al., 2013).

This prior research, however, has been limited in having people rate words or concepts, instead of actual behavior. Thus, recent work has been done to determine whether this difference in evaluation would persist when rating actual (active and inactive) behaviors. In Experiment 2 (Sunderrajan & Albarracín, 2018), participants were asked to imagine themselves eating (or not eating) broccoli. When given no additional information, results showed that participants who were asked to eat broccoli (an action) evaluated the behavior more favorably than participants who were asked not to eat broccoli (an inaction). To ensure these results were not due to any association participants may have formed between eating broccoli and healthy behaviors (or other valenced contexts), Experiment 3 was run using the trivial behavior of pressing (or not pressing) a button, replicating results. This shows that behaviors falling under the umbrella of "action" are evaluated more positively than those falling under the umbrella of "inaction."

Why are naïve evaluations of action more positive than those of inaction? The extant literature provides three possible explanations. First, our social ethics tend to prescribe work while condemning laziness (Miller, Woehr, & Hudspeth, 2002). Thus, it is feasible that any behavior falling under the overarching action umbrella might similarly be valued more, relative to those behaviors categorized as inactions. Second, there is evidence to suggest that actions are more salient than inactions, which would presumably result in actions obtaining more of our attention and thus, being evaluated to a great extent (Fazio, Sherman, & Herr, 1982; Kahneman & Miller, 1986). Third, probably because they reflect a fundamental property of goals (i.e., individuals tend to pay more attention to what to do; Albarracín, Wang, & McCulloch, 2018), actions provide a more concrete indicator of progress on a task (Ferguson & Bargh, 2008).

Actions Are Seen as More Intentional than Inactions Underlying these explanations for the action positivity bias could be the naïve belief that actions are more intentional and goal-directed than inactions (Sunderrajan & Albarracín, 2018). This would be consistent with the explanations presented above, as engagement in work and the formation of goals are often seen to be the result of intentional behaviors. Furthermore, intentionality may be a meaningful basis for evaluations of actions because social groups need to strategically direct members towards intentional actions that are necessary for the group's survival. As such, a general positivity bias for action may be driven by a corresponding intentionality bias for action.

Sunderrajan and Albarracín (2018) tested this intentionality bias possibility using the broccoli experiment mentioned previously. In the experiment, participants were not only asked to imagine eating (or not eating) broccoli but were also asked to do so in one of three conditions: high-intentionality, low-intentionality, or unspecified-intentionality. In the unspecified-intentionality condition, participants were presented with the behavioral scenario with no additional information. In the high- and low-intentionality conditions, however, participants were given further information to manipulate the level of intentionality associated with the behavior (e.g., high-intentionality: *Imagine yourself eating some broccoli ... with a goal in mind*; low-intentionality: *Imagine yourself eating some broccoli ... without a goal or purpose*).

Findings reported by Sunderrajan and Albarracín (2018) suggests that judgments of intention drive evaluations of actions and inactions. Specifically, their results found that, for the behavioral action, evaluations did not differ between the high-intentionality and unspecified-intentionality condition. However, evaluations were more positive in both of these conditions compared to the low-intentionality condition. The lack of difference between the high-intentionality and unspecified-intentionality condition thus suggests that actions are perceived to be positive, and manipulating intentionality to be high has no additional effect. For the behavioral inaction, evaluations did not differ between the unspecified-intentionality or low-intentionality condition. However, evaluations were less positive in both of these conditions compared to those in the high-intentionality condition. This finding thereby suggests that inactions are spontaneously infused with more negative evaluations, and the manipulation of intentionality is important in shifting these evaluations.

Actions Are Seen as More Effortful than Inactions Definitions of action, however, entail both high effort and commission. For example, according to Albarracín et al. (2008), behaviors involving high motor or cognitive output are characteristic of action (e.g., running), and those involving neither motor nor cognitive output are more characteristic of inaction (e.g., non-REM sleep). Therefore, action is not only associated with commission but also effort, while inaction is associated with omission and low effort.

This association between action, inaction, and effort is most transparent in McCulloch et al.'s work (2012). In Experiment 1, participants were given a list of words to rate on two scales, one measuring activity and one measuring valence, which the authors used to place these words along an activity continuum. Overall, the authors found evidence to suggest that ratings of action and inaction were more variable in the middle than at the ends—a fact which might be due to the amount of effort associated with each word. For example, "select," "walk," and "run" were three words participants characterized as actions; however, none of them had the same average rating. Instead, "select" was rated as the least active word (from this list), "run" was rated as the most active word, and "walk" was rated somewhere in between—a pattern which would be consistent with the amount of effort attributable to each behavior. While not conclusive, this suggests that lay definitions of action show them as more effortful than inaction.

Control, Intentionality, Effort, and Evaluation, However, Appear to Be Intrinsically Linked There is evidence that control, intentionality, and effort are characteristics associated with judgments of action. Yet, from the extant literature, it appears that the association between these characteristics, action, and evaluation shares a lot of overlap. For example, greater energy is ascribed to desirable behaviors via goal setting (Ryan, 2002). Furthermore, when behaviors can be controlled (i.e., when one can direct what will happen), people's motivation to perform the behavior is higher and the outcomes of the behavior are perceived as more favorable (Cornwell, Franks, & Higgins, 2014; Eitam, Kennedy, & Higgins, 2013; Franks & Higgins, 2012; Higgins, 2012). And, in fact, intentionality is normally associated with behaviors that are desirable (Fishbein & Ajzen, 2010). Thus, judgments of control, intentionality, and desirability are likely to be intricately linked.

Research has also found a strong association between labor and love, such that, the more effort placed into some pursuit, the more value is attached to it. Norton, Mochon, and Ariely (2012), for example, asked participants to either build an IKEA storage box or inspect one, and then, bid and rate how much they liked the product. Their results found that participants who built the storage box were willing to pay more for the storage box, but also for the product. This research shows that the subjective value of a behavior is determined by the effort that goes into that behavior (effort justification theory; Aronson & Mills, 1959), such that mere engagement in labor is sufficient to increase the valuation of task outcomes (the IKEA effect; Norton et al., 2012). This research reveals how interwoven control, intentionality, and effort are with each other, and with people's motivation to engage in a task, or their overall evaluation of the task.

An extension of the previously cited experiment (Sunderrajan & Albarracín, 2018) has, in fact, empirically shown that this interrelation is likely. In particular, to determine whether intentionality truly mediated the relation between action, inaction, and evaluation, the authors ran a mediation model. Results revealed a significant indirect effect of action/inaction on ratings of evaluation, mediated by intentionality. Yet, as it is conceivable that intentionality may be a byproduct of evaluation, the authors also ran a mediation model with evaluation as the mediator for the association between action, inaction, and intentionality. This model also showed a significant indirect effect. Hence, these results provide empirical support for a complex bidirectional relation between intentionality and evaluation. It will be interesting to further identify the specific roles control, intentionality, and effort play in the evaluation of actions and inactions, and just how much overlap they truly share.

We Live in an Action-Oriented Society That Favors Inaction When Outcomes Are Likely to Be Negative Action and inaction has been the focus of important decision-making research. Kahneman and Tversky (Kahneman & Miller, 1986;

Kahneman & Tversky, 1982) found that, when people experience a negative event, they value and regret commissions more than omissions. In part, this bias is because imaging a world without a committed behavior is easier than imagining a world with an omitted behavior. Research in the moral domain has thus shown that people prefer harm by omission over harm by commission (omission bias; Baron & Ritov, 2004), and in the classic notions of economy, the norm for investment decisions is pro-omission (Kahneman & Miller, 1986). According to this research, then, there exists a norm favoring inactions in our society.

Yet, recent work has revealed that the story is not as simple as it seems. In one experiment (Feldman & Albarracín, 2017), participants were presented with the classic Kahneman and Tversky (1982) investment scenarios describing two stock traders working for a financial firm: One who switched investments (action), and one who refrained from switching investments (inaction). Following the scenario, participants were asked to identify which of the two stock brokers the company would consider superior. Participants were also given a description of two investment companies, one favoring action and one favoring inaction. Participants were then asked which of these two companies was more commonly occurring in their country of residence (all participants were US residents).

Results revealed that 76% of participants indicated that the investment company would consider the inaction-oriented stock broker to be a better worker, consistent with prior research. Yet, only 12% of participants indicated that the inaction-oriented company was more commonly occurring in the USA. These data thus reveal an inconsistency between a theoretical assumption for inaction in the regret literature and the general perception of the normative behavior to take action: Although the perceived social norms in society are for taking action, the perceived norms in an investment scenario are for inaction. Additional work has revealed that, in general, there exists a strong preference for taking action. But, when presented with possible negative consequences (a common theme in the domains of morality and economic theory), people prefer norms towards not taking action. Thus, reliance on action and inaction norms fluctuates with the scenario.

Yet, even when decisions carry the potential for negative outcomes, as in the case of investments, the specific norms are highly malleable. In another series of experiments, Feldman and Albarracín (2017) assigned participants to one of three norm conditions of action, inaction, and control. They adjusted the classic Kahneman and Tversky (1982) scenario so that it described two stock traders working at a financial firm. In the scenarios, George switches investments (action), and Paul remains with his original investments (inaction). The classic scenario describes the traders as independent and participants show greater regret in the action than the inaction condition, suggesting that the norm is pro-inaction. However, Feldman and Albarracín also manipulated the company norm. In Experiment 1, the action–norm condition involved statements that the company emphasized action and proactive decision-making, and evaluated its employees based on their ability to act and actively pursue good investments. The inaction–norm condition stated that the company emphasized cautious and responsible decision-making, and evaluated its employees based on their ability to refrain from bad investments. There was also a control condition that did not indicate either preference. Following the scenario, participants indicated who was likely to experience higher regret. Participants indicated the highest probability of regret in the action–norm condition, followed by the control condition, followed by the inaction–norm condition (88%, 72%, and 56%, respectively). This supported that shifts in specific norms trigger changes in regret. Interestingly, the degree of regret was the same when participants were told that the investments were decided on intentionally by Paul and George, or by the toss of a coin (Experiment 2), and when the manipulated norms were societal (Experiment 3) or family-based (Experiment 4), rather than institutional.

Action and Inaction Goals and Active and Inactive Behavioral Means

An important distinction characterizing behaviors as actions or inactions is that of goals versus means. An inaction goal may be achieved by inhibition or by continued rest as means to the goal. When a person is sleeping, continuing to sleep requires no effortful means and is a mere continuation of the prior state. In contrast, switching to sleeping when a person is currently running involves effortful, inhibitory means. Likewise, an action goal may be achieved by inertia or by effortful behavioral means. Continuing to run when a person is running is often less effortful than stopping abruptly. In other words, changing from one state to the other is often effortful, but the degree of action or effort of the achieved state is independent of the means to arrive at that state.

General vs. Specific Action and Inaction

The construal of action and inaction operates at both general and specific levels. At a general level, action and inaction involve any behavior that can be conceptualized as involving high or low effort and engagement, respectively. For this reason, priming general action and inaction concepts has been shown to affect a variety of behaviors. Laboratory experiments have shown that when individuals have a general action (or inaction) goal, they ultimately pursue more active (or inactive) behaviors. For example, the priming procedures in Albarracín, Hepler, and Tannenbaum (2011) involved exposing participants to concepts linked to general action (e.g., "active" and "go") or general inaction (e.g., "rest" and "stop"). The assessment of activity following the primes has involved diverse tasks in the form of decision-making to political participation. For example, in Experiment 1 of Albarracín et al. (2008), participants were primed with action or inaction through a word-completion task (e.g., "Fill in the missing letter(s): ac_ive"), which was followed by a choice to participate in an active task (drawing on a piece of paper) or an inactive task (resting with eyes closed). Findings revealed that 62% of participants primed with action chose to draw instead of to rest, whereas only 36% of those primed with inaction chose to draw instead of to rest. Further, the same general action and inaction primes can influence other behaviors that also fall under the conceptual umbrella of action and inaction. For instance, experimental studies have found effects on eating, physical movement, and political participation, as well as intellectual performance, although the latter effects have not been replicated (e.g., Albarracín et al., 2008; Albarracín & Hart, 2011; Minas, Poor, Dennis, & Bartelt, 2016; Noguchi, Handley, & Albarracín, 2011).

The operation of these general action and inaction goals obeys two important principles. First, symbols and words connect with the *conceptual* representation of action and inaction. Second, these representations connect to *physiological resources* that are mobilized to meet task demands. These resources involve sympathetic regulation of adrenaline, heart rate, and bronchial dilation, which prepare organisms for fight or flight (Brehm & Self, 1989). Exposure to action words—even below the level of conscious awareness—can modulate this type of physiological activity, such that action and inaction goals, respectively, increase and decrease resource mobilization (Gendolla & Silvestrini, 2010). The generality of these mechanisms is such that general action and inaction concepts can facilitate or hinder execution of activity in a variety of specific domains.

Even though general action and inaction goals are likely to recruit relevant specific goals, specific goals are likely to drive general goals as well. For example, children who are socialized to value sports and academic activities may value those specific activities but also generalize those evaluations and appreciate action more generally. Later, however, the general goal may operate independently and seek satisfaction through other means, including impulsive ones. In fact, effects of general action and inaction goals on impulsive behavior have been demonstrated by Hepler, Albarracín, McCulloch, and Noguchi (2012). Specifically, these authors found that priming words of general action and inaction increased false alarms on a Go/No-go task, suggesting that the generality of the goals can control not only deliberative behavior but also impulsive action.

The Efficacy of Requesting Actions or Inactions

Requesting actions is likely to be more demanding than requesting inactions. As proposed by Albarracín et al. (2018), people are more likely to spontaneously form action than inaction goals. They are also more likely to experience difficulty and cognitive demands in response to multiple action demands than in response to multiple inaction demands. Compared to inactions, actions receive more attention (Kahneman & Miller, 1986) and elicit stronger emotional reactions (Landman,

1987; Zhou, Yu, & Zhou, 2010). In animal perception and learning, for example, pigeons are better able to associate rewards with video images of other pigeons that are moving than with other pigeons that are standing still (Dittrich & Lea, 1993). In humans, people who signal agreement by actively producing a response later agree with a behavior more than people who signal agreement by avoiding a response (Allison & Messick, 1988; Cioffi & Garner, 1996; Fazio et al., 1982).

The fact that action demands are greater than inaction demands is likely positive when a single behavior is requested and thus encourages attention and action preparation. However, when multiple behaviors are requested, a greater number of actions may have more detrimental effects than a greater number of inactions (Albarracín et al., 2018). Supporting this possibility, a series of experiments using a multiple Go/No-go task showed that both misses and false alarms were more frequent when participants had to press a key in response to 3 targets than when they had to not press a key in response to 3 targets. This pattern was attributable to the greater cognitive load posed by the multiple action goals and by people's natural focus on action. In fact, when participants were encouraged to focus on inaction (Experiment 4), the difference in errors decreased.

In sum, actions may be more salient, connote greater positivity, and engage greater intentionality, control, and effort. However, some interventions may seek to encourage actions (e.g., increase exercise) and others may seek to encourage inactions (e.g., sleep more). In both cases, interventions should be successful to the extent that they encourage positivity, intentionality, controllability, and effort. This is illustrated in Fig. 3.2 to emphasize that inactions must become goals that are pursued intentionally and which may require preparatory actions, or active means, to be successful. As in Albarracín et al. (2018), inaction can become a goal.

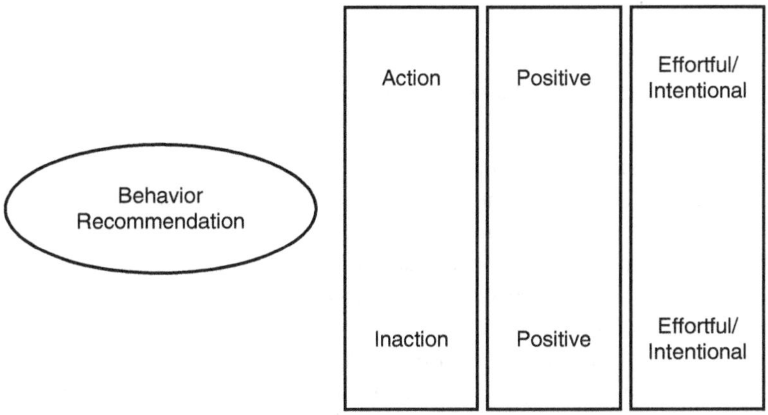

Fig. 3.2 Goal for behavior recommendations to be experienced as positive and be pursued effortfully and intentionally

Framing Inaction as Action and Action as Inaction

If action engages more effort and is generally perceived as more positive, it is only natural to try to reframe inaction recommendations by proposing substitute actions. There are several reasons for this proposal. First, at the level of cognitive change, it is easier to replace one cognition with another than it is to simply eliminate it (Chan, Jones, & Albarracín, 2017). Second, people have an easier time conceptualizing the presence of a behavior than the absence of a behavior (Albarracín et al., 2018). Third, behavioral skills programs tend to emphasize what you are going to do to change your behavior (Albarracín et al., 2005; Albarracín & Wyer, 2001; Bandura, 1986, 1997; Fisher & Fisher, 1992), so even the goal of not smoking again is likely reframed as behaviors during those models. Fourth, telling people what not to do tends to elicit psychological reactance (Brehm, 1966), thus leading us to conclude that it is better to encourage people on what to do instead of what not to do.

The degree to which recommending what to do may be more successful than recommending what not to do is illustrated by Albarracín, Cohen, and Kumkale (2003) research on abstinence and moderation. In their research, participants received a message that recommended either abstinence from, or moderation in, the use of a new type of alcohol product. After reading persuasive messages, participants either tried the product or performed a filler task before reporting their intentions to drink in the future. As predicted, participants who did not try the product reported similar intentions to drink when they received the moderation message and when they received the abstinence message. However, when participants tried the product after receiving the message, recipients of the abstinence message had significantly stronger intentions to drink than recipients of the moderation message. Apparently, trying the product after a strong recommendation led participants to the conclusion that they truly liked the forbidden product. In any case, the message anticipating some drinking was more effective than the extreme abstinence one.

Affirmed Action vs. Negated Inaction

An interesting question is whether discouraging or negating inaction is as effective at inducing active behavioral responses as is recommending action. In work conducted by Ireland, Hepler, and Albarracín (2013), participants read the political slogans used in presidential campaigns. The slogans and sources appear in Table 3.1, organized in terms of whether they affirmed action, negated inaction, and included a mix of affirmed action and belief-inducing messages as a control condition. In this experiment, both the high and moderate frequency of action conditions yielded similar intentions to vote for a political candidate that used the slogans. Thus, it appeared that moderate levels of action contents were sufficient to induce supporting intentions. More importantly, negated inaction led to much weaker intentions to vote for the candidate. Apparently, the negation, which is much more difficult to process, did not communicate action in the same way as did the affirmative statement about action.

Table 3.1 Affirmed and negated action slogans

Condition	Slogan	Source and election year
High frequency of affirmed action	*It's time to change.*	Bill Clinton (1992)
	It's time for us to get working again.	Rick Perry (2012)
	Come and take it.	Battle of Gonzales (1835)
	Stand up for your country.	George Wallace (1968)
	We're turning the corner.	Herbert Hoover (1932)
Moderate frequency of affirmed action	*It's time to renew.*	Herman Cain (2012)
	Believe in our country.	Ron Paul (2012)
	All the way.	Lyndon B. Johnson (1964)
	In your heart, you know he's right.	Barry Goldwater (1964)
	Restore our future.	Mitt Romney (2012)
High frequency of negated inaction	*You can't stop thinking about tomorrow.*	Bill Clinton (1992)
	We will not surrender.	Lyndon B. Johnson (1964)
	We can't wait.	Barack Obama (2012)
	The stakes are too high to stay home.	Lyndon B. Johnson (1964)
	Don't settle.	Michelle Bachman (2012)

Note. Slogans were adapted from Wikipedia's List of Political Slogans and other web searches. The Clinton slogan was a quote of Fleetwood Mac's (1977) "Don't Stop"

Homogeneous Action and Inaction Messages

Recommendations of action and inaction within an intervention are likely to trigger opposing processes of action initiation and inhibitory control of behavior. Action preparation entails an executive process that orchestrates a response (Jennings & Van Der Molen, 2005). Although the responses vary, the executive mechanisms of action preparation are common to a variety of tasks. Similarly, inhibitory processes generalize across tasks and behaviors. A meta-analysis of 18 experiments conducted by Tuk, Zhang, and Sweldens (2015) showed that engaging self-control in one domain (i.e., controlling thoughts, attention, food consumption, or emotions) facilitates self-control in other domains. Consistent with this finding, Berkman, Burklund, and Lieberman (2009) reported that inhibitory signals originate in the same areas of the brain across a variety of responses, suggesting a general inhibitory process.

The single process underlying action preparation in different contexts led Albarracín, Wilson, Chan, Durantini, and Sanchez (2017) to propose that a health recommendation of action would facilitate other health recommendations of action but have antagonistic effects when combined with recommendations of inaction. Furthermore, the single process underlying inhibitory control in different contexts led them to propose that a health recommendation of inaction would facilitate other inaction recommendations but hinder action recommendations. In other words, a homogeneous set of health recommendations should be more efficacious than a heterogeneous set. Recommending increases in physical activity may be more efficacious when combined with recommending increases in fruit and vegetable intake than when combined with recommending decreases in fat intake. Likewise, recommending a decrease in fat intake may be more efficacious when combined with reducing sugar intake or quitting smoking than when combined with increasing exercise.

These hypotheses were tested in a meta-analysis of reports of the effects of multiple-behavior interventions in the area of lifestyle (diet, exercise, and smoking). Reports were required to include a pretest assessment of clinical and/or behavioral outcomes, which were averaged, and the final database included 216 multiple-behavior change intervention groups (N = 74,000 participants). For coding purposes, the recommendations were the goals, or behavioral categories, targeted in the interventions. They involved specific prescribed dietary, exercise, or smoking behaviors (e.g., reducing sedentary time) made by an intervention. The total number of recommendations contained in the intervention comprised a count of the total number of primary goals (e.g., three when the recommendations were to reduce calories, to increase fruit and vegetable intake, and to increase physical activity). For each recommendation, the researchers also coded (a) the domain of the recommendation (e.g., diet, and exercise) and (b) whether the recommendation was for action (e.g., increase physical activity; increase fruit intake) or inaction (e.g., reduce fat intake; quit smoking; rest and relax).

Albarracín et al. (2017) calculated Becker's (1988) g to indicate a change in pre- to posttest measures. They subtracted the mean at the posttest from the mean at the pretest and then divided the difference by the standard deviation of the pretest measure. The sign of the effect sizes was chosen to represent improvements from a health perspective (e.g., decrease in BMI, and increase in fruit intake) as positive. Common measures of behavioral outcomes in the area of *diet* were energy intake (e.g., kcal/week); carbohydrate, protein, fiber, fat, fruit, and vegetable intake (in grams or servings); number of meals per day; whether participants achieved dietary recommendations; whether participants achieved recommendations for fruit and vegetable intake; whether participants checked their blood pressure in the past 12 months; presence of unhealthy eating; and presence of overeating. Frequent behavioral measures in the *exercise* domain entailed whether participants engaged in daily exercise; weekly hours of physical activity; whether participants engaged in occupational physical activity; whether participants had regular physical activity; whether participants achieved certain exercise recommendations; whether participants were sedentary; whether participants reported high-impact physical activity; self-monitoring of pulse and blood pressure; self-monitoring with pedometer (daily pace); time spent in physical activity; energy expenditure in physical activity (k/cal); and number of TV hours per day. Frequent behavioral measures in the *smoking* domain included current smoking status; number of cigarettes smoked per day (often via diaries); number of years of smoking; whether participants were ex-smokers, and longest quit duration. Frequent clinical measures included body weight in kilograms; body mass index; hip size; waist size; hip/waist ratio; body fat;

whether participants were overweight; whether participants were obese; systolic/diastolic blood pressure; triglycerides level; HDL/LDL cholesterol; fasting blood glucose; presence of diabetes; presence of metabolic syndrome; pulse; results from spirometer tests; results from VO_2 Max tests; results from chest X-ray; presence of nicotine in blood; lab tests to confirm right dose of medication in blood; lab tests for diabetes; results from PAP tests; results from mammogram reports; results from dental records; and results from colonoscopy reports.

Albarracín et al. (2017) used this meta-analysis to test the hypothesis that homogeneous behavioral recommendations were more efficacious than heterogeneous ones. They created a variable that classified interventions as recommending predominately action behaviors, an equal number of action and inaction behaviors, or predominately inaction behaviors. They also created a variable that averaged all behavioral and clinical measures of change available in a study. Table 3.2 presents the average effect of that variable on overall change. The table also includes Q_B statistics, which indicated a significant effect of that variable on overall change. As predicted, interventions that predominantly included recommendations for either action or action were more effective than recommendations that were equal in the inclusion of action/inaction recommendations. Further, interventions with equal numbers of action and inaction did not differ significantly from single-behavior programs or control conditions (see subscripts e and d in Table 3.2). Finally, and unexpectedly, a predominance of inaction recommendations produced more change than a predominance of action recommendations.

In this section, we have shown that an important consideration when assessing the likely impact of communications intended to change behavior is the construal of recommendations as either an action or inaction. Actions are seen as more positive, controllable, intentional, and effortful, than inactions. Yet, favorability for norms associated with actions and inactions can fluctuate and, more importantly, so can the need for action and inaction goals and recommendations in the health domain. For example, interventions may seek to encourage actions (e.g., increase fruit consumption), whereas others may seek to encourage inactions (e.g., decrease sugar intake).

Table 3.2 Overall change as a function of the action and inaction recommendations (Albarracín et al., 2017)

	Predominately inaction	Equal	Predominately action	QB_2	k
k	30	106	80		
Fixed effects $d.$	0.35_a	0.11_{bde}	0.19_c	395.84***	216
Random effects $d.$	0.48_a	0.16_b	0.23_c	35.73***	216

Note. $d.$ = weighted means. No-intervention control groups ($k = 39$, $d. = 0.06$, confidence interval $=-0.01, 0.12$) and single-behavior intervention groups ($k = 15$, $d. = 0.07$, confidence interval $=0.02, 0.13$) were excluded. Following the means, we present the QB for *the action/inaction* index. QB = homogeneity coefficient for the difference across levels of a factor, distributed as a chi-square with degrees of freedom equal to the number of factor levels—1. ds with similar subscripts a–c are not significantly different from one another. Subscript d indicates that change is not different from change in the no-intervention control group. Subscript e indicates that change is not different from change in the single-behavior control group. k number of conditions

***$p < 0.001$

Depending on factors such as intervention demand and psychological reactance, either type of communication is useful. As such, actions and inactions can both be the focus of behavioral interventions. The next step, then, is to understand what is required to achieve high levels of actual behavioral change.

Actionability

Even though successfully inducing beliefs and attitudes by means of persuasive communications is not without complications, the challenge of changing behavior is even higher. There are numerous reasons why changing behaviors is difficult. In the second part of this chapter, we propose a framework to analyze the factors that make persuasive communications actionable. We define *actionability* as the property of enabling and motivating recipients to make behavioral decisions based on the intervention content. Actionability comprises the inclusion of behavioral recommendations, the relevance of those recommendations within the context of behavior execution, and the influence of the message on the recipient's ability and motivation to carry out the recommendations. An intervention is actionable if it includes at least one behavioral recommendation, the recommendation is appropriate for the context, and the intervention promotes recipients' willingness and ability to carry out the recommendation. These premises are graphically represented in Fig. 3.3 and illustrated in the coming sections.

In our analysis, actionability varies from potential, when an intervention explicitly recommends one or more behaviors, to fully realized, when the behavior is relevant to the recipient's context and is ultimately executed. The upcoming sections cover these components of actionability and how to incorporate them in the practice of intervention design. We also review research findings and theories that have implications for our conceptualization and draw recommendations for communication and intervention design.

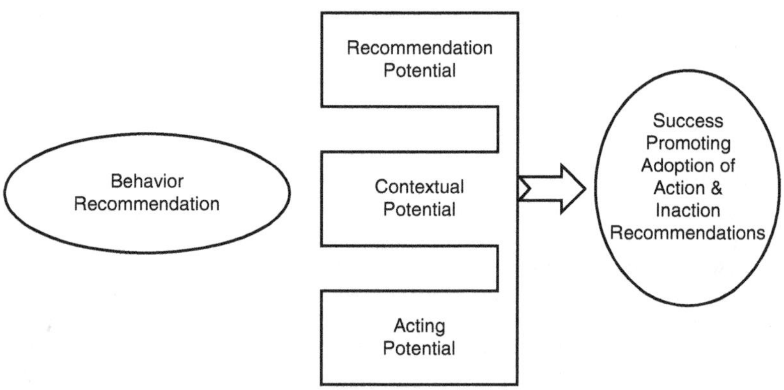

Fig. 3.3 Actionability

Table 3.3 Means (and standard deviations) of credibility and actionability as a function of message type (Dai & Albarracín, 2017)

	Credibility or strength	Actionability
High-actionability message	1.39 (0.88)	2.05 (0.71)
Low-actionability message	1.59 (0.99)	1.13 (1.11)

Distinguishing Actionability from Believability

Actionability is conceptually distinct from the believability or credibility of a persuasive communication or intervention. In theory, a message may be highly credible without having any implications for behavior. To test this possibility, we randomly assigned 28 participants to read either a positive review or a negative review of an ostensible product, a juice that could be customized to meet customer's specifications before an online order was placed (Dai & Albarracín, 2017). The high-actionability form of the message stated that the juice product offered a variety of flavors and could satisfy different needs for a wide range of customers; the low-actionability form of the message stated that the juice factor was infamous for its inefficient manufacturing process and excessive waste of fruit during manufacturing. Participants were instructed to read the message and then asked to rate their reactions on three scales. The credibility or argument strength scale included items such as "this information is persuasive" and "this information is compelling." The actionability scales include items such as "this piece of information influences my behavioral decision" and "this piece of information is relevant to my behavioral goal." The attitude scale includes items such as "this product is good" and "this product is positive." Table 3.3 summarizes participants' ratings based on each message. As shown in this table, the two messages were identical in credibility, but actionability differed.

Distinguishing Actionability from Desirability and Other Attitudinal Effects

Actionability is theoretically distinguishable from the desirability of the object or behavior promoted in an intervention. For example, a message may communicate that a future product will be more or less environmentally friendly. However, if the primary reason for purchasing the product is its low cost, arguing that it is or it is not environmentally friendly is likely to have little effect.

Even though actionability is conceptually distinct from desirability, action contents in a message tend to elicit positive feelings. For example, as mentioned previously, in research by McCulloch et al. (2012), participants were asked to rate words in terms of their action content as well as their valence. As expected, words like *action* were rated as more active than words like *freeze* or *relax*. Furthermore, words rated as active were also generally rated more positively than words rated as inactive. Given these findings, it is not surprising that many marketing campaigns are structured around active words. For example, Nike's "Just do it!" says little about the trademark's sport products but likely capitalizes on the associations between doing and positive feelings.

Recommendation Potential: Nature of Behavioral Recommendations in an Intervention

Number of Recommendations Although there are exceptions, a communication or intervention that offers no behavioral recommendation is generally unlikely to elicit behavior. Thus, the presence and number of behavioral recommendations are primary considerations in thinking about the actionability potential of any program. A meta-analysis of multiple-domain health-promotion interventions revealed that moderate numbers (2–3) of recommended behaviors produce better clinical and behavioral outcomes than both fewer (0–1) and greater (4+) numbers (Wilson et al., 2015). However, the decrease in outcome quality from 2–3 to 4+ is generally negligible, which is probably attributable to the interventions being designed to be feasible and on the basis of significant pilot testing.

Comprehension Recommendations have comprehension potential when interventions are in the language of the recipients, have a linguistic complexity appropriate for the level of education of the audience, and use language and concepts that are accessible to the level of expertise of the audience. Sheridan et al. (2011) reviewed the features that make interventions accessible to audiences with low literacy and numeracy, which are, respectively, the ability to read written verbal materials and to execute basic mathematical functions. Peters, Dieckmann, Dixon, Hibbard, and Mertz (2007), for example, found that low- and high-literacy recipients of health information about hospital quality have better comprehension when they receive only essential information. Further, presenting the essential information first when all the information was presented also improved comprehension, but this effect was present only among low-numeracy participants. Other studies have found that using higher numbers to represent the presence of a characteristic (i.e., hospital quality) (Peters et al., 2007), and presenting disease risk and treatment benefit information using the same (versus different) denominators (Garcia-Retamero & Galesic, 2009), also improved comprehension when numeracy was low. Additionally, presenting comparative information about the harms and benefits of two drugs in tables, rather than text, improved understanding, particularly for recipients with low literacy (Tait, Voepel-Lewis, Zikmund-Fisher, & Fagerlin, 2010). Finally, adding pictorial information and graphic symbols can help, although some of the findings are conflicting (Sheridan et al., 2011).

Contextual Potential

The contextual fit or appropriateness of a behavioral recommendations is an important consideration because recommendations may not apply to a context, either because of structural differences or because of an inadequate specification of the behavior. Recipients construct a mental model of what behaviors are to be executed when and where. Mismatches with reality may come in different forms, including structural discrepancies and level discrepancies. Imagine a message that states that the way to reduce the threat of influenza is to take a pill. Recipients may correctly understand the message and then proceed to go to a health clinic only to find out that the flu vaccine only comes in injectable or nasal forms.

A structural mismatch between the recommendation contained in the intervention and the contextual reality is fairly extreme, but mismatches based on level of generality are common. For example, audiences may be told to have safe sex. This recommendation is general enough to include avoiding sex with HIV-infected partners, avoiding sex with HIV-infected partners not currently on PreExposure Prophylaxis (PrEP), having sex with a condom or latex barrier, and having sex while on PrEP. Thus, having "safe sex" is too general a recommendation without specifying the spectrum of behavioral possibilities in particular contexts. Furthermore, messages and interventions that are excessively specific are likely to lose actionability potential as well. For example, a patient who only knows the commercial name of a drug may fail to identify an entire category of substitutes with a different designation.

Acting Potential

Communications and interventions become truly actionable when they instill recipients' cognitive and motivational responses in line with the message recommendation. These include (a) activation of concepts, (b) formation of beliefs and attitudes, (c) emotional feelings, (d) behavioral skills, and (e) perceptions of control. Intentions may also be involved, except that some behaviors may be relatively automatic. Many of these variables overlap with the integrative model of behavior proposed by Fishbein (Fishbein, 2000, 2008; Fishbein & Ajzen, 2010).

Activation of Concepts Prior research has shown evidence that activation of concepts through such external signals as words and pictures can influence performance of behavioral tasks completed after the signal is presented. This type of subtle influence of simple signals is also known as a priming effect (for a review, see Weingarten et al., 2016). For example, college students who unscrambled words denoting rudeness during a sentence scramble task were more likely to interrupt a conversation than those who unscrambled words about either politeness or neutral topics (Bargh, Chen, & Burrows, 1996). Similarly, in their second experiment, participants who accessed words relevant to the elderly stereotype walked down the hallway more slowly than did control participants. Despite the fact that some of these priming effects have been resistant to direct replication (Doyen, Klein, Pichon, & Cleeremans, 2012; Harris, Coburn, Rohrer, & Pashler, 2013), a large meta-analysis revealed a small but robust behavioral priming effects ($d_{FE} = 0.332$, $d_{RE} = 0.352$) (Weingarten et al., 2016). Weingarten and his colleagues also found that behavioral concepts that were valued more were associated with stronger priming effects.

The above findings suggest that interventions that can activate certain behavioral concepts, especially those that matter to the recipients, have greater potential to influence the recipients' future behaviors. For instance, a message that primes the concept "efficiency" by containing words like "fast," "speed," or "quickness" may have greater potential to speed up recipients' behaviors than a similar message without these words. Actionable interventions are often able to activate at least one, and often multiple-behavioral concepts that are relevant to the recommended behaviors. Without activating relevant behavioral concepts, messages are unlikely to have a behavioral impact. However, priming concepts alone is unlikely to exert predictable effects because the direction of the effects depends on preexisting motivations in the recipients (Hart & Albarracín, 2009; Strahan, Spencer, & Zanna, 2002). Therefore, more elaborate instructions such as belief-based messages are necessary.

Formation of Beliefs and Attitudes A belief refers to a subjective perception of the likelihood that something is true, or something will happen. Forming beliefs is one of the most mundane, yet important, capacities of the mind (Anderson, 1971; Fishbein, 1963; Wyer, 1970). It is also the foundation of most of our attitudes. Forming a belief about an object can lead to an attitude towards that object as well as an attitude towards certain behaviors related to that object. For example, a person who believes that a vaccine prevents disease tends to form a positive attitude towards both the vaccine (i.e., an attitude towards the object) and periodically receiving vaccines (i.e., an attitude towards behaviors). In contrast, a person who believes that vaccines do not prevent disease is more likely to form a negative attitude towards both the vaccine and getting vaccines.

Actionable interventions often allow recipients to form new beliefs or alter preexisting beliefs. Forming new beliefs can help with forming new attitudes and therefore developing new behavioral habits, whereas altering key prior beliefs can change preexisting attitudes towards certain objects, and therefore, change the way they interact with those objects. Messages to curb smoking emphasize that smoking is bad for health. However, such messages are likely ineffective because the primary preexisting beliefs leading to smoking concern the social image of smoking or the effects of smoking on smokers' moods. Thus, actionable messages to change behaviors require changing key beliefs at the basis of undesirable behaviors.

Emotional Feelings Another basis for attitudes is affective feelings. The question, "what do I believe about it?" is not the same as, "how do I feel about it?," and the answers to these questions may differ. For example, people might believe that the chance to win the lottery is low but still feel like purchasing a ticket each time they enter a gas station. In this case, the feelings towards the object can override the beliefs about that object and thus play a dominant role in shaping behavior.

In addition to the affect elicited directly by the attitude object, affect elicited by other relevant sources, such as experiencing a happy or sad mood, can also influence one's attitudes (Schwarz & Clore, 2007). Experimentally, induced irrelevant affect has been found to influence a wide variety of judgments, such as consuming products (Pham, 1998), risks (Gasper & Clore, 2000), and political decisions (Forgas & Bower, 1987), as long as the respondents are unaware of the true source of the affect (Gasper & Clore, 2000).

One explanation of why affects, even those that are irrelevant, can have a big influence on judgments is proposed by the Affect-as-Information model. Schwarz and Clore (1983) proposed that the embodied information of feelings can itself influence judgments. In one of their studies, they found that people were more satisfied with their lives when in a good mood (induced by sunny days) rather than when in bad mood (induced by rainy days). However, this effect would go away if people were instructed to attribute the affect information to its true source. The effect is thus unlikely when people have high knowledge in the judgment domain (Averbeck, Jones, & Robertson, 2011).

One of the more investigated emotional aspects in the area of persuasion and behavioral interventions is the use of fear. Fear appeals are persuasive attempts at arousing fear by highlighting a threat or danger (Dillard, Plotnick, Godbold, Freimuth, & Edgar, 1996; Maddux & Rogers, 1983). Tannenbaum et al. (2015) meta-analyzed the effects of fear appeals and found a moderate significant effect. In fact, fear appeals facilitated the recommended behavior in all of the conditions under which the effects were examined. Clearly, actionable interventions often elicit emotional responses among the recipients. In some cases, as in the case of fear appeals, the emotion is directly relevant to the recommended behavior. Other times, these emotions are not necessarily relevant to the target object or behavior but still prepare the recipients for the intended behaviors. For example, if a message is intended to encourage a positive attitude towards the purchase of a certain product, subtly inducing positive emotions using irrelevant stimuli can succeed at producing misattribution of those feelings to the product. Usually, the more intense emotions a message can elicit, the greater its potential to influence behavioral decisions among recipients is.

Behavioral Skills Atkinson (1964) introduced a formula to calculate the tendency to act using three determinants: (a) the motivation to act, (b) incentive for success, and (c) the probability of success, which is often based on behavioral skills. Based on Atkinson's model, even when a person has both a strong motivation and incentive to act, behavioral skills to ensure success are key for the person to perform the behavior. That is, a person whose significant other jumps off a bridge is likely to jump to their rescue only when the person knows how to swim.

There is considerable support for the importance of behavioral skills in changing behaviors. For example, Albarracín et al. (2005) found that interventions to promote condom use were more successful when they included behavioral skills training than when they did not. A lack of behavioral skills predicted failures to quit smoking (Tait et al., 2007), but training smokers in skills increased smoking abstinence at a 4-year follow-up (Conner & Higgins, 2010). Similar results have been found in the area of alcohol use, where skills training reduced alcohol use at a 4-year follow-up (Koning, van den Eijnden, Verdurmen, Engels, & Vollebergh, 2013). Therefore, actionable interventions must focus on altering recipients' beliefs and feelings about the behavior but also the skills necessary to execute a behavior.

Perceptions of Control In general, perceptions of control refer to a person's perception that he or she can influence the occurrence of an event (Wallston, Wallston, Smith, & Dobbins, 1987). A number of studies have shown that taking into account perceived behavioral control improves the prediction of behavior (Aizen, Fishbein, Lohmann, & Albarracín, n.d.). Meta-analyses have found that, on average, perceived behavioral control explains approximately 2% of the variance in behavior over and above behavioral intentions (Armitage & Conner, 2001; Cheung & Chan, 2000). However, the contribution of perceived behavioral control depends largely on the degree to which the behavior is under volitional control. When volitional control is high, intentions are good predictors of behavior and perceived behavioral control adds very little. In contrast, when a behavior is not under complete volitional control, perceptions of control become more important (Madden, Ellen, & Ajzen, 1992).

As such, perceptions of control are another important factor that can influence the perceived chance of success, increasing or decreasing a person's tendency to act. Smokers, for example, perceive a low probability of success for any attempt at quitting and therefore must change these perceptions to increase their chances of success. According to Bandura and Wood (1989), having perceived control, or having a high sense of self-efficacy, is key to human agency and attempts at changing one's circumstances and behaviors. Furthermore, there is evidence that persuasive communications designed to promote condom use are more successful when they include arguments designed to persuade recipients that they have control over their behavior (Albarracín, McNatt, et al., 2003).

In this section, we introduced actionability as the potential for intervention content to change behaviors. Actionability is conceptually different from credibility or desirability, although they tend to be correlated. To fully realize its actionability, an intervention needs to provide at least one behavioral recommendation, which are context appropriate, elicit recipients' cognitive responses (i.e., activation of concepts, formation of beliefs and attitudes, and perceptions of control) and affective responses (i.e., experience of emotions) in line with the desired behaviors, and teach necessary skills to implement the recommended behaviors. Readers can use our advice as guidelines in designing better intervention content to change behaviors.

Action/Inaction and Actionability

In this chapter, our objective has been to provide a framework and integration of our work of judgments of behavior and on behavioral change interventions and mechanisms of change. Both actions and inactions can be the focus of behavioral interventions, and in both cases the interventions require high levels of actionability to be successful. As more research accumulates, readers should be able to further test these ideas and implement our advice in the development of successful programs to change behavior. We look forward to assess progress in this critical field in the next decade.

References

Aizen, I., Fishbein, M., Lohmann, S., & Albarracín, D. (n.d.). The influence of attitudes on behaviors. In D. Albarracín & B. T. Johnson (Eds.), *Handbook of attitudes: Basic principles* (2nd ed.).

Albarracín, D., Cohen, J. B., & Kumkale, G. T. (2003). When communications collide with recipients' actions: Effects of post-message behavior on intentions to follow the message recommendation. *Personality & Social Psychology Bulletin*. https://doi.org/10.1177/0146167203029007003

Albarracín, D., Gillette, J. C., Earl, A. N., Glasman, L. R., Durantini, M. R., & Ho, M. H. (2005). A test of major assumptions about behavior change: A comprehensive look at the effects of passive and active HIV-prevention interventions since the beginning of the epidemic. *Psychological Bulletin, 131*(6), 856–897. https://doi.org/10.1037/0033-2909.131.6.856

Albarracín, D., Handley, I. M., Noguchi, K., McCulloch, K. C., Li, H., Leeper, J., … Hart, W. P. (2008). Increasing and decreasing motor and cognitive output: A model of general action and inaction goals. *Journal of Personality and Social Psychology*. https://doi.org/10.1037/a0012833

Albarracín, D., & Hart, W. (2011). Positive mood + action = negative mood + inaction: Effects of general action and inaction concepts on decisions and performance as a function of affect. *Emotion*. https://doi.org/10.1037/a0024130

Albarracín, D., Hepler, J., & Tannenbaum, M. (2011). General action and inaction goals: Their behavioral, cognitive, and affective origins and influences. *Current Directions in Psychological Science*. https://doi.org/10.1177/0963721411402666

Albarracín, D., McNatt, P. S., Klein, C. T. F., Ho, R. M., Mitchell, A. L., & Kumkale, G. T. (2003). Persuasive communications to change actions: An analysis of behavioral and cognitive impact in HIV prevention. *Health Psychology, 22*(2), 166–177. https://doi.org/10.1037/0278-6133.22.2.166

Albarracín, D., Wang, W., & McCulloch, K. C. (2018). Action dominance: The performance effects of multiple action demands and the benefits of an inaction focus. *Personality & Social Psychology Bulletin, 44,* 996–1007.

Albarracín, D., Wilson, K., Chan, M. S., Durantini, M., & Sanchez, F. (2017). Action and inaction in multi-behaviour recommendations: A meta-analysis of lifestyle interventions. *Health Psychology Review*, 1–24. https://doi.org/10.1080/17437199.2017.1369140

Albarracín, D., & Wyer, R. S. (2001). Elaborative and nonelaborative processing of a behavior-related communication. *Personality and Social Psychology Bulletin, 27*(6), 691–705. https://doi.org/10.1177/0146167201276005

Allison, S. T., & Messick, D. M. (1988). The feature-positive effect, attitude strength, and degree of perceived consensus. *Personality and Social Psychology Bulletin*. https://doi.org/10.1177/0146167288142002

Anderson, N. H. (1971). Integration theory and attitude change. *Psychological Review, 78*(3), 171–206. https://doi.org/10.1037/h0021465

Armitage, C. J., & Conner, M. (2001). Efficacy of the theory of planned behaviour: A meta-analytic review. *British Journal of Social Psychology, 40*(4), 471–499. https://doi.org/10.1348/014466601164939

Aronson, E., & Mills, J. (1959). The effect of severity of initiation on liking for a group. *The Journal of Abnormal and Social Psychology, 59*(2), 177.

Atkinson, J. W. (1964). *An introduction to motivation* (Vol. 9). Princeton, NJ: Van Nostrand.
Averbeck, J. M., Jones, A., & Robertson, K. (2011). Prior knowledge and health messages: An examination of affect as heuristics and information as systematic processing for fear appeals. *Southern Communication Journal, 76*(1), 35–54. https://doi.org/10.1080/10417940902951824
Bandura, A. (1986). *Social foundations of thought and action: A social cognitive theory, Prentice-Hall series in social learning theory* (Vol. 1). Englewood Cliffs, NJ: Prentice Hall.
Bandura, A. (1997). *Self-efficacy: The exercise of control*. New York, NY: Macmillan.
Bandura, A., & Wood, R. (1989). Effect of perceived controllability and performance standards on self-regulation of complex decision making. *Journal of Personality and Social Psychology, 56*(5), 805–814. https://doi.org/10.1037/0022-3514.56.5.805
Bargh, J. A., Chen, M., & Burrows, L. (1996). Automaticity of social behavior: Direct effects of trait construct and stereotype activation on action. *Journal of Personality and Social Psychology, 71*(2), 230–244. https://doi.org/10.1037/0022-3514.71.2.230
Baron, J., & Ritov, I. (2004). Omission bias, individual differences, and normality. *Organizational Behavior and Human Decision Processes*. https://doi.org/10.1016/j.obhdp.2004.03.003
Becker, B. J. (1988). Synthesizing standardized mean change measures. *British Journal of Mathematical and Statistical Psychology, 41*, 257–278. https://doi.org/10.1111/j.2044-8317.1988.tb00901.x
Berkman, E. T., Burklund, L., & Lieberman, M. D. (2009). Inhibitory spillover: Intentional motor inhibition produces incidental limbic inhibition via right inferior frontal cortex. *NeuroImage, 47*(2), 705–712. https://doi.org/10.1016/j.neuroimage.2009.04.084
Brehm, J. W. (1966). *A theory of psychological reactance*. New York, NY: Academic Press. https://doi.org/10.1002/hrdq.20027
Brehm, J. W., & Self, E. A. (1989). The intensity of motivation. *Annual Review of Psychology, 40*(1), 109–131. https://doi.org/10.1146/annurev.ps.40.020189.000545
Chan, M. S., Jones, C. R., & Albarracín, D. (2017). Countering false beliefs: An analysis of the evidence and recommendations of best practices for the retraction and correction of scientific misinformation. In *Handbook of the science of science communication*. https://doi.org/10.1093/oxfordhb/9780190497620.013.37
Cheung, S.-F., & Chan, D. K.-S. (2000). *The role of perceived behavioral control in predicting human behavior: A meta-analytic review of studies on the theory of planned behavior*. Unpublished manuscript, Chinese University of Hong Kong.
Cioffi, D., & Garner, R. (1996). On doing the decision: Effects of active versus passive choice on commitment and self-perception. *Personality & Social Psychology Bulletin, 22*, 133–147.
Conner, M., & Higgins, A. R. (2010). Long-term effects of implementation intentions on prevention of smoking uptake among adolescents: A cluster randomized controlled trial. *Health Psychology, 29*(5), 529–538. https://doi.org/10.1037/a0020317
Cornwell, J. F. M., Franks, B., & Higgins, E. T. (2014). Truth, control, and value motivations: The "what" "how" and "why" of approach and avoidance. *Frontiers in Systems Neuroscience, 8*. https://doi.org/10.3389/fnsys.2014.00194
Dai, W., & Albarracín, D. (2017). *Action and inaction content in message*. Unpublished raw data, University of Illinois Urbana Champaign.
Dillard, J. P., Plotnick, C. A., Godbold, L. C., Freimuth, V. S., & Edgar, T. (1996). The multiple affective outcomes of AIDS PSAs: Fear appeals do more than scare people. *Communication Research, 23*(1), 44–72. https://doi.org/10.1177/009365096023001002
Dittrich, W. H., & Lea, S. E. (1993). Motion as a natural category for pigeons: Generalization and a feature-positive effect. *Journal of the Experimental Analysis of Behavior*. https://doi.org/10.1901/jeab.1993.59-115
Doyen, S., Klein, O., Pichon, C. L., & Cleeremans, A. (2012). Behavioral priming: It's all in the mind, but whose mind? *PLoS One, 7*(1). https://doi.org/10.1371/journal.pone.0029081
Eitam, B., Kennedy, P. M., & Higgins, E. T. (2013). Motivation from control. *Experimental Brain Research, 229*(3), 475–484. https://doi.org/10.1007/s00221-012-3370-7
Fazio, R. H., Sherman, S. J., & Herr, P. M. (1982). The feature-positive effect in the self-perception process: Does not doing matter as much as doing? *Journal of Personality and Social Psychology*. https://doi.org/10.1037/0022-3514.42.3.404

Feldman, G., & Albarracín, D. (2017). Norm theory and the action-effect: The role of social norms in regret following action and inaction. *Journal of Experimental Social Psychology*. https://doi.org/10.1016/j.jesp.2016.07.009

Ferguson, M. J., & Bargh, J. A. (2008). Evaluative readiness: The motivational nature of automatic evaluation. In A. J. Elliot (Ed.), *Handbook of approach and avoidance motivation* (pp. 289–306). New York, NY: Psychology Press. https://doi.org/10.4324/9780203888148.ch17

Fishbein, M. (1963). An investigation of the relationships between beliefs about an object and the attitude toward that object. *Human Relations, 16*(3), 233–239. https://doi.org/10.1177/001872676301600302

Fishbein, M. (2000). The role of theory in HIV prevention. *AIDS Care, 12*(3), 273–278. https://doi.org/10.1080/09540120050042918

Fishbein, M. (2008). A reasoned action approach to health promotion. *Medical Decision Making, 28*(6), 834–844. https://doi.org/10.1177/0272989X08326092

Fishbein, M., & Ajzen, I. (2010). *Predicting and changing behaviour: The reasoned action approach*. New York, NY: Psychology Press. https://doi.org/10.4324/9780203937082

Fisher, J. D., & Fisher, W. A. (1992). Changing AIDS-risk behavior. *Psychological Bulletin, 111*(3), 455–474. https://doi.org/10.1037/0033-2909.111.3.455

Forgas, J. P., & Bower, G. H. (1987). Mood effects on person-perception judgments. *Journal of Personality and Social Psychology, 53*(1), 53–60. https://doi.org/10.1037/0022-3514.53.1.53

Franks, B., & Tory Higgins, E. (2012). Effectiveness in humans and other animals. A common basis for well-being and welfare. *Advances in Experimental Social Psychology*. https://doi.org/10.1016/B978-0-12-394281-4.00006-4

Garcia-Retamero, R., & Galesic, M. (2009). Communicating treatment risk reduction to people with low numeracy skills: A cross-cultural comparison. *American Journal of Public Health, 99*(12), 2196–2202. https://doi.org/10.2105/AJPH.2009.160234

Gasper, K., & Clore, G. L. (2000). Do you have to pay attention to your feelings to be influenced by them? *Personality and Social Psychology Bulletin, 26*(6), 698–711. https://doi.org/10.1177/0146167200268005

Gendolla, G. H. E., & Silvestrini, N. (2010). The implicit "go": Masked action cues directly mobilize mental effort. *Psychological Science*. https://doi.org/10.1177/0956797610384149

Harris, C. R., Coburn, N., Rohrer, D., & Pashler, H. (2013). Two failures to replicate high-performance-goal priming effects. *PLoS One, 8*(8). https://doi.org/10.1371/journal.pone.0072467

Hart, W., & Albarracín, D. (2009). The effects of chronic achievement motivation and achievement primes on the activation of achievement and fun goals. *Journal of Personality and Social Psychology, 97*, 1129–1141.

Hepler, J., Albarracín, D., McCulloch, K. C., & Noguchi, K. (2012). Being active and impulsive: The role of goals for action and inaction in self-control. *Motivation and Emotion*. https://doi.org/10.1007/s11031-011-9263-4

Higgins, E. T. (2012). Motivation science in social psychology: A tale of two histories. In A. W. Kruglanski & W. Stroebe (Eds.), *Handbook of the history of social psychology* (pp. 199–218). New York, NY: Psychology Press.

Ireland, M. E., Hepler, J., & Albarracín, D. (2013). Unpublished data, University of Illinois at Urbana Champaign.

Ireland, M. E., Hepler, J., Li, H., & Albarracín, D. (2015). Neuroticism and attitudes toward action in 19 countries. *Journal of Personality*. https://doi.org/10.1111/jopy.12099

Jennings, J. R., & Van Der Molen, M. W. (2005). Preparation for speeded action as a psychophysiological concept. *Psychological Bulletin, 131*(3), 434–459. https://doi.org/10.1037/0033-2909.131.3.434

Kahneman, D., & Miller, D. T. (1986). Norm theory: Comparing reality to its alternatives. *Psychological Review*. https://doi.org/10.1037/0033-295X.93.2.136

Kahneman, D., & Tversky, A. (1982). The psychology of preferences. *Scientific American, 246*(1), 160–173. https://doi.org/10.1038/scientificamerican0182-160

Koning, I. M., van den Eijnden, R. J. J. M., Verdurmen, J. E. E., Engels, R. C. M. E., & Vollebergh, W. A. M. (2013). A cluster randomized trial on the effects of a parent and student intervention on alcohol use in adolescents four years after baseline; no evidence of catching-up behavior. *Addictive Behaviors, 38*(4), 2032–2039. https://doi.org/10.1016/j.addbeh.2012.12.013

Landman, J. (1987). Regret and elation following action and inaction: Affective responses to positive versus negative outcomes. *Personality and Social Psychology Bulletin.* https://doi.org/10.1177/0146167287134009

Madden, T. J., Ellen, P. S., & Ajzen, I. (1992). A comparison of the theory of planned behavior and the theory of reasoned action. *Personality and Social Psychology Bulletin, 18*(1), 3–9. https://doi.org/10.1177/0146167292181001

Maddux, J. E., & Rogers, R. W. (1983). Protection motivation and self-efficacy: A revised theory of fear appeals and attitude change. *Journal of Experimental Social Psychology, 19*(5), 469–479. https://doi.org/10.1016/0022-1031(83)90023-9

McCulloch, K. C., Li, H., Hong, S., & Albarracín, D. (2012). Naïve definitions of action and inaction: The continuum, spread, and valence of behaviors. *European Journal of Social Psychology.* https://doi.org/10.1002/ejsp.860

Miller, M. J., Woehr, D. J., & Hudspeth, N. (2002). The meaning and measurement of work ethic: Construction and initial validation of a multidimensional inventory. *Journal of Vocational Behavior, 60*(3), 451–489. https://doi.org/10.1006/jvbe.2001.1838

Minas, R. K., Poor, M., Dennis, A. R., & Bartelt, V. L. (2016). A prime a day keeps calories away: The effects of supraliminal priming on food consumption and the moderating role of gender and eating restraint. *Appetite, 105*, 494–499. https://doi.org/10.1016/j.appet.2016.05.022

Noguchi, K., Handley, I. M., & Albarracín, D. (2011). Participating in politics resembles physical activity: General action patterns in international archives, United States archives, and experiments. *Psychological Science.* https://doi.org/10.1177/0956797610393746

Norton, M. I., Mochon, D., & Ariely, D. (2012). The IKEA effect: When labor leads to love. *Journal of Consumer Psychology, 22*(3), 453–460. https://doi.org/10.1016/j.jcps.2011.08.002

Peters, E., Dieckmann, N., Dixon, A., Hibbard, J. H., & Mertz, C. K. (2007). Less is more in presenting quality information to consumers. *Medical Care Research and Review, 64*(2), 169–190. https://doi.org/10.1177/10775587070640020301

Pham, M. T. (1998). Representativeness, relevance, and the use of feelings in decision making. *Journal of Consumer Research, 25*(2), 144–159. https://doi.org/10.1086/209532

Ryan, J. J. (2002). Work values and organizational citizenship behaviors: Values that work for employees and organizations. *Journal of Business and Psychology, 17*(1), 123–132. https://doi.org/10.1023/A:1016246103190

Schwarz, N., & Clore, G. L. (1983). Mood, misattribution, and judgments of well-being: Informative and directive functions of affective states. *Journal of Personality and Social Psychology, 45*(3), 513–523. https://doi.org/10.1037/0022-3514.45.3.513

Schwarz, N., & Clore, G. L. (2007). Feelings and phenomenal experiences. In *Social psychology: Handbook of basic principles* (pp. 385–407). https://doi.org/10.1023/A:1021223113233

Sheridan, S. L., Halpern, D. J., Viera, A. J., Berkman, N. D., Donahue, K. E., & Crotty, K. (2011). Interventions for individuals with low health literacy: A systematic review. *Journal of Health Communication, 16*, 30–54. https://doi.org/10.1080/10810730.2011.604391

Strahan, E. J., Spencer, S. J., & Zanna, M. P. (2002). Subliminal priming and persuasion: Striking while the iron is hot. *Journal of Experimental Social Psychology, 38*(6), 556–568. https://doi.org/10.1016/S0022-1031(02)00502-4

Sunderrajan, A., & Albarracín, D. (2018). *Perceived intentionality and evaluations of mundane commissions and omissions* (Submitted for publication).

Tait, A. R., Voepel-Lewis, T., Zikmund-Fisher, B. J., & Fagerlin, A. (2010). Presenting research risks and benefits to parents: Does format matter? *Anesthesia and Analgesia, 111*(3), 718–723. https://doi.org/10.1213/ANE.0b013e3181e8570a

Tait, R. J., Hulse, G. K., Waterreus, A., Flicker, L., Lautenschlager, N. T., Jamrozik, K., & Almeida, O. P. (2007). Effectiveness of a smoking cessation intervention in older adults. *Addiction (Abingdon, England), 102*, 148–155. https://doi.org/10.1111/j.1360-0443.2006.01647.x

Tannenbaum, M. B., Hepler, J., Zimmerman, R. S., Saul, L., Jacobs, S., Wilson, K., & Albarracín, D. (2015). Appealing to fear: A meta-analysis of fear appeal effectiveness and theories. *Psychological Bulletin, 141*(6), 1178–1204. https://doi.org/10.1037/a0039729

Tuk, M. A., Zhang, K., & Sweldens, S. (2015). The propagation of self-control: Self-control in one domain simultaneously improves self-control in other domains. *Journal of Experimental Psychology: General, 144*(3), 639–654. https://doi.org/10.1037/xge0000065

Wallston, K. A., Wallston, B. S., Smith, S., & Dobbins, C. J. (1987). Perceived control and health. *Current Psychological Research & Reviews, 6*(1), 5–25. https://doi.org/10.1007/BF02686633

Weingarten, E., Chen, Q., McAdams, M., Yi, J., Hepler, J., & Albarracín, D. (2016). From primed concepts to action: A meta-analysis of the behavioral effects of incidentally presented words. *Psychological Bulletin, 142*(5), 472–497. https://doi.org/10.1037/bul0000030

Wilson, K., Senay, I., Durantini, M., Sánchez, F., Hennessy, M., Spring, B., & Albarracín, D. (2015). When it comes to lifestyle recommendations, more is sometimes less: A meta-analysis of theoretical assumptions underlying the effectiveness of interventions promoting multiple behavior domain change. *Psychological Bulletin, 141*(2), 474–509. https://doi.org/10.1037/a0038295

Wyer, R. S. (1970). Quantitative prediction of belief and opinion change: A further test of a subjective probability model. *Journal of Personality and Social Psychology, 16*(4), 559–570. https://doi.org/10.1037/h0030064

Zell, E., Su, R., Li, H., Ho, M. H. R., Hong, S., Kumkale, T., … Albarracín, D. (2013). Cultural differences in attitudes toward action and inaction: The role of dialecticism. *Social Psychological and Personality Science, 4*(5), 521–528. https://doi.org/10.1177/1948550612468774

Zhou, Z., Yu, R., & Zhou, X. (2010). To do or not to do? Action enlarges the FRN and P300 effects in outcome evaluation. *Neuropsychologia*. https://doi.org/10.1016/j.neuropsychologia.2010.08.010

Chapter 4
Change and Maintaining Change in School Cafeterias: Economic and Behavioral-Economic Approaches to Increasing Fruit and Vegetable Consumption

Gregory J. Madden, Joseph Price, and Heidi Wengreen

Introduction

There are indisputable health benefits of a diet rich in fruits and vegetables (FV). They are high in water and have a high nutrient-to-calorie ratio, thereby providing important vitamins, minerals, fiber, and phytochemicals important to human health (Darmon, Darmon, Maillot, & Drewnowski, 2005). Phytochemicals such as carotenoids, polyphenols, and flavonoids are noteworthy as antioxidants and anti-inflammatory agents contributing to health. Diets rich in fruits and vegetables are associated with reduced risk of chronic health conditions and mortality from all causes (Ovesen, 2005). For example, an additional serving of FV consumed per day is associated with a 5% reduced risk of mortality (Wang et al., 2014). Higher intakes of a *variety* of FVs is important in lowering the risk of cardiovascular disease (Dauchet, Amouyel, Hercberg, & Dallongeville, 2006; Hu, Huang, Wang, Zhang, & Qu, 2014; Savica, Bellinghieri, & Kopple, 2010), asthma (Hosseini, Berthon, Wark, & Wood, 2017), and cognitive decline in the elderly (Jiang et al., 2017).

The contribution of FV consumption to obesity is more difficult to evaluate. The cause of obesity is multifactorial and FV consumption is often confounded with behaviors that impact body weight (e.g., physical activity; Grosso et al., 2017; Hobbs, Pearson, Foster, & Biddle, 2014). Most, but not all, studies of adults reveal an inverse association between FV consumption and either being overweight or

G. J. Madden (✉)
Department of Psychology, Utah State University, Logan, UT, USA
e-mail: greg.madden@usu.edu

J. Price
Department of Economics, Brigham Young University, Provo, UT, USA

H. Wengreen
Department of Nutrition Dietetics and Food Science, Utah State University, Logan, UT, USA

D. A. Hope, R. A. Bevins (eds.), *Change and Maintaining Change*, Nebraska Symposium on Motivation 65, https://doi.org/10.1007/978-3-319-96920-6_4

gaining weight over time (Ledoux, Hingle, & Baranowski, 2011). However, simply eating more FV will not reduce weight (Fulton, McKinley, Young, Cardwell, & Woodside, 2016); FV consumption must *displace* consumption of other foods to achieve an energy deficit (Mytton, Nnoaham, Eyles, Scarborough, & Mhurchu, 2014; Smith-Warner et al., 2000). The high fiber and water content of FV can produce satiety supporting that energy-deficit goal. Experimental trials manipulating FV intake without changing other dietary behaviors are rare (Whigham et al., 2012). In an exception to this rule, Tapsell et al. (2014) randomized overweight adults to energy-deficit groups who either consumed standard or double-sized portions of vegetables. Weight loss was positively correlated with proportion of energy consumed as vegetables; supporting the position that the satiety induced by FV consumption helps to displace the intake of higher-energy foods and leads to weight loss (Newby, 2009).

The same general patterns appear to be true of children, although less empirical evidence is available. Overweight children and adolescents consume less fruit and more french fries than normal-weight children (Lorson, Melgar-Quinonez, & Taylor, 2009). Early childhood patterns of eating FV appear to be important. For example, children who consumed few FV in early childhood were more likely to be severely or morbidly overweight in later childhood than were their peers who often consumed FV from an early age (Fletcher, Wright, Jones, Parkinson, & Adamson, 2017). However, what is true of adults is also true for children—if FV intake is to reduce the risk of obesity, these foods must displace consumption of energy-dense nutrient-poor foods (Looney & Raynor, 2012).

In sum, there are many life span health benefits to motivate policy makers to explore ways to increase children's FV consumption. Additional motivation is provided by longitudinal studies, which suggest eating habits developed in childhood continue into adolescence (Lytle, Seifert, Greenstein, & McGovern, 2000) and beyond (Freedman, Khan, Dietz, Srinivasan, & Berenson, 2001). Therefore, effective interventions designed to increase habitual FV consumption in children can impact public health for decades to come.

Unfortunately, few US children consume the USDA-recommended five or more servings of FV each day (Coulthard & Blissett, 2009; Kim et al., 2014). Recent National Health and Nutrition Examination Surveys suggest US children consume less than half of the recommended amount of vegetables, and this number is even lower when white potatoes were excluded (Kim et al., 2014; Storey & Anderson, 2016). Rendering the picture more-dire is the possibility that parents and children over-estimate their FV consumption in these surveys (cf. Brug & Van Assema, 2001).

Elementary schools are an ideal setting in which to begin addressing this behavioral deficit impacting public health. Over 30 million US children eat school-provided lunch (USDA, 2016) and National School Lunch Program (NSLP) guidelines require that FV be available as part of reimbursable meals in the school, every day. Thus, the minimum requirements are in place for behavior change—large numbers of children with frequent low- or no-cost access to FV. At present, however, most children who participate in the NSLP under-consume these foods (Cullen & Dave, 2017).

This chapter begins by evaluating the naturally occurring economic factors that have conspired to reduce FV consumption among US children. In response to these factors, the National School Lunch Program recently redesigned public-school lunches. Larger portions and a greater variety of FV are now on the menu. Below, we survey the limited evidence evaluating the efficacy of this policy change. The remainder of the chapter provides a non-comprehensive survey of studies using traditional-economic (e.g., price changes) or behavioral-economic (e.g., defaults) strategies to positively influence healthy eating in elementary schools. We conclude with policy recommendations supported by the studies reviewed.

Change vs. Believable Change

Because the studies appearing in this chapter were reviewed with policy recommendations in mind, our inclusion criteria were stricter than is the norm. Studies exclusively using self-report measures are not reviewed because of the likelihood of social desirability bias; i.e., a tendency to stretch the truth about our actions in order to make it appear that we conform to, or exceed social norms (Eckmanns, Bessert, Behnke, Gastmeier, & Rüden, 2006; Nichols & Maner, 2008; Orne, 1962). Just as people tend to under-report their energy and fat intake (Archer, Hand, & Blair, 2013; Heitmann, Lissner, & Osler, 2000) and over-report their physical activity and healthy-eating episodes (Nix & Wengreen, 2017; Shuval et al., 2015), parents and children may over-report how many FVs they consume each day. While some self-report measures may be validated against directly observed levels of consumption (e.g., Lytle et al., 1993), these validations are not established in the context of intervention research, where children are exposed to the intervention and inherent demand characteristics can induce prevarication in a direction that exaggerates the intervention effect. We agree with Archer, Pavela, and Lavie (2015) that basing policy advice on potentially biased self-report data is ill advised.

Our review also avoids studies in which obvious demand characteristics might be expected to increase healthy eating. For example, demand characteristics may exist when a teacher, or other adult, administers the intervention and then obtrusively measures the child's behavior. In such cases, it may be clear to the child what the adult wants (eat your FV), and the child may feel compelled to comply with the authority figure's apparent wishes (Eckmanns et al., 2006). Those familiar with the Stanley Milgram experiments[1] will recall how demand characteristics can increase conformity to the expectation of an authority figure.

The present review also favored studies that measured FV more than once or twice because the health benefits of this behavior can only be realized if it becomes

[1] In Milgram's experiments, adult participants were led to believe they were administering electric shocks to a "learner" when he made errors. Most participants complied with the experimenter's expectation that shocks be administered, and many administered what they believed to be potentially lethal shocks.

a temporally extended pattern of behavior. Finally, we preferred studies that used objective measures of FV consumption (e.g., weights of plate waste). Taking FV from the cafeteria line is important, but if these foods are not consumed, then this benefits the farming industry, but not public health. Where objective measurement was impossible (e.g., human observers were used to record what children consumed), we favored studies that evaluated and established good (>85%) inter-observer agreement scores. Doing so reduces the probability of experimenter expectancies biasing the data collected, particularly when human observers are not blinded to the study design.

Economic Factors Influencing FV Consumption

A core microeconomic principle is the law of demand: All else being equal, as the price of a commodity increases its consumption will decline. We are all familiar with this law when applied to gasoline. As the price increases, we drive a little slower, make a few less discretionary trips, and carpool more often. The demand law is well established under controlled laboratory condition both with humans and nonhuman animals (Bickel & Madden, 1999; Kagel, Battalio, & Green, 1995).

When applied to food, the law of demand predicts that if the price of FV increases, its consumption will decline. And, indeed, since 1980 the inflation adjusted price of FVs has risen (Monsivais & Drewnowski, 2007). The decline in FV consumption predicted by this price increase is compounded by a concurrent decrease in the price of unhealthy foods (Wright & Aronne, 2012). Because unhealthy foods can substitute for the satiety-producing effects of eating FV, this increase in the *relative* price of FV is expected to produce a large decrease in FV consumption (Madden, 2000).

As FV prices were increasing and processed food decreasing, there were other economic factors influencing FV consumption. As more women entered the workforce, home-cooked meals declined in frequency, often replaced by prepared foods (e.g., TV dinners) and eating out in restaurants (Nicklas et al., 2004). These alternatives to the home-cooked meal are much less likely to include FVs (Boutelle, Fulkerson, Neumark-Sztainer, Story, & French, 2007). To overcome the concerns of parents about the well-being of their children, restaurants and prepared food producers prolifically advertised (Story & French, 2004) highlighting their convenience, taste, and establishing the appearance of a new social norm for the family meal.

Changes in price may help explain why children consume fewer FVs at home, but it does not explain why they eat so few FVs at school. Nearly all low-income children in the USA have access to free FVs as part of their school-provided meals. Even for children whose parent pay for school lunch, the price of the lunch is a non-factor in the child's decision to eat the FVs—since the child did not pay for the FVs, the monetary price is irrelevant. Instead, relative *non-monetary* price factors are important. That is, if foods are available that are better tasting, more attractively packaged, or easier to eat, then they are more competitive in the marketplace of children's dietary decision-making. Support for this comes from schools in which unhealthy foods are available in the cafeteria or in vending machines. These are the schools at which FV consumption tends to be lowest (Kubik, Lytle, Hannan, Perry, & Story, 2003). In sum, price, relative price, and the availability of more convenient, better promoted, and better tasting alternatives to FV have combined to reduce children's consumption of these healthy foods at home and at school.

Impact of Changes to the US National School Lunch Program

The National School Lunch program (NSLP) seeks to address this deficit in FV consumption by creating a food oasis in which healthy foods are available for the millions of children who take lunch in school cafeterias. Schools participating in the NSLP receive cash subsidies and commodity foods from the USDA if they offer lunch to all children, provide free or reduced-price lunch to eligible children, and serve meals that meet specific nutritional requirements. These requirements were updated in 2010 under the Healthy, Hunger-Free Kids Act (USDA, 2012). The legislation better aligned what was served in schools with the recommendations found in the Dietary Guidelines for Americans (Health.gov, 2010).

Under the Act, school lunches were redesigned to include more whole grains, a wider variety of FV, larger portions of FV, less saturated fat, gradually reduced sodium levels, and meal sizes that met age-specific calorie limits. With respect to FV, schools were to serve students a minimum of 0.5 cup of fruit and 0.75–1 cup of vegetables each day; more than doubling the FV offered prior to the Act. The most salient initial effect of the policy change was an increase in the amount of FVs that were thrown away rather than consumed. This garnered the policy change some rather bad press (e.g., Watanabe, 2014). Concerns about the increased cost of providing school lunches that were being thrown away led, in 2015, to implementation of the USDA's "Offer vs. Serve" policy (USDA, 2013). Under this amendment to the Act, children must select a serving of fruit, vegetable, *or* a mix of the two.

The impact of these policy changes is not yet well established. In an experimental study conducted before the roll-out of the Act, when children were served larger portions of FV each day, the fraction of children eating FVs increased by 20%, but there was also a dramatic increase in food waste (Just & Price, 2013a; see also Byker, Farris, Marcenelle, Davis, & Serrano, 2014). Because of the latter, the schools had to spend an additional $1.72 in food costs to encourage one additional child to eat one additional serving for 1 day, thus making the approach less cost-effective than other approaches.

Since the roll-out of the new school lunches there have been only four peer-reviewed studies evaluating its effect. The studies paint a mixed picture (see review by Cullen & Dave, 2017). Where some studies reported an increase in one category of fruit (e.g., diced fruit cups served with juice) no study reported an increase in total fruit consumption. The effects of the policy change on vegetable consumption have also been mixed. Some studies report an increase in total vegetable consumption

(Cohen, Richardson, Parker, Catalano, & Rimm, 2014; Schwartz, Henderson, Read, Danna, & Ickovics, 2015 but inconsistently across years in the latter study), where others report no change (Cullen, Chen, & Dave, 2015) or a decrease in vegetable consumption (Amin, Yon, Taylor, & Johnson, 2015).

Thus far, no studies have examined FV consumption after the "Offer vs. Serve" policy was implemented. Anecdotal observations of children in the cafeterias in which we have worked suggest the policy change has dramatically decreased the number of children taking vegetables; indeed, some schools have liberally interpreted the guideline to mean that all children are served fruit, with vegetables available for those who request a serving. These findings suggest additional measures will be needed to increase FV consumption to the levels needed to positively impact public health.

Education and Messaging

From a classical economics perspective, if perfect knowledge of the costs and benefits of an action are known, the rational decision-maker will optimize his behavior (Rice, Hanoch, & Barnes, 2017). This perspective underlies public-information campaigns which assume consumers make suboptimal menu choices because they are not fully aware of the health benefits of adhering to the Dietary Guidelines for Americans. From this perspective, children given more perfect knowledge of the health benefits of eating FV should consume more of these foods.

From a behavioral-economic perspective, however, nutrition-education interventions are likely to have limited effects because they point to utilitarian benefits that are of little interest to a present-biased consumer. To unpack this position, consider what are the consequences experienced by a child who is convinced to take a bite of vegetables. As these foods are often disliked (e.g., Brug, Tak, te Vedle, Bere, & de Bourdeaudhuji, 2008; Cooke & Wardle, 2005), the immediate consequence is an aversive taste and an unfamiliar food texture in the mouth (Lautenschlager & Smith, 2007). These consequences were not mentioned in Health class, but they are immediate and highly salient when FV are consumed. Thus, the immediate consequences of tasting vegetables are often negative.

The benefits of FV consumption most often discussed in Health classes are to be experienced in the distant future, probabilistically, and only if a consistent pattern of FV consumption occurs. Because children steeply discount the value of delayed consequences (Green, Myerson, Lichtman, Rosen, & Fry, 1996; Read & Read, 2004), these promised outcomes will be nearly valueless, and will factor little into their dietary decision-making. Instead, consistent with decades of research on choice between substitutable commodities (e.g., Herrnstein, 1970; Madden & Perone, 1999), the *immediate* relative consequences of eating healthy and unhealthy foods (i.e., their tastes and textures) will play a dominant role. Again, this is a difficult marketplace in which to compete. Where the taste and texture of vegetables are often disliked, the competition foods have been engineered for taste, texture, and ease of consumption (e.g., Zampini & Spence, 2004).

Although education may be the most common component of school-based interventions, very little objective data are available to evaluate if this strategy increases FV consumption. The vast majority of education-based interventions evaluate only self-reported FV consumption. Those that objectively measure consumption typically implement multi-component interventions that make it impossible to evaluate the unique contribution of education to positive outcomes (e.g., Perry et al., 1998, 2004). Two exceptions are the education-alone interventions evaluated by Wardle et al. (2003) and Auld, Romaniello, Heimendinger, Hambidge, and Hambidge (1999). The former arranged very brief educational opportunities and found no positive impact on FV intake. The latter provided more substantive education opportunities. This approach did not increase FV consumption above baseline levels, but it appeared to protect children against the declines in consumption observed in control schools. Beyond these two studies, we identified only one education-based multi-component study that objectively measured FV consumption and did not either incentivize this behavior (incentives are known to positively influence FV consumption, see below) or arrange a school garden. Despite substantial amounts of nutrition education, Reynolds et al. (2000) found no increase in objectively measured FV consumption; although self-reported intake increased (see Beccarelli et al. (2016) for comparable results).

Education-based interventions that include school gardening opportunities also rarely objectively measure FV intake, but when they do include such measures the outcomes are mixed. Three studies revealed no positive effect of school gardens on objectively measured FV consumption (Christian, Evans, Nykjaer, Hancock, & Cade, 2014; Ratcliffe, Merrigan, Rogers, & Goldberg, 2011; Wright & Rowell, 2010) and one reported a significant decrease in skin carotenoid levels (a biomarker of carotenoid-containing FV consumption; Beccarelli et al., 2016). Where a fifth study showed more promising outcomes (Parmer, Salisbury-Glennon, Shannon, & Struempler, 2009), the direct-observation methodology was open to experimenter bias.[2]

An alternative approach to education is motivational point-of-purchase messaging such as signs or videos in the cafeteria. These messages are designed to highlight the benefits of eating FV, and to do it in a way that children will find entertaining. For example, Wansink, Just, Payne, and Klinger (2012) used such fun messaging when they labeled carrots as "X-ray vision carrots." This small change produced a 66% increase in the fraction of children choosing carrots from the cafeteria line. However, a longer-term evaluation of the labeling reported somewhat smaller increases in taking (20%), suggesting perhaps that some children were dissatisfied

[2] Children were allowed to take as many FV as they wanted from the cafeteria line. The observer, who was not blind to study design, did not record the amount taken as children exited the cafeteria line (only whether some FV were taken). After lunch, the observer estimated if half or more of the FV were consumed; but without a measure of the amount taken, there was no way to estimate this fraction (Sondra Parmer, personal communication, July 13, 2016).

with the actual vision-enhancing effects of the carrots (Wansink, Just, & Smith, 2011). The Wansink lab has been accused of scientific misconduct, so these outcomes should be viewed skeptically. In another study, pictures of vegetable superheroes were featured on the school salad bar and/or a nearby video display, along with the "super powers" that each vegetable promotes (Hanks, Just, & Brumberg, 2016). While the combination of these messages more than doubled the fraction of children taking vegetables, this and the Wansink et al. studies are limited in that vegetable *consumption* was not reported. Given the low-cost and potential impact of these interventions, it will be important for future studies to measure FV consumption, lest programs that further increase FV waste be disseminated.

Another point-of-purchase approach omits health-benefit messaging, but instead simply prompts children to take a serving of FV from the cafeteria line. In a study conducted before the NSLP revisions, asking every child if he/she would like a serving of fruit increased its consumption by 86% (Schwartz, 2007). This finding is interesting in light of the above-referenced reports that fruit consumption has not increased under the revised NSLP. Perhaps children are more likely to consume a freely chosen food than a food placed on their tray by mandate. Now that the USDA "Offer vs. Serve" policy is in place, the replicability of the Schwartz finding should be evaluated, as should the efficacy of prompting children to take vegetables as they move through the cafeteria line. If increased consumption proves robust with fruit and vegetable prompts, it would be an effective no-cost intervention that could be widely disseminated in schools.

A promising choice-preserving nonverbal-prompt is to embed a picture of vegetables in one of the compartments of children's lunch trays. This conveys the message that this area of the tray is for vegetables, which may simultaneously displace other, less healthy, foods from being placed in that area of the tray. One study implementing this approach found that it increased vegetable consumption by about 4 g (Reicks, Redden, Mann, Mykerezi, & Vickers, 2012). While this is a modest increase (about half a baby carrot), it suggests a low-cost intervention that may enhance the beneficial effects of other, concurrently deployed interventions designed to increase healthy eating in schools.

Another mechanism that may underlie the impact of prompts is social norms; i.e., the tendency to behave in accord with the actions of others in the in-group (Bikhchandani, Hirshleifer, & Welch, 1992). These effects are particularly salient when children observe high-status peers participating in the activity. Applied to FV consumption, one study enlisted the help of four slightly older peers in a laboratory setting and randomized the reaction of these older peers when tasting a new food (Greenhalgh et al., 2009). Children observing a positive reaction in these peers were more likely to consume the new food themselves, while children observing a negative reaction to the novel food were more likely to refuse it; both of these effects proved to be long-lasting. These results suggest an important target for FV interventions: If FV consumption can be increased among the older children attending the school (e.g., fourth and fifth graders), younger children may be more likely to adhere to this social norm.

Variety, Substitutes, and Defaults

Some evidence suggests that children will consume more FV if they are offered a wider variety of these foods from which they can choose (Adams, Pelletier, Zive, & Sallis, 2005). Children vary in which specific FVs they enjoy or are willing to eat, so when more options are available there is, in theory, an increased probability of consumption. Increasing the variety of FVs offered also increases the possibility of benefitting from a complementary relation between two of these foods. For example, children may be more likely to consume broccoli if served with lettuce, as consuming them together (in a salad) simultaneously reduces the bitter taste of the broccoli and improves the crunchiness of the lettuce. One study reported that providing a larger variety of FV during lunch increased consumption of fruit by 28% and vegetables by 19% (Hakim & Meissen, 2013). Another found that each additional FV option offered increased the fraction of children eating at least one serving of fruits or vegetables by 12% (Just, Lund, & Price, 2012). Most of this increase was fruit consumption, with some evidence suggesting that offering more fruit options decreased vegetable consumption.

This displacement of consumption of a less preferred food (vegetables) by a more preferred food (fruit) is, again, in accord with decades old quantitative models of choice between substitutable goods (Herrnstein, 1970). When different goods serve the same function, they can substitute for one another. Children raised in homes that rarely serve unhealthy foods consume more FV than those in which substitutes are readily available (Ong, Ullah, Magarey, Miller, & Leslie, 2017). Thus, an economic-inspired approach to increasing vegetable consumption at school is to serve these foods without concurrent competitor foods. For example, USDA's Fresh Fruit and Vegetable Program provides FVs in the classroom prior to lunch as a mid-morning snack. Children generally consume these foods in the classroom (e.g., Jamelske & Bica, 2014) but positive effects on total at-school consumption of FV are less clearly established (Huang et al., 2013).

A similar strategy, and one that takes no classroom time away from academics, is to serve vegetables as a first course, before serving other foods in the cafeteria. In one study, this doubled the consumption of vegetables (Spill, Birch, Roe, & Rolls, 2010) and similarly impressive increases have been observed when raw vegetables are made available to children while waiting in the cafeteria line for their meal (Elsbernd et al., 2016; Redden et al., 2015). A similar tactic is to serve fruit as dessert, after the main course. When Zellner and Cobuzzi (2016) piloted this technique in a 2-day pre-post comparison study, the percentage of children consuming all of their kale salad increased by 175% relative to pre-intervention levels. In addition, where 40% of children consumed no kale salad when fruit was served with the meal, all children took at least one bite of the salad when fruit was provided as dessert.

Behavioral economists have found that defaults can have a large impact on decision-making (Johnson & Goldstein, 2003). A default intervention opts the consumer into a choice unless they take action to opt out. The classic example is the very large increase in organ donors after a policy change that made donation the default option (Johnson & Goldstein, 2003). Consistent with the philosophy of *Libertarian Paternalism*, the consumer can opt out of the default option, but must take action to do so. In practice, few consumers opt out of the default option unless it is highly non-preferred. Defaults appear to work through an endorsement effect (i.e., the consumer trusts the agency who set the default option) or a status-quo bias (i.e., reluctance to change because opting out may result in a loss, relative to the status quo).

Applied to the cafeteria, a policy might be implemented in which children are served white milk by default, but they can request chocolate milk. While O'Bryan, Price, and Riis (2017) found that default placement of lettuce and tomatoes on hamburgers nearly tripled the fraction of college students who ate them, the effects of adding default servings of FV to school lunch has produced less encouraging results (Cullen & Dave, 2017). Defaults may have limited, or no impact when the consumer has a strong aversion to the default option. For example, Wansink and Just (2016) reported that 87% of children opted out of a default serving of apples when french fries were the alternative choice.

Decreasing Price

As noted above, the law of demand holds that when the price of a commodity increases, consumption of that commodity should decrease. The converse is also true. If the price of FV were to decrease, then consumption of these foods should increase. Because elementary-school children do not decide, as a consumer, to spend their own money on FV, we must look to non-monetary variables that affect price.

It is helpful to conceptualize price as a cost-benefit ratio. Doing so clarifies that there are two ways to reduce price: decrease the cost (e.g., from $2.50 to $1.50 per gallon) or increase the benefit (improved mileage, reduced emissions). Both of these price-impacting manipulations should alter consumption. The next section of this chapter will discuss methods for increasing the benefits of FV consumption. Here we discuss FV cost reductions.

When we purchase gasoline, we do not work at the gas station for several hours in exchange for a tank of gas. Instead, we use money as a medium of exchanging our past efforts (at our jobs) for gasoline. Thus, effort expended to procure a commodity may be conceptualized as a cost. Applied to FV consumption, a school-based intervention might take steps to reduce the procurement costs of obtaining a serving of FV. This cost-decreasing strategy, in part, underlies the smart-lunchroom interventions in which healthy foods are placed in convenient locations. These placements reduce search and travel costs, and may have a social-norm function (i.e., we place these foods here because consumers frequently choose them). Although the smart-lunchroom approach has been widely adopted in cafeterias, little empirical research has evaluated its effect on objectively measured FV consumption in elementary schools.

On the positive side, one study of the smart-lunchroom arrangement reported that fruit consumption increased by at least 32% and vegetable consumption by at least 43% (Hanks, Just, & Wansink, 2013). However, in that study employees prompted children to take a serving of FV and, as noted above, prompting alone can increase FV consumption. Thus, it is difficult to evaluate the independent contribution of the smart-lunchroom design on FV consumption in the Hanks et al. (2013) study. In a 1-day study of increasing the convenience of the salad bar, Adams, Bruening, Ohri-Vachaspati, and Hurley (2016) reported an impressive five-fold increase in FV consumption. Evaluating the long-term impact of this intervention will be important, because a 4-month evaluation of smart-lunchroom techniques revealed an increase in FV taking but not consumption (Cohen et al., 2015).

An alternative cost-decreasing approach is to reduce the handling costs of FV. For example, the time, effort, and mess incurred in peeling an orange represent a high price on consuming this food. Likewise, young children pay large handling costs to eat whole fruits such as apples, which are difficult for children with loose teeth or limited gapes, making it harder to bite into the fruit. When elementary-school cafeterias reduced these costs by serving sliced instead of whole apples, consumption increases by 62% (McCool, Myung, & Chien, 2006). Less encouraging, in a 1-day study, Swanson, Bransum, and Nakayima (2009) reported that approximately 8% more children ate sliced oranges, but there was no effect on apple consumption.

Anecdotally, we have noted that, for hygiene or freshness reasons, FVs are often served in packages that children must open in order to eat their contents. For example, baby carrots and apple slices are served in small plastic pouches that young children find difficult to open. This packaging makes it easier for food service employees who don't have to slice apples and mix them with lemon juice to prevent browning, but they appear to be increasing the price of these foods and, according to the law of demand, decreasing their consumption. Likewise, for schools to ensure that they are serving children the minimum amounts of FV required under the NSLP, they prepare measured servings in plastic cups with lids. Relative to the tater tots and corn dogs that appear on their plate and may be consumed without opening anything, including cutlery, these cups must be opened. Thus, the prices of FV appear to be inadvertently increased by concerns about hygiene and remaining in compliance with federal mandates.

A final cost-decreasing strategy that elementary-school cafeterias can employ is to reduce the opportunity costs of eating FV. Opportunity costs refer to that which is forgone when one chooses to spend income on a particular commodity. In the cafeteria, time is income and it is fixed each day. Time spent consuming FV is, in some schools, time not spent at recess. Scheduling lunch to occur after recess removes this potential opportunity cost, and in one study this scheduling change increased FV consumption by 54% (Just & Price, 2015). A related strategy is to increase children's income—give them more time to eat lunch. Setting a fixed amount of time to eat, with no one released to recess earlier, appears to have a beneficial effect on FV consumption. In one study, children given <20 min to eat consumed 12% fewer vegetables than children given >25 min to eat (Cohen et al., 2016).

Increasing Benefits

As children are temporally myopic discounters of future events, interventions designed to increase the *immediate* benefits of FV consumption are anticipated to produce robust effects. As the literature on repeated tasting of FV suggests, if children can be induced to consume FV a sufficient number of times, their liking of these foods can increase (Anzman-Frasca, Savage, Marini, Fisher, & Birch, 2012; Lakkakula et al., 2011).

One approach to increasing the immediate benefits of FV consumption is to improve their taste. At least two studies have evaluated the impact of this approach on objectively measured FV consumption. Cohen et al. (2012) had chefs train cafeteria staff in two middle-schools, helping them to prepare better tasting FV offerings. Relative to control schools, vegetable consumption increased by 200% but fruit intake was unchanged. In a larger and more comprehensive evaluation of chef-prepared meals, Cohen et al. (2015) used plate-waste methods to objectively measure FV consumption in low-income elementary- and middle-schools. Three months into the intervention, more children attending the chef schools were taking vegetables, but there was no increase in vegetable consumption; likewise, there was no change in fruit taking or consumption. By the end of the 7-month study, children attending the chef schools were consuming ~82% more fruit and ~115% more vegetables than they did during baseline. Adding a smart-lunchroom arrangement to the chef schools did not enhance the efficacy of this program.

The other, and most often employed, approach to increasing the benefits of FV consumption is to provide an incentive contingent upon eating these foods. This contingent-reinforcement approach has been extensively investigated in other areas of clinical research, where behavior change is difficult; most notably in the treatment of substance use disorders. Early research showed that incentivizing cocaine abstinence could produce quit rates that were substantially higher than treatment as usual (e.g., Higgins et al., 1994; Silverman et al., 1996) and a large body of research now reveals incentives are among the most effective approach to encouraging abstinence from cigarettes and illicit drugs, and for encouraging weight loss and medication adherence (see Bickel, Moody, & Higgins, 2016 for review).

These findings are relevant for at least two reasons. First, children, like substance-dependent adults, steeply discount the delayed consequences of their behavior (Madden, Petry, Badger, & Bickel, 1997); thus, there is good reason to expect incentives can improve difficult-to-change behavior in impulsive populations. Second, sustained drug abstinence and FV consumption are critical to improving public health in their respective domains. Thus, those contingencies of incentive delivery that have proven most effective, and most cost-effective in treating substance-dependence might profitably be imported into school-based FV incentive programs (Peirce et al., 2006; Roll, Higgins, & Badger, 1996).

While incentives have a proven record of health behavior change, they are not without controversy (e.g., Pink, 2011). When designed to influence children's behavior, teachers and parents may object to the cheating that incentives can induce

(Just & Price, 2013b) and may object philosophically to paying children to engage in positive behaviors such as healthy eating. Within the social and economic sciences, one of the most common objections to the use of incentives is variously referred to as the "overjustification," "boomerang," or "crowding out" effect. Such terms refer to a possible decline to below-baseline levels when the incentive is suspended (Lepper, Greene, & Nisbett, 1973). According to self-determination theory (Deci & Ryan, 2012), this effect occurs because intrinsic motivation to engage in the behavior is "crowded out" by extrinsic incentives. When the latter are suspended, the intrinsic benefits of the behavior are no longer sufficient to maintain it.

Applied to healthy eating, incentives can increase FV consumption, but when the intervention ends the overjustification effect predicts children will consume less than they did before. Several thoughtful discussions have accompanied meta-analyses of the overjustification effect, and some of these are relevant to the topic at hand (Cameron, Banko, & Pierce, 2001; Cerasoli, Nicklin, & Nassrelgrgawi, 2016; Gneezy, Meier, & Rey-Biel, 2011). These authors suggest incentives can be appropriate for simple behaviors that are not inherently enjoyable (e.g., abstaining from a preferred drug), and for which creative problem-solving is not required. Given children's frequent disliking of vegetables, and the simplicity of eating them, incentivizing FV consumption may be appropriate. Incentives can be a powerful tool in convincing children to repeatedly taste FV. Doing so allows them to contact foods that they already like, or to develop a liking of foods they once feared (i.e., to identify new intrinsic sources of motivation).

Several studies illustrate the powerful effects that brief incentive-based interventions can have on healthy eating in elementary schools. Just and Price (2013b), for example, employed small monetary incentives to encourage FV consumption in 15 schools. Consistent with the substance-abuse treatment literature (e.g., Silverman, Chutuape, Bigelow, & Stitzer, 1999) larger incentives ($0.25) produced larger increases in consumption of FV, and consistent with the temporal myopathy of youth, providing the incentive immediately produced a larger effect than providing the same reward in 2 weeks. Across schools and the variety of incentives and delays they employed, the number of children eating fruits or vegetables at lunch increased by 82%.

Long-duration incentive-based interventions typically include other intervention components, which makes it difficult to isolate the unique contribution of incentives to behavior change. For example, the Food Dudes program combines incentives with default servings of FV and video role-modeling. The program yields increases in fruit (from 27 to 245%) and vegetable (from 23 to 197%) consumption in preschool (Horne et al., 2011) and elementary-school settings (Horne et al., 2004, 2009; Lowe, Horne, Tapper, Bowdery, & Egerton, 2004; Morrill, Madden, Wengreen, Fargo, & Aguilar, 2016; Wengreen, Madden, Aguilar, Smits, & Jones, 2013). The exception to these findings is Upton, Upton, and Taylor (2013), who took a naturalistic approach to implementation of the Food Dudes program. Specifically, they provided the program to the schools but did not take steps to ensure that all components of the program were properly implemented. In this case, they reported no positive effect of the program on FV consumption.

In a laboratory study, Cooke, Chambers, Añez, Croker, et al. (2011) isolated the effects of incentives in a 12-session program targeting consumption of a non-preferred vegetable. Tangible incentives (stickers) and social praise produced large, and statistically comparable increases in vegetable consumption. Following up on the Cooke et al. findings, Morrill et al. (2016) found that social praise produced comparable increases in FV consumption only in the short term. At 6-month follow-up, only those whose FV consumption was tangibly incentivized continued to consume more FV. The substance-abuse literature offers one possible explanation for this finding. When incentives are used to encourage drug abstinence, better long-term outcomes are observed among those who sustain abstinence for a longer continuous duration during the incentive phase (Higgins, Heil, Rogers, & Chivers, 1999). Similarly, tangible incentives may be necessary to sustain FV consumption over a continuous duration sufficiently long to shift the behavior from conscious control to habit (Lally, van Jaarsveld, Pttos, & Wardle, 2010).

Because long-duration incentive-based interventions often evaluate FV consumption long after incentives are withdrawn, we can return to concerns about the overjustification effect. Cooke, Chambers, Añez, and Wardle (2011) reviewed the available research and found evidence for the overjustification effect only when consumption of *palatable* foods was incentivized; importantly, the effect was confined to food-liking, not consumption. The same review revealed that incentives arranged for consuming *less palatable* foods (like vegetables) produced no decrement in any measure of intrinsic motivation.

In the ten relevant studies published after the Cooke, Chambers, Añez, and Wardle (2011) review (Belot, James, & Nolen, 2016; Cooke, Chambers, Añez, Croker, et al., 2011; Hoffman et al., 2011; Horne et al., 2011; Just & Price, 2013b; List & Samek, 2015; Loewenstein, Price, & Volpp, 2016; Morrill et al., 2016; Remington, An, Croker, Wardle, & Cooke, 2012; Upton et al., 2013), all but one reported that incentives increased FV consumption during the intervention and in no way reduced intrinsic motivation to consume these foods after incentives were removed. The exception (Upton et al., 2013) failed to produce an incentive effect on FV consumption, and the post-incentive decline in consumption was observed in both the incentive and control schools; thus, it would be inappropriate to refer to the post-incentive decline as an overjustification effect. In those nine studies that showed a positive effect of incentives on FV consumption, six reported that the significant increases in FV consumption were still evident months after the incentives had been terminated (Cooke, Chambers, Añez, Croker, et al., 2011; Horne et al., 2011; List & Samek, 2015; Loewenstein et al., 2016; Morrill et al., 2016; Remington et al., 2012). In sum, there is no published evidence that incentivizing FV consumption in schools will crowd out children's intrinsic motivation to consume these foods. To the contrary, the modal effect of incentives is the opposite.

The primary obstacle to adoption and long-term implementation of any school-based intervention is cost (Appleton et al., 2016). Schools' primary mission is education and their budgets leave little room to purchase tangible incentives that might be used to promote the repeated tasting and daily consumption of FV. An additional expense of incentive systems is the labor required to administer them. This typically involves verifying if each child has eaten their serving of FV and providing the incentive only when they did. Verification is important because incentives can induce cheating (Just & Price, 2013b). In our experience, the prevalence of cheating appears proportional to the amount of the reward. A large reward is likely to induce a host of cheats, including dropping vegetables on the floor, stuffing them into a pocket, or holding them in the mouth just long enough for an adult to be fooled into giving them a reward. Providing an incentive for these behaviors will undermine the intervention.

There are also the labor costs associated with transporting incentives to the schools and classrooms, and having teachers pass them out. These labor costs are serious impediments to the adoption of an incentive-based intervention. Much of the incentive-based research reviewed above is grant-funded, and so many of these materials and labor costs are not paid by schools. If they were, there seems little chance that schools would adopt these programs.

Low-Cost Game-Based Incentives

If the materials and labor costs of existing incentive programs are a barrier to their widespread adoption in schools, then reducing these costs should be a direction for future research and innovation. One such direction is to arrange no-cost virtual incentives that will establish patterns of healthy eating in children. A challenge is in giving virtual rewards enough value to influence real-world behavior. One context in which virtual incentives can strongly influence human actions is in videogames. These games have a rich narrative and immersive environment in which the player will expend considerable efforts to acquire virtual rewards such as in-game currency, which may be used to purchase items that aid in winning the game (Reeves &Read, 2009).

Some attempts have been made to create videogames designed to positively influence healthy eating. Many of these efforts have taken an education approach (e.g., Lew, Alviando, Kwon, & Camba, 2017), where others have more comprehensively incorporated goal-setting, feedback, and self-efficacy building (e.g., Thompson et al., 2015). Two significant hurdles must be overcome if this gaming approach is to be successful. First, if the games are played on a computer, smartphone, or gaming platform, they will need to effectively compete against the large array of concurrently available highly entertaining games that include no healthy behavior messaging. Simply put, health-promoting games will need to be engaging. Second, the games must include a means of objectively measuring FV consumption. At present, serious games targeting healthy eating have relied heavily on self-reported outcomes (e.g., Baranowski et al., 2003) and this may inadvertently encourage cheating (Thompson, 2017).

Our research group has begun to address some of these challenges by arranging low-cost game-based incentives to increase FV consumption in elementary schools. Jones, Madden, Wengreen, Aguilar, and Desjardins (2014) developed a rudimentary episode-based adventure game. Within the game's narrative, heroic characters fought the forces of evil and enlisted the aid of the school—if they met a daily FV consumption goal, the heroes continued to make progress toward the object of the game: capturing a band of villains. When consumption goals were met, teachers would read the next episode; when the school fell short of their goal, they were encouraged to try again tomorrow. This rudimentary low-cost, no-tech game increased objectively measured fruit and vegetable consumption by 66% and 44%, respectively over a 13-day period (Jones, Madden, Wengreen, Aguilar, et al., 2014). Relative to our previous work using tangible incentives (Morrill et al., 2016; Wengreen et al., 2013), the game was far less expensive (no materials costs), did not induce cheating, and produced comparable increases in FV consumption.

The game was refined in a follow-up study conducted in a second school (Jones, Madden, & Wengreen, 2014). The revised game was designed using five rudimentary game-design principles (see Reeves & Read, 2009; Schell, 2015). First, and consistent with the prior version, there was a clear object of the game—locate and capture the villains. Second, the narrative was expanded and enriched to improve its entertainment value. A good vs. evil narrative formed the core archetype, and episodes included periodic surprises, humor, and cliff-hanger endings designed to better motivate meeting the daily FV-consumption goals. Third, children playing the game were occasionally given autonomy to choose the direction of the narrative. Fourth, the game included a virtual economy—when children exceeded their daily FV consumption goal, they earned virtual currency that could be exchanged for goods and services within the game (e.g., repairing the ship or purchasing a tool). Finally, the daily goal was set to a level that only slightly exceeded recent median levels of FV consumption. Because the incentives were judged to be small in benefit, their acquisition price was low. By gradually increasing the goal as the school succeeded in meeting it, the difficulty of the game matched the skills of the player. This redesigned version of the game increased fruit and vegetable consumption by 39% and 33%, respectively (Jones, Madden, & Wengreen, 2014).[3]

A third iteration of the game was designed to further reduce its operating costs. Where previously the game asked teachers to read the episodes to children, Joyner et al. (2017) presented them as comic-book panels displayed in large format on a cafeteria wall. This change relieved teachers of a duty and served as a prompt, reminding children to meet their healthy-eating goal in the location in which this behavior was to occur. Only vegetable consumption was targeted for improvement and plate-waste measures were used, as above. In two participating elementary schools, the game nearly doubled vegetable consumption (fruit consumption was unchanged).

A shortcoming of these three game-based studies is their short duration (usually less than 1 month) and the lack of follow-up evaluations of FV consumption after

[3] The smaller percentage increase relative to Jones, Madden, Wengreen, Aguilar, et al. (2014) is due to higher baseline levels of FV consumption. The latter may be due to the increased variety of FV offerings (Adams et al., 2005) and chef-quality offerings (Cohen et al., 2015) available at the school throughout the study.

the game has been won. Future research should expand game duration to evaluate if this approach can produce the long-lasting increases in FV consumption that are associated with tangible reward programs (e.g., Morrill et al., 2016).

Concise Policy Recommendations

This chapter has reviewed intervention research conducted in elementary-school cafeterias that has objectively measured changes in FV consumption. The latter standard provides the most rigorous evidence for the efficacy of an intervention. Programs that have not provided such evidence cannot be recommended to policy makers. With the exception of incentives, there are, at present, only small numbers of mostly short-duration studies available in any of the intervention categories summarize above. Thus, the recommendations below should be viewed as tentative, pending replications in the future research.

As noted above, the widespread adoption of healthy-eating interventions in schools will be facilitated by low- (or no-) cost programs that are easy to implement. Several such programs may be initiated by food-service personnel without involvement of the school's faculty. The available evidence suggests that slicing fruits before serving them to children will increase their consumption. Serving them directly to the child's plate (instead of serving wrapped portions) reduces the handling cost of accessing these foods. Large increases in vegetable consumption can be achieved by either serving these foods to children while they wait in the cafeteria line, or by serving fruit after the main course, as dessert. Making a wider variety of vegetables available to children each day increases the probability they will find one they will eat. Two final simple policy changes include scheduling lunch after recess and giving children at least 25 min to eat their lunch.

Should more involved interventions prove necessary, increasing the benefits of eating FV is in order. This can be accomplished by improving the taste of these foods and/or incentivizing their daily consumption. Cohen et al. (2015) reported large increases in vegetable consumption when the taste of these foods was improved, but the effects were not observed for several months after the new menus were introduced. Children may have been afraid to try these new foods, and may have done so only when they saw their peers try them and report that they tasted good. If so, the uptake of these new foods could be expedited if tasting them were briefly incentivized. If a no-cost game could be employed to motivate children to repeatedly try these better tasting vegetable offerings, the children may discover several foods that they like to eat, facilitating the acquisition of healthy-eating habits at school and home, and maintained well after the game has been won.

Acknowledgements The first and third authors' efforts were supported, in part, by a grant from the Eunice Kennedy Shriver National Institute of Child Health and Development; R21 HD083702-01.

References

Adams, M. A., Bruening, M., Ohri-Vachaspati, P., & Hurley, J. C. (2016). Location of school lunch salad bars and fruit and vegetable consumption in middle schools: A cross-sectional plate waste study. *Journal of the Academy of Nutrition and Dietetics, 116*(3), 407–416.

Adams, M. A., Pelletier, R. L., Zive, M. M., & Sallis, J. F. (2005). Salad bars and fruit and vegetable consumption in elementary schools: A plate waste study. *Journal of the American Dietetic Association, 105*(11), 1789–1792.

Amin, S. A., Yon, B. A., Taylor, J. C., & Johnson, R. K. (2015). Impact of the National School Lunch Program on fruit and vegetable selection in northeastern elementary schoolchildren, 2012–2013. *Public Health Reports, 130*(5), 453–457.

Anzman-Frasca, S., Savage, J. S., Marini, M. E., Fisher, J. O., & Birch, L. L. (2012). Repeated exposure and associative conditioning promote preschool children's liking of vegetables. *Appetite, 58*(2), 543–553.

Appleton, K. M., Hemingway, A., Saulais, L., Dinnella, C., Monteleone, E., Depezay, L., … Hartwell, H. (2016). Increasing vegetable intakes: Rationale and systematic review of published interventions. *European Journal of Nutrition, 55*(3), 869–896.

Archer, E., Hand, G. A., & Blair, S. N. (2013). Validity of U.S. nutritional surveillance: National healthy and nutrition examination survey caloric energy intake data, 1971-2010. *PLoS One*. https://doi.org/10.1371/journal.pone.0076632

Archer, E., Pavela, G., & Lavie, C. J. (2015). The inadmissibility of what we eat in America and NHANES dietary data in nutrition and obesity research and the scientific formulation of national dietary guidelines. *Mayo Clinic Proceedings, 90*, 911–926.

Auld, G. W., Romaniello, C., Heimendinger, J., Hambidge, C., & Hambidge, M. (1999). Outcomes from a school-based nutrition education program alternating special resource teachers and classroom teachers. *Journal of School Health, 69*(10), 403–408.

Baranowski, T., Baranowski, J., Cullen, K. W., Marsh, T., Islam, N., Zakeri, I., … deMoor, C. (2003). Squire's Quest! Dietary outcome evaluation of a multimedia game. *American Journal of Preventive Medicine, 24*, 52–61.

Beccarelli, L. M., Scherr, R. E., Dharmar, M., Ermakov, I. V., Gellermann, W., Jahns, L., … Zidenberg-Cherr, S. (2016). Using skin carotenoids to assess dietary changes in students after 1 academic year of participating in the shaping healthy choices program. *Journal of Nutrition Education and Behavior*. https://doi.org/10.1016/j.jneb.2016.09.007

Belot, M., James, J., & Nolen, P. (2016). Incentives and children's dietary choices: A field experiment in primary schools. *Journal of Health Economics, 50*, 213–229.

Bickel, W. K., & Madden, G. J. (1999). The behavioral economics of smoking. In *The economic analysis of substance use and abuse: An integration of econometrics and behavioral economic research* (pp. 31–74). Chicago, IL: University of Chicago Press.

Bickel, W. K., Moody, L., & Higgins, S. T. (2016). Some current dimensions of the behavioral economics of health-related behavior change. *Preventive Medicine, 92*, 16–23.

Bikhchandani, S., Hirshleifer, D., & Welch, I. (1992). A theory of fashion, custom, and cultural change. *Journal of Political Economy, 100*, 992–1026.

Boutelle, K. N., Fulkerson, J. A., Neumark-Sztainer, D., Story, M., & French, S. A. (2007). Fast food for family meals: Relationships with parent and adolescent food intake, home food availability and weight status. *Public Health Nutrition, 10*(1), 16–23.

Brug, J., Tak, N. I., te Vedle, S. J., Bere, E., & de Bourdeaudhuji, I. (2008). Taste preferences, liking and other factors related to fruit and vegetable intakes among schoolchildren: Results from observational studies. *British Journal of Nutrition, 99*, S7–S14.

Brug, J., & Van Assema, P. (2001). Belief about fat: Why do we hold beliefs about fat and why and how do we study these beliefs. In L. Frewer, E. Risvikk, & H. Schifferstein (Eds.), *Food, people and society: A European perspective of consumers'food choices*. Heidelberg, Germany: Springer.

Byker, C. J., Farris, A. R., Marcenelle, M., Davis, G. C., & Serrano, E. L. (2014). Food waste in a school nutrition program after implementation of new lunch program guidelines. *Journal of Nutrition Education and Behavior, 46*(5), 406–411.

Cameron, J., Banko, K. M., & Pierce, W. D. (2001). Pervasive negative effects of rewards on intrinsic motivation: The myth continues. *The Behavior Analyst, 24*, 1–44.

Cerasoli, C. P., Nicklin, J. M., & Nassrelgrgawi, A. S. (2016). Performance, incentives, and needs for autonomy, competence, and relatedness: A meta-analysis. *Motivation and Emotion, 40*(6), 781–813.

Christian, M. S., Evans, C. E., Nykjaer, C., Hancock, N., & Cade, J. E. (2014). Evaluation of the impact of a school gardening intervention on children's fruit and vegetable intake: A randomised controlled trial. *International Journal of Behavioral Nutrition and Physical Activity, 11*(1), 99.

Cohen, J. F., Richardson, S., Parker, E., Catalano, P. J., & Rimm, E. B. (2014). Impact of the new U.S. Department of Agriculture school meal standards on food selection, consumption, and waste. *American Journal of Preventive Medicine, 46*, 388–394.

Cohen, J. F., Richardson, S. A., Cluggish, S. A., Parker, E., Catalano, P. J., & Rimm, E. B. (2015). Effects of choice architecture and chef-enhanced meals on the selection and consumption of healthier school foods. *JAMA Pediatrics, 169*(5), 431–437.

Cohen, J. F., Smit, L. A., Parker, E., Austin, S. B., Frazier, A. L., Economos, C. D., & Rimm, E. B. (2012). Long-term impact of a chef on school lunch consumption: Findings from a 2-year pilot study in Boston middle schools. *Journal of the Academy of Nutrition & Dietetics, 112*, 927–933.

Cohen, J. F. W., Jahn, J. L., Richardson, S. A., Cluggish, S. A., Parker, E., Catalano, P. J., & Rimm, E. B. (2016). Amount of time to eat lunch is associated with children's selection and consumption of school meal entrée, fruits, vegetables, and milk. *Journal of the Academy of Nutrition and Dietetics, 116*, 123–128.

Cooke, L. J., Chambers, L. C., Añez, E. V., Croker, H. A., Boniface, D., Yeomans, M. R., & Wardle, J. (2011). Eating for pleasure or profit: The effects of incentives on children's enjoyment of vegetables. *Psychological Science, 22*, 190–196.

Cooke, L. J., Chambers, L. C., Añez, E. V., & Wardle, J. (2011). Facilitating or undermining? The effect of reward on food acceptance. A narrative review. *Appetite, 57*(2), 493–497.

Cooke, L. J., & Wardle, J. (2005). Age and gender differences in children's food preferences. *British Journal of Nutrition, 93*, 741–746.

Coulthard, H., & Blissett, J. (2009). Fruit and vegetable consumption in children and their mothers. Moderating effects of child sensory sensitivity. *Appetite, 52*(2), 410–415.

Cullen, K. W., Chen, T. A., & Dave, J. M. (2015). Changes in foods selected and consumed after implementation of the new National School Lunch Program meal patterns in southeast Texas. *Preventive Medicine Reports, 2*, 440–443.

Cullen, K. W., & Dave, J. M. (2017). The new Federal School Nutrition Standards and meal patterns: Early evidence examining the influence on student dietary behavior and the school food environment. *Journal of the Academy of Nutrition and Dietetics, 117*(2), 185–191.

Darmon, N., Darmon, M., Maillot, M., & Drewnowski, A. (2005). A nutrient density standard for vegetables and fruits: Nutrients per calorie and nutrients per unit cost. *Journal of the American Dietetic Association, 105*(12), 1881–1887.

Dauchet, L., Amouyel, P., Hercberg, S., & Dallongeville, J. (2006). Fruit and vegetable consumption and risk of coronary heart disease: A meta-analysis of cohort studies. *The Journal of Nutrition, 136*(10), 2588–2593.

Deci, E. L., & Ryan, R. M. (2012). Self-determination theory. In P. A. M. Van Lange, A. W. Kruglanski, & E. T. Higgins (Eds.), *Handbook of theories of social psychology* (Vol. 1, pp. 416–433). Thousand Oaks, CA: Sage.

Eckmanns, T., Bessert, J., Behnke, M., Gastmeier, P., & Rüden, H. (2006). Compliance with antiseptic hand rub use in intensive care units the Hawthorne Effect. *Infection Control, 27*, 931–934.

Elsbernd, S. L., Reicks, M. M., Mann, T. L., Redden, J. P., Mykerezi, E., & Vickers, Z. M. (2016). Serving vegetables first: A strategy to increase vegetable consumption in elementary school cafeterias. *Appetite, 96*, 111–115.

Fletcher, S., Wright, C., Jones, A., Parkinson, K., & Adamson, A. (2017). Tracking of toddler fruit and vegetable preferences to intake and adiposity later in childhood. *Maternal & Child Nutrition, 13*(2), 1–13.

Freedman, D. S., Khan, L. K., Dietz, W. H., Srinivasan, S. R., & Berenson, G. S. (2001). Relationship of childhood obesity to coronary heart disease risk factors in adulthood. The Bogalusa heart study. *Pediatrics, 108*, 712–718.

Fulton, S. L., McKinley, M. C., Young, I. S., Cardwell, C. R., & Woodside, J. V. (2016). The effect of increasing fruit and vegetable consumption on overall diet: A systematic review and meta-analysis. *Critical Reviews in Food Science and Nutrition, 56*(5), 802–816.

Gneezy, U., Meier, S., & Rey-Biel, P. (2011). When and why incentives (don't) work to modify behavior. *The Journal of Economic Perspectives, 25*(4), 191–209.

Green, L., Myerson, J., Lichtman, D., Rosen, S., & Fry, A. (1996). Temporal discounting in choice between delayed rewards: The role of age and income. *Psychology and Aging, 11*(1), 79.

Greenhalgh, J., Dowey, A. J., Horne, P. J., Lowe, C. F., Griffiths, J. H., & Whitaker, C. J. (2009). Positive- and negative peer modelling effects on young children's consumption of novel blue foods. *Appetite, 52*, 646–653.

Grosso, G., Micek, A., Godos, J., Pajak, A., Sciacca, S., Galvano, F., & Boffetta, P. (2017). Health risk factors associated with meat, fruit and vegetable consumption in cohort studies: A comprehensive meta-analysis. *PLoS One, 12*(8), e0183787.

Hakim, S. M., & Meissen, G. (2013). Increasing consumption of fruits and vegetables in the school cafeteria: The influence of active choice. *Journal of Health Care for the Poor and Underserved, 24*(supplement), 145–157.

Hanks, A. S., Just, D. R., & Brumberg, A. (2016). Marketing vegetables in elementary school cafeterias to increase uptake. *Pediatrics, 138*, e20151720.

Hanks, A. S., Just, D. R., & Wansink, B. (2013). Smarter lunchrooms can address new school lunchroom guidelines and childhood obesity. *The Journal of Pediatrics, 162*(4), 867–869.

Health.gov. (2010). *Dietary guidelines for Americans*. Retrieved from https://health.gov/dietaryguidelines/2010/

Heitmann, B. L., Lissner, L., & Osler, M. (2000). Do we eat less fat, or just report so? *International Journal of Obesity and Related Metabolic Disorders, 24*, 435–442.

Herrnstein, R. J. (1970). On the law of effect. *Journal of the Experimental Analysis of Behavior, 13*(2), 243–266.

Higgins, S. T., Budney, A. J., Bickel, W. K., Foerg, F. E., Donham, R., & Badger, G. J. (1994). Incentives improve outcome in outpatient behavioral treatment of cocaine dependence. *Archives of General Psychiatry, 51*(7), 568–576.

Higgins, S. T., Heil, S. H., Rogers, R. E., & Chivers, L. (1999). Contingency management in the treatment of cocaine dependence. In S. T. Higgins & K. Silverman (Eds.), *Motivating behavior change among illicit-drug abusers*. Washington, DC: American Psychological Association.

Hobbs, M., Pearson, N., Foster, P. J., & Biddle, S. J. (2014). Sedentary behaviour and diet across the lifespan: An updated systematic review. *British Journal of Sports Medicine, 49*, 1179–1188.

Hoffman, J. A., Thompson, D. R., Franko, D. L., Power, T. J., Leff, S. S., & Stallings, V. A. (2011). Decaying behavioral effects in a randomized, multi-year fruit and vegetable intake intervention. *Preventive Medicine, 52*, 370–375. https://doi.org/10.1016/j.ypmed.2011.02.013

Horne, P. J., Greenhalgh, J., Erjavec, M., Lowe, C. F., Viktor, S., & Whitaker, C. J. (2011). Increasing pre-school children's consumption of fruit and vegetables. A modelling and rewards intervention. *Appetite, 56*, 375–385.

Horne, P. J., Hardman, C. A., Lowe, C. F., Tapper, K., Le Noury, J., Madden, P., … Doody, M. (2009). Increasing parental provision and children's consumption of lunchbox fruit and vegetables in Ireland: The Food Dudes intervention. *European Journal of Clinical Nutrition, 63*, 613–618.

Horne, P. J., Tapper, K., Lowe, C. F., Hardman, C. A., Jackson, M. C., & Woolner, J. (2004). Increasing children's fruit and vegetable consumption: A peer-modelling and rewards-based intervention. *European Journal of Clinical Nutrition, 58*, 1649–1660.

Hosseini, B., Berthon, B. S., Wark, P., & Wood, L. G. (2017). Effects of fruit and vegetable consumption on risk of asthma, wheezing and immune responses: A systematic review and meta-analysis. *Nutrients, 9*(4), 341.

Hu, D., Huang, J., Wang, Y., Zhang, D., & Qu, Y. (2014). Fruits and vegetables consumption and risk of stroke. *Stroke, 45*, 1613–1619.

Huang, L., Lin, Y. C., Foland, E., Bai, Y., Liu, Y., & Fly, A. D. (2013). 2010–2011 USDA fresh fruit and vegetable program (FFVP) improved Indiana elementary students' consumption of fruit. *The FASEB Journal, 27*(1 Supplement), 1063–1065.

Jamelske, E. M., & Bica, L. A. (2014). The USDA fresh fruit and vegetable program: A case study of implementation and consumption in Wisconsin. *Journal of Child Nutrition & Management, 38*(2), n2.

Jiang, X., Huang, J., Song, D., Deng, R., Wei, J., & Zhang, Z. (2017). Increased consumption of fruit and vegetables is related to a reduced risk of cognitive impairment and dementia: Meta-analysis. *Frontiers in Aging Neuroscience, 9*, 18.

Johnson, E. J., & Goldstein, D. (2003). Do defaults save lives? *Science, 302*, 1338–1339.

Jones, B. A., Madden, G. J., & Wengreen, H. J. (2014). The FIT Game: Preliminary evaluation of a gamification approach to increasing fruit and vegetable consumption in school. *Preventive Medicine, 68*, 76–79. https://doi.org/10.1016/j.ypmed.2014.04.015

Jones, B. A., Madden, G. J., Wengreen, H. J., Aguilar, S. S., & Desjardins, E. A. (2014). Gamification of dietary decision-making in elementary school cafeteria. *PLoS One, 9*(4), e93872. https://doi.org/10.1371/journal.pone.0093872

Joyner, D., Wengreen, H. J., Aguilar, S., Anderson Spruance, L., Morrill, B. A., & Madden, G. J. (2017). The FIT Game III: Reducing the operating expenses of a game-based approach to increasing healthy eating in elementary schools. *Games for Health Journal: Research, Development, and Clinical Applications, 6*, 111–118.

Just, D., & Price, J. (2013a). Default options, incentives and food choices: Evidence from elementary-school children. *Public Health Nutrition, 16*(12), 2281–2288.

Just, D., & Price, J. (2013b). Using incentives to encourage healthy eating in children. *Journal of Human Resources, 48*, 855–872.

Just, D. R., Lund, J., & Price, J. (2012). The role of variety in increasing the consumption of fruits and vegetables among children. *Agricultural and Resource Economics Review, 41*, 72–81.

Just, D. R., & Price, J. (2015). Lunch, recess and nutrition: Responding to time incentives in the cafeteria. *Preventive Medicine, 71*, 27–30.

Kagel, J. H., Battalio, R. C., & Green, L. (1995). *Economic choice theory*. Cambridge, England: Cambridge University Press.

Kim, S. A., Moore, L. V., Galuska, D., Wright, A. P., Harris, D., Grummer-Strawn, L. M., … Rhodes, D. G. (2014). Vital signs: Fruit and vegetable intake among children—United States, 2003–2010. *Morbidity and Mortality Weekly Report, 63*(31), 671–676.

Kubik, M. Y., Lytle, L. A., Hannan, P. J., Perry, C. L., & Story, M. (2003). The association of the school food environment with dietary behaviors of young adolescents. *American Journal of Public Health, 93*(7), 1168–1173.

Lakkakula, A., Geaghan, J. P., Wong, W. P., Zanovec, M., Pierce, S. H., & Tuuri, G. (2011). A cafeteria-based tasting program increased liking of fruits and vegetables by lower, middle and upper elementary school-age children. *Appetite, 57*(1), 299–302.

Lally, P., van Jaarsveld, C. H. M., Pttos, H. W. W., & Wardle, J. (2010). How are habits formed: Modeling habit formation in the real world. *European Journal of Social Psychology, 40*, 998–1009.

Lautenschlager, L., & Smith, C. (2007). Beliefs, knowledge, and values held by inner-city youth about gardening, nutrition, and cooking. *Agriculture and Human Values, 24*(2), 245–258.

Ledoux, T., Hingle, M., & Baranowski, T. (2011). Relationship of fruit and vegetable intake with adiposity: A systematic review. *Obesity Reviews, 12*, e143–e150.

Lepper, M., Greene, D., & Nisbett, R. (1973). Undermining children's intrinsic interest with extrinsic reward: A test of the 'overjustification' hypothesis. *Journal of Personality and Social Psychology, 28*, 129–137.

Lew, E., Alviando, J., Kwon, E., & Camba, J. D. (2017). Gamifying the eating experience: An interactive companion for children's nutrition education and behavior. In P. Zaphiris & A. Ioannou (Eds.), *Learning and collaboration technologies: Novel learning ecosystems* (pp. 462–473). Cham: Springer.

List, J. A., & Samek, A. S. (2015). The behavioralist as nutritionist: Leveraging behavioral economics to improve child food choice and consumption. *Journal of Health Economics, 39*, 135–146.

Loewenstein, G., Price, J., & Volpp, K. (2016). Habit formation in children: Evidence from incentives for healthy eating. *Journal of Health Economics, 45*, 47–54.

Looney, S. M., & Raynor, H. A. (2012). Are changes in consumption of "healthy" foods related to changes in consumption of "unhealthy" foods during pediatric obesity treatment? *International Journal of Environmental Research and Public Health, 9*(4), 1368–1378.

Lorson, B. A., Melgar-Quinonez, H. R., & Taylor, C. A. (2009). Correlates of fruit and vegetable intakes in US children. *Journal of the American Dietetic Association, 109*(3), 474–478.

Lowe, C. F., Horne, P. J., Tapper, K., Bowdery, M., & Egerton, C. (2004). Effects of a peer modeling and rewards-based intervention to increase fruit and vegetable consumption in children. *European Journal of Clinical Nutrition, 58*, 510–522.

Lytle, L. A., Nichaman, M. Z., Obarzanek, E., Glovsky, E., Montgomery, D., Nicklas, T., … Feldman, H. (1993). Validation of 24-hour recalls assisted by food records in third-grade children. *Journal of the American Dietetic Association, 93*(12), 1431–1436.

Lytle, L. A., Seifert, S., Greenstein, J., & McGovern, P. (2000). How do children's eating patterns and food choices change over time? Results from a cohort study. *American Journal of Health Promotion, 14*(4), 222.

Madden, G. J. (2000). A behavioral-economics primer. In W. K. Bickel & R. Vuchinich (Eds.), *Reframing health behavior change with behavioral economics* (pp. 3–26). Mahwah, NJ: Lawrence Erlbaum & Associates.

Madden, G. J., & Perone, M. (1999). Human sensitivity to concurrent schedules of reinforcement: Effects of observing schedule-correlated stimuli. *Journal of the Experimental Analysis of Behavior, 71*(3), 303–318.

Madden, G. J., Petry, N., Badger, G. J., & Bickel, W. K. (1997). Impulsive and self-control choices in opiate-dependent patients and non-drug-using control participants: Drug and monetary rewards. *Experimental and Clinical Psychopharmacology, 5*, 256–262.

McCool, A. C., Myung, E., & Chien, T. (2006). Modification of the form in which fresh fruit is served as a possible means of increasing the consumption of fruit offered to elementary and middle school students. *Journal of Foodservice Business Research, 8*, 73–85.

Monsivais, P., & Drewnowski, A. (2007). The rising cost of low-energy-density foods. *Journal of the American Dietetic Association, 107*(12), 2071–2076.

Morrill, B. A., Madden, G. J., Wengreen, H. J., Fargo, J., & Aguilar, S. S. (2016). A randomized-control trial of the Food Dudes program: Tangible rewards are more effective than social rewards for increasing short- and long-term fruit and vegetable consumption. *Journal of the Academy of Nutrition and Dietetics, 116*, 618–629.

Mytton, O. T., Nnoaham, K., Eyles, H., Scarborough, P., & Mhurchu, C. N. (2014). Systematic review and meta-analysis of the effect of increased vegetable and fruit consumption on body weight and energy intake. *BMC Public Health, 14*(1), 886.

Newby, P. K. (2009). Plant foods and plant-based diets: Protective against childhood obesity? *American Journal of Clinical Nutrition, 89*, 1572S–1587S.

Nichols, A. L., & Maner, J. K. (2008). The good-subject effect: Investigating participant demand characteristics. *The Journal of General Psychology, 135*(2), 151–165.

Nicklas, T. A., Morales, M., Linares, A., Yang, S. J., Baranowski, T., De Moor, C., & Berenson, G. (2004). Children's meal patterns have changed over a 21-year period: The Bogalusa Heart Study. *Journal of the American Dietetic Association, 104*(5), 753–761.

Nix, E., & Wengreen, H. J. (2017). Social approval bias in self-reported fruit and vegetable intake after presentation of a normative message in college students. *Appetite, 116*, 552–558.

O'Bryan, A., Price, J., & Riis, J. (2017). Using default options to increase healthy add-ons to a meal. *Journal of Marketing Behavior, 3*, 39–50.

Ong, J. X., Ullah, S., Magarey, A., Miller, J., & Leslie, E. (2017). Relationship between the home environment and fruit and vegetable consumption in children aged 6–12 years: A systematic review. *Public Health Nutrition, 20*(3), 464–480.

Orne, M. T. (1962). On the social psychology of the psychological experiment: With particular reference to demand characteristics and their implication. *American Psychologist, 17*(11), 776–783.

Ovesen, L. F. (2005). Is a high intake of fruits and vegetables related to a lowered risk of cerebrovascular disease? *Ugeskr Laeger, 167*, 2748–2752.

Parmer, S. M., Salisbury-Glennon, J., Shannon, D., & Struempler, B. (2009). School gardens: An experiential learning approach for a nutrition education program to increase fruit and vegetable knowledge, preference, and consumption among second-grade students. *Journal of Nutrition Education and Behavior, 41*(3), 212–217.

Peirce, J. M., Petry, N. M., Stitzer, M. L., Blaine, J., Kellogg, S., Satterfield, F., … Kirby, K. C. (2006). Effects of lower-cost incentives on stimulant abstinence in methadone maintenance treatment: A National Drug Abuse Treatment Clinical Trials Network study. *Archives of General Psychiatry, 63*(2), 201–208.

Perry, C. L., Bishop, D. B., Taylor, G., Murray, D. M., Mays, R. W., Dudovitz, B. S., … Story, M. (1998). Changing fruit and vegetable consumption among children: The 5-a-Day Power Plus program in St. Paul, Minnesota. *American Journal of Public Health, 88*(4), 603–609.

Perry, C. L., Bishop, D. B., Taylor, G. L., Davis, M., Story, M., Gray, C., … Harnack, L. (2004). A randomized school trial of environmental strategies to encourage fruit and vegetable consumption among children. *Health Education & Behavior, 31*(1), 65–76.

Pink, D. H. (2011). *Drive: The surprising truth about what motivates us*. New York: Penguin.

Ratcliffe, M. M., Merrigan, K. A., Rogers, B. L., & Goldberg, J. P. (2011). The effects of school garden experiences on middle school-aged students' knowledge, attitudes, and behaviors associated with vegetable consumption. *Health Promotion Practice, 12*(1), 36–43.

Read, D., & Read, N. L. (2004). Time discounting over the lifespan. *Organizational Behavior and Human Decision Processes, 94*, 22–32.

Redden, J. P., Mann, T., Vickers, Z., Mykerezi, E., Reicks, M., & Elsbernd, S. (2015). Serving first in isolation increases vegetable intake among elementary school children. *PLoS One, 10*, e0121283.

Reeves, B., & Read, J. L. (2009). *Total engagement*. Boston, MA: Harvard Business School Press.

Reicks, M., Redden, J. P., Mann, T., Mykerezi, E., & Vickers, Z. (2012). Photographs in lunch tray compartments and vegetable consumption among children in elementary school cafeterias. *JAMA, 307*, 784–785.

Remington, A., An, E., Croker, H., Wardle, J., & Cooke, L. (2012). Increasing food acceptance in the home setting: A randomized controlled trial of parent-administered taste exposure with incentives. *The American Journal of Clinical Nutrition, 95*, 72–77.

Reynolds, K. D., Franklin, F. A., Binkley, D., Raczynski, J. M., Harrington, K. F., Kirk, K. A., & Person, S. (2000). Increasing the fruit and vegetable consumption of fourth-graders: Results from the high 5 project. *Preventive Medicine, 30*(4), 309–319.

Rice, T., Hanoch, Y., & Barnes, A. J. (2017). A brief overview of behavioral economics. In Y. Hanoch, A. J. Barnes, & T. Rice (Eds.), *Behavioral economics and healthy behaviors: Key concepts and current research* (pp. 14–29). New York, NY: Routledge.

Roll, J. M., Higgins, S. T., & Badger, G. J. (1996). An experimental comparison of three different schedules of reinforcement of drug abstinence using cigarette smoking as an exemplar. *Journal of Applied Behavior Analysis, 29*(4), 495–505.

Savica, V., Bellinghieri, G., & Kopple, J. D. (2010). The effect of nutrition on blood pressure. *Annual Review of Nutrition, 30*, 365–401.

Schell, J. (2015). *The art of game design*. Boca Raton, FL: CRC Press.

Schwartz, M. B. (2007). The influence of a verbal prompt on school lunch fruit consumption: A pilot study. *International Journal of Behavioral Nutrition and Physical Activity, 4*, 1–5.

Schwartz, M. B., Henderson, K. E., Read, M., Danna, N., & Ickovics, J. R. (2015). New school meal regulations increase fruit consumption and do not increase total plate waste. *Childhood Obesity, 11*, 242–247.

Shuval, K., Barlow, C. E., Finley, C. E., Gabriel, K. P., Schmidt, M. D., & DeFina, L. F. (2015). Standing, obesity, and metabolic syndrome: Findings from the Cooper Center longitudinal study. *Mayo Clinic Proceedings, 90*, 1524–1532.

Silverman, K., Chutuape, M. A., Bigelow, G. E., & Stitzer, M. L. (1999). Voucher-based reinforcement of cocaine abstinence in treatment-resistant methadone patients: Effects of reinforcement magnitude. *Psychopharmacology, 146*(2), 128–138.

Silverman, K., Higgins, S. T., Brooner, R. K., Montoya, I. D., Cone, E. J., Schuster, C. R., & Preston, K. L. (1996). Sustained cocaine abstinence in methadone maintenance patients through voucher-based reinforcement therapy. *Archives of General Psychiatry, 53*(5), 409–415.

Smith-Warner, S. A., Elmer, P. J., Tharp, T. M., Fosdick, L., Randall, B., Gross, M., … Potter, J. D. (2000). Increasing vegetable and fruit intake: Randomized intervention and monitoring in an at-risk population. *Cancer Epidemiology and Prevention Biomarkers, 9*(3), 307–317.

Spill, M. K., Birch, L. L., Roe, L. S., & Rolls, B. J. (2010). Eating vegetables first: The use of portion size to increase vegetable intake in preschool children. *The American Journal of Clinical Nutrition, 91*, 1237–1243.

Storey, M. L., & Anderson, P. A. (2016). Nutrient intakes and vegetable and white potato consumption by children aged 1 to 3 years. *Advances in Nutrition, 7*(1), 241S–246S.

Story, M., & French, S. (2004). Food advertising and marketing directed at children and adolescents in the US. *International Journal of Behavioral Nutrition and Physical Activity, 1*, 1–13.

Swanson, M., Bransum, A., & Nakayima, P. J. (2009). Promoting consumption of fruit in elementary school cafeterias. The effects of slicing apples and oranges. *Appetite, 53*, 264–267.

Tapsell, L. C., Batterham, M. J., Thorne, R. L., O'shea, J. E., Grafenauer, S. J., & Probst, Y. C. (2014). Weight loss effects from vegetable intake: A 12-month randomised controlled trial. *European Journal of Clinical Nutrition, 68*(7), 778–785.

Thompson, D. (2017). Incorporating behavioral techniques into a serious videogame for children. *Games for Health Journal: Research, Development, and Clinical Applications, 6*, 75–86.

Thompson, D., Bhatt, R., Vazquez, I., Cullen, K. W., Baranowski, J., Baranowski, T., & Liu, Y. (2015). Creating action plans in a serious video game increases and maintains fruit-vegetable intake: A randomized controlled trial. *International Journal of Behavioral Nutrition and Physical Activity, 12*, 1–10.

United States Department of Agriculture. (2012). *Nutrition standards in the National School Lunch and School Breakfast Programs: Final rule* (Vol. 7, pp. 4088–4167). FNS 2007-0038. CFR Parts 210 and 220. Federal Register.

United States Department of Agriculture. (2013). *Food and Nutrition Service. Offer versus serve: Guidance for the national school lunch program and the school breakfast program*. Washington, DC: Government Printing Office.

United States Department of Agriculture. (2016). *Food and Nutrition Service. National school lunch program: Participation and lunches served*. Retrieved from https://fns-prod.azureedge.net/sites/default/files/pd/slsummar.pdf

Upton, D., Upton, P., & Taylor, C. (2013). Increasing children's lunchtime consumption of fruit and vegetables: An evaluation of the Food Dudes programme. *Public Health Nutrition, 16*, 1066–1072. https://doi.org/10.1017/S1368980012004612

Wang, X., Ouyang, Y., Liu, J., Zhu, M., Zhao, G., Bao, W., & Hu, F. B. (2014). Fruit and vegetable consumption and mortality from all causes, cardiovascular disease, and cancer: Systematic review and dose-response meta-analysis of prospective cohort studies. *British Medical Journal, 349*, g4490.

Wansink, B., Just, D., Hanks, A. S., & Smith, L. (2013). Pre-sliced fruit in school cafeterias: Children's selection and intake. *American Journal of Preventive Medicine, 44*, 477–480.
Wansink, B., Just, D., & Smith, L. (2011). What is in a name? Giving descriptive names to vegetables increases lunchroom sales. *Journal of Nutrition Education and Behavior, 43*, S1.
Wansink, B., & Just, D. R. (2016). The limits of defaults: Why french fries trump apple slices. *BMC Research Notes, 9*, 1.
Wansink, B., Just, D. R., Payne, C. R., & Klinger, M. Z. (2012). Attractive names sustain increased vegetable intake in schools. *Preventive Medicine, 55*, 330–332.
Wardle, J., Cooke, L. J., Gibson, E. L., Sapochnik, M., Sheiham, A., & Lawson, M. (2003). Increasing children's acceptance of vegetables; a randomized trial of parent-led exposure. *Appetite, 40*(2), 155–162.
Watanabe, T. (2014, April 1). Solutions sought to reduce food waste at schools. *Los Angeles Times*. Retrieved from http://www.latimes.com/local/la-me-lausd-waste-20140402-story.html
Wengreen, H. J., Madden, G. J., Aguilar, S. S., Smits, R. R., & Jones, B. A. (2013). Incentivizing children's fruit and vegetable consumption: Results of a United States pilot study of the food dudes program. *Journal of Nutrition Education and Behavior, 45*, 54–59.
Whigham, L. D., Valentine, A. R., Johnson, L. K., Zhang, Z., Atkinson, R. L., & Tanumihardjo, S. A. (2012). Increased vegetable and fruit consumption during weight loss effort correlates with increased weight and fat loss. *Nutrition & Diabetes, 2*(10), e48.
Wright, S. M., & Aronne, L. J. (2012). Abdom imaging. *Causes of Obesity, 37*(5), 730–732.
Wright, W., & Rowell, L. (2010). Examining the effect of gardening on vegetable consumption among youth in kindergarten through fifth grade. *Wisconsin Medical Journal, 109*(3), 125.
Zampini, M., & Spence, C. (2004). The role of auditory cues in modulating the perceived crispness and staleness of potato chips. *Journal of Sensory Studies, 19*(5), 347–363.
Zellner, D. A., & Cobuzzi, J. L. (2016). Just dessert: Serving fruit as a separate "dessert" course increases vegetable consumption in a school lunch. *Food Quality and Preference, 48*, 195–198.

Chapter 5
Understanding Social Structural Barriers and Facilitators to Behavioral Change: The Case of Cisgender Women Diagnosed with HIV

Martha E. Lang and Chloe E. Bird

Introduction

Researchers and clinicians have reached a broad consensus that the sooner individuals with the human immunodeficiency virus (HIV) start combination antiretroviral therapy (cART), the more likely they are to remain healthy and avoid transmitting HIV to others (Günthard et al., 2016). Early and consistent treatment also ensures preservation of the immune system and minimizes the risk of other complications of HIV infection. Therefore, the US medical community considers it a best medical practice to place people on cART soon after diagnosis (Günthard et al., 2016; Insight Start Study Group, 2015). However, beginning and remaining on cART requires a wide array of social, medical, structural, and financial supports, to which those individuals vulnerable to HIV infection are also least likely to have access (Adimora & Auerbach, 2010; Messer et al., 2013).

Modern cART effectively preserves the health of people living with HIV (PLHIV) and most cART regimens currently available in the USA are relatively simple with once daily dosing and low pill burdens. However, people newly diagnosed with HIV must still come to terms with having a serious, stigmatizing medical condition which results in ongoing public health surveillance while simultaneously embarking on a lifelong course of medical change. To preserve their health, people with HIV are expected to take daily medication, to remain in medical care for HIV, to get screened and treated for other co-occurring health problems, learn to live with side effects, and to cope with the ongoing stigma associated with

M. E. Lang
Providence College, Providence, RI, USA

C. E. Bird (✉)
RAND Corporation, Santa Monica, CA, USA
e-mail: chloe@rand.org

D. A. Hope, R. A. Bevins (eds.), *Change and Maintaining Change*, Nebraska Symposium on Motivation 65, https://doi.org/10.1007/978-3-319-96920-6_5

the diagnosis. Indeed, although achieving an undetectable viral load[1] is thought to be possible for most who maintain at least 90–95% cART adherence, within the USA only an estimated 30% of people with HIV are in care and virally suppressed. Moreover, among people living with HIV (PLHIV), cisgender women (i.e., individuals assigned a female sex at birth who also identify as female) utilize HIV care more than do cisgender men (i.e., individuals assigned a male sex at birth who also identify as male), yet have lower rates of adherence and viral suppression (Centers for Disease Control and Prevention, 2016c). Furthermore, the life expectancy for cisgender women living with HIV (referred to hereafter as cWLHIV) is at least 5 years less than the life expectancy of cisgender men living with HIV (referred to hereafter as cMLHIV) (Samji et al., 2013), although cisgender women have longer life expectancy than do cisgender men in the general population (Bird & Rieker, 2008).

In particular, cisgender women who are at the margins of society face social, medical, financial, and structural barriers that render them uniquely vulnerable to contracting HIV, and those same barriers impede diagnosis, beginning care, and staying in care. Most interventions to ensure that PLHIV maintain cART adherence and remain in medical care are biomedically focused and therefore centered on individual-level, behavioral-based interventions (Chesney, 2006; Magnus et al., 2013). Yet, there are numerous structural barriers that interfere with individual behaviors. This chapter serves as an introduction to HIV/AIDS epidemiology, treatment, and policy for PLHIV with a specific focus on cWLHIV. In it we utilize a constrained choice approach to systematically examine how decisions made and actions taken at the levels of family, workplace, community, and governmental policy can create barriers to initiating and maintaining cART adherence for PLHIV generally and cWLHIV specifically. While this introduction to cART adherence barriers is primarily focused on the USA, we also use occasional draw on examples from other countries to situate the US epidemic in its international context. The chapter includes the following sections: (1) an exploration of the paradigm of constrained choice and its use as a tool for understanding how decisions made and actions taken at different levels of society can enhance or limit the health and well-being of cWLHIV; (2) a discussion of the current epidemiology of HIV in the USA and how it is impacted by gender, socioeconomic, and racial inequalities; (3) an exploration of the current HIV treatment and population-level cART adherence, how these relate to HIV prevention, and the implications for cWLHIV; (4) an analysis of some of the most common barriers to cART adherence for cWLHIV, and finally a discussion of implications, including how a constrained choice approach can be used to inform future HIV/AIDS policy for cWLHIV.

Transgender women (i.e., individuals assigned a male sex at birth who identify as female) are one of the most profoundly marginalized groups of PLHIV and face

[1]The term *viral load* refers to the amount of HIV virus within the body. The goal of cART is an undetectable viral load. In the USA, this is generally defined as less than 50 copies of the HIV virus per cubic milliliter of blood with current tests which is the goal of cART. The terms *virally suppressed* or *viral suppression* are also used to describe maintenance of an undetectable viral load.

marked disparities in HIV care, support, research, and survival (see Baral et al., 2013; Operario & Nemoto, 2010; Poteat et al., 2015; Reisner et al., 2016). We do not include transgender women in this analysis because the disparities and experiences they face are markedly different from cWLHIV and worthy of their own, separate, in-depth analysis. For similar reasons, we also do not address the experiences of transgender men (i.e., individuals assigned a female sex at birth who identify as male), nonbinary, or genderqueer people living with HIV. Although we have not addressed the experiences of these individuals here, we acknowledge their importance.

Among cWLHIV, the overwhelming majority contract HIV through heterosexual transmission (Centers for Disease Control and Prevention, 2017d). Therefore, cisgender women in this transmission category are the primary focus of this chapter. While those with mental illness are also at increased risk both of HIV and of barriers to care and behavioral change, here we focus on those without mental illness, in part because we want to understand the impacts of policy decisions on individuals' choice and the constraints on their *personal agency*, the capacity of individuals to act on their own behalf and make free choices. We touch only briefly on other transmission categories, such as perinatal transmission and intravenous drug use. Finally, we are indebted to the theoretical paradigm of intersectionality in informing much of our discussion in this chapter. Both constrained choice theory and the work presented here build on the theory and research on how multiple social statuses, particularly gender, race/ethnicity, and socioeconomic status, interact in their influence on men's and women's lives and experiences. However, in contrast to our focus here on cisgender women, a full application of intersectionality would go on to explore the impact of additional social statuses.

Section 1: Constrained Choice

In this section, we address the model of constrained choice and how it can be used to understand the particular health challenges faced by cWLHIV at the individual, family, workplace, community, and governmental policy levels of society.

Health behavior is often perceived as an individual decision or choice. As a result, most models for initial and ongoing engagement of newly diagnosed PLHIV in medical care focus on individual behavior and motivation (Marks, Gardner, Craw, & Crepaz, 2010). However, social structure is an important driver in medical care engagement (Andersen, Davidson, & Baumeister, 2014). As shown in the figure below, the constrained choice model illustrates how decisions made and actions taken at the level of family/work community and government/social policy can either impede or enhance an individual's health status (Bird & Rieker, 2008). Furthermore, this model is helpful in understanding gender differences in health outcomes. The constrained choice model demonstrates the interplay between biological factors and social influences to create burdens to allostatic load. Allostasis is the normal process of activation of the immune, neural, and neuroendocrine systems in response to stress in which each of these systems returns to normal after the stressor is removed or the stressful event passes (McEwen, 1998). However, exposure to repeated or chronic stress can increase allostatic load via the dysregulation of blood pressure, blood lipids, and blood sugar and higher waist to hip ratio (Geronimus, Hicken, Keene, & Bound, 2006, p. 826). At the population level, women and people of color generally have demonstrably higher allostatic loads than men and whites, with black women having the highest (Geronimus et al., 2006; Krieger, 2001). This pattern itself suggests that the larger intersecting forces of sexism and racism directly impact the body (Bird, Lang, & Rieker, 2012). While the impact of allostatic load on the progression of HIV is not well-researched or understood, particularly among women, it is possible that cWLHIV who have health problems or conditions as the result of a high allostatic load will require more complex HIV care. In addition, the stress of living with HIV may add to allostatic load, creating additional health problems that challenge long-term adherence (U.S. Department of Health and Human Services, Health Resources & Services Administration [HRSA], 2014) (Fig. 5.1).

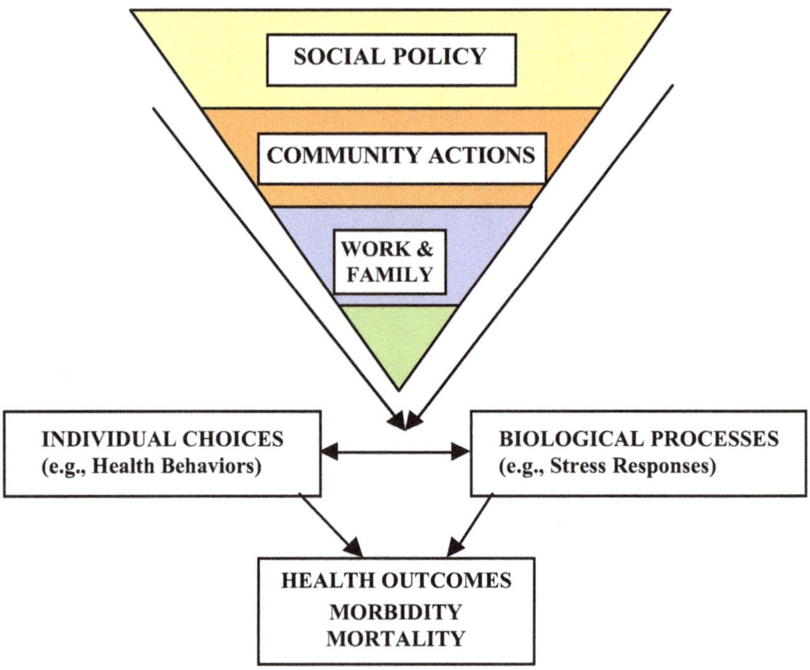

Fig. 5.1 Constrained choice conceptual model. From Bird, C. E., & Rieker, P. P. (2008). *Gender and Health: The Effects of Constrained Choices and Social Policies*. New York, NY: Cambridge University Press

Individual Level

Personal agency directly impacts health (Bird & Rieker, 2008). To address its effects on health, the constrained choice model focuses on individual everyday choices that influence health and the ways in which decisions at the levels of family, work, community, and broader public policy operate to limit or increase the options available and their relative cost or burden to the individual. Personal agency may also be impeded or empowered at times by social position and status including gender, class, race/ethnicity, or sexual orientation and the larger society, state, or community in which the person lives. A particular status may profoundly impact both health and personal status if that status is stigmatized (Bird & Lang, 2014). For example, the stigma surrounding HIV is persistent and well documented (Alonzo & Reynolds, 1995; Earnshaw, Smith, Chaudoir, Amico, & Copenhaver, 2013; Mahajan et al., 2008) as are its negative impacts on timely diagnosis, treatment, cART adherence, and continued engagement in care for cWLHIV. We will address these in greater detail in our discussion of barriers to adherence.

Each day, individuals must balance numerous obligations and priorities and therefore health-based decisions, including but not limited to those regarding smoking, diet, and exercise. For people in good health, most of these decisions may have little or no effect on a day-to-day basis but can yield major cumulative health effects over time (Bird & Lang, 2014). However, people with serious illnesses, such as HIV/AIDS, may not have that luxury and therefore may face significant consequences if unable to continuously balance life obligations with health priorities.

Family Level

Social roles and role expectations create and amplify broader gender patterns in individuals' lives, even within family roles and role expectations contribute to gender differences in stress exposure, related coping mechanisms, and health behaviors (Bird & Lang, 2014). For example, women in the USA and around the world typically do a disproportionate amount of household labor (Ridgeway, 2011), and time spent managing a household is often time taken away from self-care activities such as exercise, sleep, and stress management. For cWLHIV specifically, family can be a source of support in maintaining both health and adherence (Ciambrone, 2003; Kempf et al., 2010). Conversely, some families shun cWLHIV due to stigma, creating both stress and isolation (Carr & Gramling, 2004; Vanable, Carey, Blair, & Littlewood, 2006). The social structural forces that limit a woman's personal agency within her family (i.e., gender inequality and patriarchy) also limit her agency within intimate relationships, increasing risk for HIV and potentially impacting adherence to cART as well (Campbell et al., 2008; Lopez, Jones, Villar-Loubet, Arheart, & Weiss, 2010).

Workplace Level

Gender stratification across occupations contributes to differences in pay and benefits as well as occupational stress (Reskin & Roos, 2009). PLHIV already face multiple physical stressors (Deeks, 2011; Leserman, 2008), and, therefore, occupational stress is even more impactful. For women of color, who are impacted disproportionately by HIV, these stressors can be compounded by issues of institutional and individual racism. Furthermore, women typically receive lower wages than their male colleagues and are more likely to have fewer benefits, including health insurance (Bird & Lang, 2014). Women are less likely to have private insurance than are men and cWLHIV are no exception (Kaiser Family Foundation, 2017). Therefore, they often must rely on public insurance programs such as Medicaid and Ryan White that have variable eligibility requirements across states as well as coverage (Kates & Dawson, 2017). As discussed further below, insurance coverage can affect cART use and adherence.

Community Level

At the community level, constrained choice addresses the impact of local policy and built environment on individual health and the ability of individuals to make healthful choices (Bird & Lang, 2014). While other aspects of society, such as social capital, may also shape individual health, addressing these is markedly different from assessing the impact of written policies and their impact on health. Moreover, policies that affect health are not limited to health policies. For example, condom distribution in schools, restaurants, and/or bars lowers risk of HIV as well as other sexually transmitted infections (Bedimo, Pinkerton, Cohen, Gray, & Farley, 2002; Kirby, 2002). In fact, policies on education, housing, or public safety impact health directly and indirectly, and all of these typically have a local component or authority.

Similarly, state commitments to public health also have direct impact on the health of people with HIV. For example, states that have been included in Medicaid expansion have larger percentages of their HIV-positive populations engaged in care, on cART and with undetectable viral loads and thus have enhanced the health of PLHIV and may have protected the health of the larger population as well (Kates & Dawson, 2017).

Social Policy Level

Social policies at the state and federal level profoundly impact individual health and health decisions and therefore HIV care and cART adherence. For example, comparative cross-national research on the health gradient demonstrates that the US population, regardless of gender, is less healthy than that of other high-income countries with universal coverage (Marmot, 2005). Not surprisingly, in countries with strong commitments to public health such as universal health care coverage, PLHIV generally have higher levels of engagement in their care as well as better health outcomes. For example, Denmark and Great Britain both have universal health care coverage with free cART access and have an estimated 60% and 59%, respectively, of their populations of PLHIV engaged in care and maintaining viral suppression (Raymond, Hill, & Pozniak, 2013). Conversely, in the USA, which lacks universal health care and inconsistent cART access, that percentage is only 30% (Bradley et al., 2014). State commitments to public health also have a direct impact on the health status of PLHIV. For example, states that have adopted Medicaid expansion have larger percentages of their PLHIV engaged in care, on ARVs, and with undetectable viral loads and have thereby enhanced the health of PLHIV and may have protected the health of the larger population as well (Henry J. Kaiser Family Foundation, 2017). Conversely, deficits beyond health care also impact the lives of PLHIV. For example, poverty and housing instability both make cisgender women more vulnerable to contracting HIV (Denning & DiNenno, 2017) and decrease cART adherence for those living with HIV (Riley, Gandhi, Hare, Cohen, & Hwang, 2007). Therefore, federal programs to alleviate poverty, such as Temporary Assistance for Needy Families (TANF) or Supplemental Food Assistance Program (SNAP) , or to ensure housing through the housing choice assistance program also decrease population-level HIV risk and improve the health of cWLHIV.

Section 2: Epidemiology of HIV in the USA

In this section, we begin with a discussion of the biological processes of HIV and AIDS, address general HIV prevalence and incidence, and then move into a more detailed discussion of specific aspects of HIV/AID epidemiology, including race and ethnicity, regional effects, and economic status. Finally, we explore HIV in cisgender women, including incidence, prevalence, biological and social structural risk factors for infection, and gaps in research on cWLHIV.

Biological Processes and Social Epidemiology of HIV and AIDS

HIV, the virus that causes AIDS, attacks both CD4 cells, the white blood cells that control immune system activation and regulation, and other components of the immune system (Whiteside, 2016). If left untreated, HIV lowers the level of CD4 cells until PLHIV progress to AIDS and become increasingly susceptible to AIDS-defining medical conditions; a variety of life threatening bacterial, viral, fungal, and parasitic infections; as well as cancers (Whiteside, 2016). In addition, the amount of HIV in an untreated person's blood, tissues, and organs, commonly referred to as viral load, will increase. Higher viral loads increase associated chronic inflammation and make an individual vulnerable to neurocognitive disorders, cardiovascular disease, and cancers that are not HIV- or AIDS-specific (Deeks, 2011; Hunt, 2012).[2] Without treatment, PLHIV nearly always face dramatic declines in health and develop AIDS, eventually resulting in death.

While the disease process for HIV is largely similar across sexes, there are several distinct differences for cisgender women. At the onset of HIV infection, cWLHIV tend to have lower viral loads and higher CD4 counts than do males even when controlling for age, race, mode of infection, and cART use (Addo & Altfeld, 2014; Donnelly et al., 2005; Gandhi et al., 2002). However, in comparison to males with untreated HIV and similar viral loads, cWLHIV who do not receive treatment show faster disease progression and higher mortality (Curno et al., 2016). Overall, cWLHIV in the USA and Canada have higher mortality and lower life expectancy than do cMLHIV (Health Resources & Services Administration, 2013; Samji et al., 2013; Siddiqi, Hall, Hu, & Song, 2016). However, in other high-income countries, cWLHIV have higher life expectancies than do cMLHIV (Antiretroviral Therapy Cohort Collaboration, 2008).

There are additional medical complications for cWLHIV that are sex specific and require specialized care. These include pelvic inflammatory disease, yeast infections, and invasive cervical cancer, which is an AIDS-defining medical condition (Health Resources & Services Administration, 2013). This form of cancer is caused by human papilloma virus (HPV), a virus that creates elevated cancer risk for numerous populations impacted by HPV (Health Resources & Services Administration, 2013). In cWLHIV, HPV requires continual monitoring through regular gynecological exams, cervical pap smears, anal pap smears, and other medical procedures, creating a greater burden of specialized care (Health Resources & Services Administration, 2013).

Without treatment, AIDS results in death. HIV and AIDS are clearly demarcated in the epidemiological discussion that follows because high AIDS prevalence indicates more people with advanced disease and suggests structural problems with access to care.

General HIV Prevalence and Incidence In 2014 in the USA, an estimated 1.2 million people were living with HIV for a prevalence rate of about 0.45% of the adult population (Centers for Disease Control and Prevention, 2016b). This prevalence rate is defined as a low-level epidemic, at less than 1% of the general population (World Health Organization, 2013). However, in certain geographic regions, such as Washington DC and impoverished areas of other US cities, the rate of HIV in heterosexual populations is 2% or higher, indicating a generalized epidemic by the WHO definition (Denning & DiNenno, 2017; District of Columbia Department of Health HIV/AIDS, Hepatitis, STD, and TB Administration, 2016; World Health Organization, 2013). In 2015, approximately 39,500 people in the USA were diagnosed with HIV and 18,300 with AIDS (Centers for Disease Control and Prevention, 2017f).

[2] Without treatment, PLHIV nearly always face dramatic declines in health and develop AIDS. AIDS is defined by the CDC as having a CD4 count of 200 cells or less per cubic milliliter of blood, an AIDS-defining medical condition, or both (Health Resources & Services Administration, 2014).

Race/Ethnicity and HIV People of color are disproportionately impacted by HIV. Latinos represent 18% of the population but make up 24% of people living with HIV, and African Americans represent 12% of the population but make up 45% of people living with HIV (Centers for Disease Control and Prevention, 2017f). Of those diagnosed with AIDS, 48% were African American and African Americans represented 53% of all deaths from AIDS (Centers for Disease Control and Prevention, 2017a). Among people with HIV, African Americans disproportionately die of HIV. Their age adjusted death rate is 8.3 per 100,000, while for whites it is 1.1 (Centers for Disease Control and Prevention, 2016a).

Region and HIV When AIDS first appeared as a national problem, most cases were concentrated in major urban centers, with especially high rates in the big cities of the Northeast and West Coast. However, increasingly HIV and AIDS are concentrated in the South. Southern states make up only 37% of the national population, yet 44% of all PLHIV live in this region. In 2015, the South accounted for 52% of new AIDS diagnoses with the Northeast, West, and Midwest regions accounting for 18%, 17%, and 12%, respectively (Centers for Disease Control and Prevention, 2016a). Prevalence rates for HIV remain highest in the Northeast followed by the South, the West, and then the Midwest. African Americans are disproportionately affected by HIV in all regions of the country, except for the West, where Latinos have the highest percentage (Centers for Disease Control and Prevention, 2017b). The South also consistently has the lowest rate of linkages to care within 3 months of diagnosis. In 2015, 53% of the deaths directly attributable to HIV/AIDS were located in the South. In fact, in some southern states PLHIV are three times more likely to die compared to PLHIV in all other regions of the USA (Centers for Disease Control and Prevention, 2016a). The CDC also notes that states with the highest death rate among people diagnosed with HIV in 2012 were, respectively, from highest to lowest Louisiana, Delaware, Alabama, Mississippi, and South Carolina. High death rates for HIV suggest a lack of HIV care or unsuccessful linkage to care (Centers for Disease Control and Prevention, 2016d).

Economic Status and HIV Increasingly, economic status is a powerful predictor of HIV status among the urban poor. Denning and DiNenno (2017) surveyed heterosexuals in low-income areas with high HIV prevalence rates of 23 major urban areas of the USA and found that 75% of PLHIV lived at or below the federal poverty threshold and that the lower one's SES the higher the likelihood that one would be HIV positive, regardless of race or ethnicity. In addition, the seroprevalence rate, at 2.1%, constituted a generalized epidemic, on par with Ethiopia, Burundi, and Haiti. Like the generalized epidemic in low-income countries, the percentage of PLWHIV who are women was at 55%. Therefore, it appears that geographic location and poverty in this context are stronger drivers of HIV risk than are individual behaviors. These include the prevalence and incidence of HIV within sexual networks. Sexual networks are social networks of people who are also connected with one another sexually. Individuals' sexual partners tend to be limited to their social networks, which are often based on their geographic location; therefore, having sex in a network with high HIV prevalence already increases risk. Also, for women at risk for HIV, problems associated with poverty, such as housing instability, may result in entry into exchange relationships with men that leave them unable to negotiate condom use and therefore place them at further risk for HIV (Aidala et al., 2016; Riley et al., 2007). Food insecurity, a situation in which an individual or household has limited or uncertain access to adequate nutritious or safe food, can also drive women to enter into exchange relationships that increase HIV risk (Weiser et al., 2011).

Cisgender Women and HIV Worldwide, over half of the people diagnosed with HIV are cisgender women (UNAIDS, 2016). In the USA, about 24% of PLHIV are cisgender women (Centers for Disease Control and Prevention, 2017f). They represent 19% of all new HIV diagnoses, and the vast majority of cisgender women who contract HIV do so through heterosexual intercourse (86%), and a much smaller percentage acquire it through intravenous (IV) drug use (13%). White cWLHIV are disproportionately represented in this population with 32% acquired the virus through IV drug use (Centers for Disease Control and Prevention, 2017f). Women also accounted for 24% of all new AIDS diagnoses in 2015 and make up 19% of all people with AIDS (Centers for Disease Control and Prevention, 2017f). Of the total number of cisgender women diagnosed with HIV in the USA in 2014, 60% were African American, 17% were white, and 17% Latina (Centers for Disease Control and Prevention, 2017d). In recent years, the number of new cases of HIV has seen marked declines in cWLHIV. African-American women have seen the steepest decline in cases since 2005 at 44% with a 25% decline from 2009 to 2014 (Centers for Disease Control and Prevention, 2016d). This has been the fastest decline for any group within that time period, regardless of gender. Despite this, HIV is the fourth leading cause of death for black cisgender women aged 35–44 (Centers for Disease Control and Prevention, 2017g).

For many cWLHIV of childbearing age, a fundamental concern is being able to conceive, carry, and deliver a baby who is HIV negative. Without prenatal care with prophylaxis, the chances of perinatal HIV transmission are around 25%, but with proper, HIV-specific prenatal care, this risk is lowered to less than 1% (Centers for Disease Control and Prevention, 2017c; Townsend et al., 2014). Instances where perinatal transmission did occur indicate larger problems of health disparity. For all cases of perinatal HIV transmission in the USA from 2004–2007, a significant majority of mothers were of low SES, from southern states, and women of color, and fewer than half of the mothers had received prenatal care or cART prophylaxis (Centers for Disease Control and Prevention, 2010; Taylor et al., 2017).

Biological Risk Factors Many studies have documented that cisgender women are more biologically susceptible to HIV infection through heterosexual transmission than are cisgender men, due to the large surface area of the vagina, endocervical vulnerabilities, and generally high levels of immune activation in the female genital tract (Pomerantz et al., 1988; Royce, Seña, Cates, & Cohen, 1997). Moreover, adolescents and younger women whose bodies are still developing are at even higher risk for HIV infection because they are more susceptible to genital injury during heterosexual intercourse (Mojola, 2014).

Social Structural Risk Factors Cisgender heterosexual women also face disproportionate social risk for HIV in comparison to cisgender heterosexual men which is rooted in larger structural inequalities. These limit the decisions and personal agency at multiple levels within the constrained choice framework. For example, within sexual relationships, being able to negotiate condom use in particular is crucial to lowering HIV risk and preventing infection. However, cisgender women are on average at a marked disadvantage due to unequal SES and social power relative to their partner(s). Pulerwitz, Amaro, Jong, Gortmaker, and Rudd (2002) found that women who reported lower levels of social power in their relationships were significantly less likely to insist that their male partners wear condoms. Other researchers have found that women who report domestic violence are also less likely to be able to insist that their male partner(s) wear condoms due to nonconsensual sex and because they fear the violent reprisals that may result (Kalichman, Williams, Cherry, Belcher, & Nachimson, 1998; Swan & O'Connell, 2012).

Beyond individual social power, HIV risk is also shaped by structural factors that deeply and directly shape HIV risk for women of color. Specifically, sexual networks and social contexts have been demonstrated to drive the disproportionate impact of HIV on African-American communities (Adimora, Schoenbach, & Doherty, 2006) especially in the southern USA (Adimora et al., 2006; Adimora, Ramirez, Schoenbach, & Cohen, 2014) and among cisgender women (Adimora, Hughes, et al., 2014; Messer et al., 2013). The reasons for elevated risk within African-American heterosexual sexual networks are complex. The first is geographic, in that many women of color live in areas with high levels of HIV which drives up risk (Adimora et al., 2006; Denning & DiNenno, 2017). In addition, although social norms are changing, people tend to have sexual partners of their same racial/ethnic group, and if HIV occurs disproportionately within that group, risk is disproportionate as well (Adimora et al., 2006; Adimora, Hughes, et al., 2014). Moreover, the number of African-American male sexual partners is limited because of high rates of death due to violence as well as high incarceration rates (Adimora et al., 2006). With smaller numbers of men within the network at any given time, African-American women have limited choices of sexual partners of the same race/ethnicity, and patterns of sexual concurrency emerge, where one man may have several sexual partners at the same time. With this smaller, concurrent sexual network, "bridging," where a sexual partner with other HIV risk behaviors (such as IV drug use or male same-sex partners) can inadvertently expose multiple partners to HIV. PLHIV are most contagious during and immediately after seroconversion (Colfax et al., 2002). Thus, if one partner is in that stage of infection, HIV can be spread easily within the network.

In addition, sexual concurrency leads to the easy spread of sexually transmitted infections, which also increases HIV risk (Adimora, Hughes, et al., 2014). Untreated sexually transmitted infections are quite common in people without access to primary medical care and are even more common among African Americans due to concurrency (Adimora, Hughes, et al., 2014). These infections greatly increase the risk of contracting HIV due to the presence of inflammatory cells susceptible to

HIV and the breakdown of mucosal barriers to HIV infection (Fleming & Wasserheit, 1999). While these networks and their consequences may be complex, they are driven by constrained choice and are the result of state and federal policies that lead to the mass incarceration of men of color as well as a removal of state and federal social safety nets to protect people from poverty and its consequences.

Gaps in Research on cWLHIV In general, women have often been omitted from clinical trials and other forms of research due to the possibility of pregnancy, concerns about hormonal fluctuations invalidating results, and, until recently, a general lack of understanding of the biological differences between men and women (Raz & Miller, 2013). Curno et al. (2016) found that HIV research is no exception. For example, they discovered that women made up a median of 19.2% of subjects in antiretroviral drug (ARV) clinical trials and that the proportion of female subjects in these trials was directly related to private funding with publically funded research having much lower median participation. They also found that women were underrepresented in vaccine studies and HIV cure studies, making up only 38.1% and 11.1%, of research subjects, respectively. In fact, some studies lacked transparency in this regard, in that they did not report the sex of participants, and about 3% of antiretroviral studies and 28% of cure studies reported no female participants (Curno et al., 2016). For PLHIV, the current cART regimens are prescribed in fixed doses regardless of age, weight, or gender. In addition, we do know that many forms of cART have different pharmacokinetic effects on women than men and that in observational studies, women report different and higher rates of side effects (Loutfy et al., 2013).

Section 3: cART, Adherence, and Prevention

In this section, we address the current state of cART treatment recommendations and discuss the concept of treatment as prevention and its implications for PLHIV. We then move into analysis of the treatment cascade, a population-level measure of engagement in HIV care and cART adherence to explore the challenges of treatment as prevention. We also address gender disparities in the treatment cascade and their implications for cWLHIV.

In the mid-1990s, the development of combination antiretroviral therapy, the practice of using three or more ARVs together to treat HIV, revolutionized treatment for HIV and made long-term survival possible for the first time. Prior to this innovation, a hard, painful death from AIDS was the typical illness experience for nearly all PLHIV. To achieve an undetectable viral load, PLHIV must achieve at least 90–95% adherence to their cART (Bangsberg, Ragland, Monk, & Deeks, 2010; Chesney, 2006). Adherence is defined as taking cART at the same time of day, every day.

Current HIV Treatment Recommendations and Treatment as Prevention

The goal of cART is to get PLHIV to an undetectable status and continue to be virally suppressed. Doing so will restore or maintain the immune system and prevent inflammatory damage from HIV. In addition to improving individual health, ongoing, effective cART may have public health benefits as well: If a person achieves and maintains an undetectable viral load, the chances of that person transmitting HIV sexually are extremely low, regardless of the gender or type of sexual act. The PARTNER study, a longitudinal study based in 14 European countries, reports no HIV transmission for serodiscordant couples after approximately 58,000 reported acts of condomless sex (Rodger et al., 2016). A second study, HPTN-052, involving 1763 serodiscordant couples from nine countries on four continents, yielded similar results (Cohen et al., 2016). Many researchers believe that these results could have population-level implications and that if a large enough percentage of PLHIV are engaged in medical care and maintaining an undetectable viral load, the number of new infections will drop, and treatment can be used as prevention (Dieffenbach & Fauci, 2009; Gardner, McLees, Steiner, Del Rio, & Burman, 2011).

HIV activists, physicians, and researchers have recently begun a campaign, "Undetectable = Untransmittable" to educate PLHIV on this research (Prevention Access Campaign, 2017). Activists and medical professionals suggest that this message holds the potential to undo stigma. For example, Dr. Rich Wolitski in the closing plenary for the 2016 United States Conference on AIDS stated, "We are not dirty, we are not a threat, and we are not disease vectors. In fact, we are the solution. People living with HIV who achieve viral suppression, who become undetectable, are the solution to the end of new HIV infections in the United States" (as cited in King, 2016). Activists also offer the promise of condomless sex as an added benefit to maintaining undetectable viral loads (Grindley, 2014; King, 2016). However, this discussion is largely centered in among men who have sex with men. It is unclear how much of an incentive condomless sex may be to cWLHIV to stay in care and adherent to cART.

While these findings may have profound significance for individuals, evidence for population-level success of treatment as prevention is limited: Montaner et al. (2014) reported statistically significant declines in new HIV infections as well as AIDS diagnoses and HIV-related mortality in one province of Canada over a 16-year period. However, some of these declines may reflect improvements in cART and better primary prevention, rather than a direct relationship with treatment as prevention. There is more promising evidence of reduction in the community viral load in San Francisco creating reductions in new HIV infections (Das et al., 2010) and mathematical models (for example, Dodd, Garnett, & Hallett, 2010; Granich, Gilks, Dye, De Cock, & Williams, 2009) also demonstrate the possibility that declines in new HIV infections could occur in populations if enough people are on cART and have undetectable viral loads. However, there is still very limited population-level evidence of the effectiveness of treatment as prevention. One reason for this is the difficulty of engaging and retaining people with HIV in care, as evidenced by the treatment cascade.

Treatment Cascade

A treatment cascade is a paradigm for visualizing engagement in medical care and treatment for a variety of medical conditions including HIV (Gardner et al., 2011). In the USA in 2011, 1.2 million people were living with HIV. Of these, 86% had been diagnosed, 40% were engaged in medical care, 37% were prescribed cART, and 30% achieved an undetectable viral load (Bradley et al., 2014). At each stage of the cascade, the percentage shrinks, and therefore only a fraction of PLHIV have achieved an undetectable viral load. While the relatively low percentage of people at the optimum end of the cascade challenges the larger public health goal of treatment as prevention (Hull, Wu, & Montaner, 2012), it also means that 70% of the population of PLHIV are at risk for health problems associated with untreated or undertreated HIV and AIDS. When considering adherence, of particular concern are those who are "lost to care," people who test positive for HIV and either are never connected to medical care or do not stay in medical care. People in this group have demonstrably higher mortality and worse health. For example, Mugavero et al. (2009) found that patients who missed visits in their first year of care had more than twice the rate of long-term mortality.

Treatment Cascade for cWLHIV According to Bradley et al. (2014), of cWLHIV in the USA, 88% had been diagnosed, 45% engaged in medical care, 41% prescribed ART, and 32% had achieved an undetectable viral load. However, the CDC indicates that while cWLHIV are more likely to know their status and have higher rates of engagement in care, they also are more likely than men to have detectable viral loads and to receive an AIDS diagnosis at the time they are first diagnosed with HIV (Centers for Disease Control and Prevention, 2016c). In addition, cWLHIV are less likely to be prescribed cART and/or prophylaxis for opportunistic infections than are cMLHIV (Agency for Healthcare Research and Quality, 2014a). Indeed, in certain clinical contexts women have lower engagement in care. For example, Mugavero et al. (2009) found that women in a clinical setting in the Deep South were significantly more likely to miss appointments during their first year of HIV care and that these missed visits were a significant predictor of later mortality. Messer et al. (2013) found that women of color faced multiple personal, provider, community, and clinic-level barriers to entry into care.

Adherence and the Treatment Cascade

If a person with HIV is unable to maintain 90% adherence to their medication, their virus may become resistant to one or more ARVs in their cART regimen; resulting in *virologic failure*, a failure of the cART regimen to suppress HIV to undetectable levels. In addition, even PLHIV who are adherent to their medication can develop resistance to cART and virologic failure after taking the regimen for a long time (Clavel & Hance, 2004). However, this form of virologic failure is less likely with modern first line cART (Rocheleau, Brumme, Shoveller, Lima, & Harrigan, 2018). Those who have been on many medications over the long term, the "treatment-experienced" find that they have fewer cART options with each subsequent medication switch. When comparing virologic failure across white, black, and Hispanic women, McFall et al. (2013) found that African-American women were significantly more likely to experience treatment failure than Hispanic and white women and that low annual income was predictive of virologic failure for all three groups.

Section 4: Barriers to cART Adherence for cWLHIV

In this section, we address common barriers to cART adherence. We begin with an examination of medical considerations such as preexisting health problems coping with an HIV diagnosis, starting HIV care, gender differences in responses to treatment and side effects, and anticipating and coping with adverse effects. We close this section with an exploration of treatment fatigue. We then move into discussion of how role conflict as well as unmet basic needs such as housing and adequate food impact cWLHIV adherence. Next, we turn to the psychological issues that impact cART adherence, including trauma, posttraumatic stress disorder (PTSD), stigma, and intimate partner violence. We then address how the payment for HIV treatment and care impacts cART adherence with an examination of pubic insurance programs such as Medicaid and the Ryan White HIV/AIDS program, Private insurance programs and the impact of the Affordable Care Act (ACA), and pharmaceutical company assistance programs. We end with a discussion of the impact of HIV criminalization on cART adherence for PLHIV generally and cWLHIV specifically.

Within the USA, it is recommended that people with HIV begin treatment shortly after diagnosis. There are several reasons for this. Early treatment ensures that immune function will be preserved through maintaining a high CD4 count and limiting other forms of damage that HIV does to the immune system. While doing so may improve their health and potentially prevent transmission of HIV to others, it is a biomedical solution to an epidemic that is driven by social inequalities (Nguyen, Bajos, Dubois-Arber, O'Malley, & Pirkle, 2011). It therefore may be at odds with individual needs or be impractical in consideration of the complexity of psychosocial, biomedical, social structural, and financial needs, which must be addressed in order to ensure that treatment is successful. Indeed, the structural barriers to cWLHIV beginning and staying in care include the same disparities that place them at risk for contracting HIV in the first place. Women with HIV face additional, compound challenges due to intersectional drivers of race, class, and gender. Here are the major areas that are addressed with diagnosis and commencement of HIV cART.

Medical Considerations

Preexisting Health Problems Primary health care provides multiple functions. It allows doctors to detect and treat medical conditions such as high blood pressure, hyperlipidemia, and impaired glucose tolerance before they lead to serious complications such as heart attack, stroke, kidney failure, and type II diabetes (Wilper et al., 2009). Primary care also includes vaccinations for diseases that can damage organ systems, such as hepatitis A and hepatitis B, as well as screening for other infectious diseases and cancer. However, unlike most other high-income countries, the USA does not have universal health care coverage. As a result, large portions of the population forgo primary preventative care, and those who are in poor health have even less access to care as well as increased mortality (Ayanian, Weissman, Schneider, Ginsburg, & Zaslavsky, 2000; Wilper et al., 2009).

Without regular access to primary care, individuals are less likely to be tested for HIV, and early indications of compromised immunity will go undetected. This pattern is particularly pronounced in the southern USA, where black cWLHIV have been disproportionately impacted by HIV (Krawczyk, Funkhouser, Kilby, & Vermund, 2006; Reif, Safley, McAllaster, Wilson, & Whetten, 2017). As a result, people without primary health care access who have undiagnosed HIV will face two likely health challenges when finally diagnosed. The first is that they are more likely to have advanced HIV and may receive a concurrent AIDS diagnosis; the second is that their immune and organ systems will bear greater damage from opportunistic infections and untreated viremia. These may limit their chances of survival, the response of their bodies to cART, and result in a permanently lowered CD4 count (Hall, McDavid, Ling, & Sloggett, 2006; Health Resources & Services Administration, 2014).

Preexisting health problems may limit the types of ARVs available to newly diagnosed PLHIV. For example, Stribild, a single pill combination regimen, must not be initiated in people with low creatinine clearance because of the burden it places on the kidneys (Health Resources & Services Administration, 2014, p. 372). Similarly, Nevirapine, a drug commonly used in low-income countries to prevent mother to child transmission, is contraindicated for people with liver disease or liver damage (Health Resources & Services Administration, 2013). Protease inhibitors, an older class of ARVs with high efficacy, are often contraindicated for people with a history of cardiovascular disease because they tend to cause marked hyperlipidemia (Health Resources & Services Administration, 2013). While it is still possible to find effective cART regimens for people with preexisting health problems, it is less likely that the single pill regimens preferred by both patients and providers for their ease of use will be available to them. Furthermore, their HIV care will likely be more complicated, requiring coordination of care by an infectious disease doctor and one or more specialists, and additional treatments, monitoring, and doctors' visits. All of these factors can make it harder to stay in care and stay adherent.

Coping with an HIV Diagnosis Simply receiving the news that one is HIV positive can be emotionally devastating. Indeed, there is growing evidence that finding out that one has HIV, like other life-threatening diseases, can lead to posttraumatic stress disorder (PTSD) (Kelly et al., 1998; Martin & Kagee, 2011). For example, in a study of women recently diagnosed with HIV in South Africa, Martin and Kagee found that 40% experienced PTSD as a direct result of the diagnosis itself. In their study of men who have sex with men, Kelly and colleagues found that an HIV diagnosis resulted in PTSD for over 30% of their sample. Illness-related PTSD is also reported in cisgender women who have survived other life-threatening illnesses, but the rates are not nearly as high. For example, PTSD in women as a result of breast cancer diagnosis runs at about 4–6% (Andrykowski, Cordova, Studts, & Miller, 1998). One likely reason for the higher incidence of PTSD in cWLHIV is the high level of stigma associated with living with HIV. The shock and grief that many women experience with learning that they are HIV positive must be processed and the diagnosis accepted in order for treatment to be successful (Brezing, Ferrara, & Freudenreich, 2015; Ciambrone, 2003). However, the model of "test and treat" may not necessarily provide clinical space or support for that process.

Beginning HIV Care When a person is newly diagnosed with HIV, a multiplicity of complex processes must take place in order to ensure the success of treatment. A patient in good health and in the early stages of HIV infection will require multiple blood tests, ongoing monitoring by medical providers, self-monitoring, and at least five medical appointments in the first year of treatment (Health Resources & Services Administration, 2014). While the appointment burden is dramatically reduced in the first year of treatment for someone who is in good health, multiple medical appointments with additional specialists will be necessary for someone who is not in good health. Furthermore, treatment of multiple medical conditions increases pill burden which makes adherence more difficult.

Gender Differences in Response to Treatment For adults, HIV medications are prescribed in fixed doses, regardless of age, weight, gender, or other health issues. However, the pharmacokinetics of cART are different for cisgender men and cisgender women, with cisgender women being more likely to encounter toxicity from some cART medications (Floridia, Giuliano, Palmisano, & Vella, 2008; Loutfy et al., 2013).

Side Effects One major reason for lack of adherence is coping with side effects of ART. Side effects can range from transient adjustments when starting ART, ongoing minor side effects that can be managed with appropriate medical and social supports, to major side effects that can be debilitating or even life threatening. The most common side effects found across different ARVs include nausea, gastrointestinal side effects, fatigue, and problems with concentration. Overall, cWLHIV report more side effects than do cMLHIV. This may be the result of women better articulating discomfort. However, clinical evidence indicates that cWLHIV are significantly more likely to have rashes and liver toxicity from medications; lipodystrophy, a disfiguring form of fat redistribution; and hyperlipidemia (Loutfy et al., 2013) than cMLHIV. Experiencing side effects plays a significant role in cWLHIV switching medications, and many choose nonadherence as a way to improve their day-to-day well-being, even if this has negative long-term health consequences (Kempf et al., 2009).

In addition to minor side effects, more serious adverse events can also occur. While these events are less common with newer ARVs, they can still occur and require cWLHIV to be constantly vigilant for signs of emergent issues such as hepatic failure, renal failure, and lactic acidosis (Montessori, Press, Harris, Akagi, & Montaner, 2004).

Serious complications from cART and long-term HIV infection often emerge over time for cWLHIV, which can create new challenges to adherence. Three well-documented conditions of PLHIV are renal disease, bone disease, and cancer. Long-term use of tenofovir disoproxil fumarate (TDF), a nucleoside reverse transcriptase inhibitor, is associated with elevated kidney disease risk.[3] In addition to causing renal issues, TDF can also lower bone mineral density, making PLHIV susceptible to osteopenia and osteoporosis (Yin et al., 2011). Women are already vulnerable to these conditions as they age, which further complicates their treatment and prognosis.

In 2015, Gilead pharmaceuticals released tenofovir alafenamide fumarate (TAF), which delivers the drug more efficiently and safely to the cells and is therefore thought to remove renal and osteoporosis risks. Although TDF is currently being phased out as a form of cART in the USA, it is still used for pre-exposure prophylaxis (PrEP) and continues to impact the health of cWLHIV who have been on it for years, limiting treatment options and complicating adherence.

Additionally, PLHIV are at elevated risk for multiple forms of cancer (Grulich, van Leeuwen, Falster, & Vajdic, 2007), and women with HIV are at increased risk for breast and reproductive organ cancers (Grulich et al., 2007; Loutfy et al., 2013). Cancer treatment makes cART adherence even more difficult because of additional side effects and drug interactions.

Pill Fatigue/Treatment Fatigue People living with HIV who have been on cART for years often report increasing "treatment fatigue," defined by Claborn and colleagues as "decreased desire and motivation to maintain vigilance in adhering to a treatment regimen among patients prescribed long-term protocol" (Claborn, Meier,

---

[3] Scherzer et al. (2012) found that with each additional year of TDF exposure patients faced a 33% increase in chronic kidney disease and that risk of adverse kidney events did not disappear after ceasing TDF use. Cisgender women absorb TDF at higher levels than do cisgender men (Loutfy et al., 2013) which places cWLHIV at particular risk for TDF-associated renal problems (Poizot-Martin et al., 2013).

Miller, & Leffingwell, 2015, p. 255). Treatment fatigue is more likely to occur in PLHIV who have been on cART for a long period of time (Claborn et al., 2015), have to take a high number of pills (Bangsberg et al., 2010), report significant side effects, and/or have other psychosocial stressors (Gay et al., 2011).

Role Conflict

Gendered role expectations that women will serve as primary caregivers within family systems can be a source of stress and may lead to lower adherence to ART; Merenstein et al. (2009) found that the odds of cWLHIV remaining adherent to treatment dropped significantly with increased child care burdens, regardless of the number of other adults living in the household. In qualitative research, cWLHIV report that taking care of children and/or grandchildren was a major and ongoing source of stress (see, for example, Brown, Vanable, Naughton, & Carey, 2015) or a barrier to keeping medical appointments (Kempf et al., 2010).

Basic Needs

Housing The level of regimentation required for cART adherence is difficult for cWLHIV who are homeless or unstably housed (Riley et al., 2007). Furthermore, when people are struggling to meet basic survival needs, medications and medical care become a low priority. For PLHIV, being homeless or unstably housed is a barrier to medical care, medical access, ARV adherence, and viral suppression, and it increases the risk of transmission of HIV to others (Aidala et al., 2016). In the USA, approximately 12% of all PLHIV are homeless or have an unmet housing need (Aidala et al., 2016). Housing Opportunities for People with AIDS is a federal program administered at the state level that provides rental assistance, mortgage assistance, and emergency housing assistance to PLHIV and their families. The program is administered through grants, and therefore the quality and coverage varies widely from state to state and even from county to county.

Food Insecurity Food insecurity is defined in part as "having uncertain or limited availability of nutritionally adequate food or the inability to acquire personally acceptable foods in socially acceptable ways" (Weiser et al., 2011, p. 1729s). Having insufficient nutritional intake is directly related to lowered cART adherence for PLHIV. Indeed, Kalichman and colleagues found that in their sample, food insecurity was the strongest predictor of cART nonadherence (Kalichman et al., 2010, p. 631). In addition to lowered treatment adherence, food insecurity is also associated with lowered CD4 count, wasting, lowered body mass index (BMI), more HIV symptoms, higher viral load, and decreased survival (Kalichman et al., 2010; Weiser et al., 2011).

Psychosocial Issues

Issues of trauma, PTSD, and stigma are consistent and significant barriers to cART adherence for cWLHIV. In this section, we explore trauma incidence, PTSD prevalence, HIV diagnosis resulting in PTSD, stigma, and how these issues combine to create barriers to adherence.

Trauma PLHIV, regardless of gender, report histories of trauma at significantly higher rates than the general population (Brezing et al., 2015; Whetten, Reif, Whetten, & Murphy-McMillan, 2008). Trauma and the PTSD that often accompanies it often lead to anxiety, depression, and other disorders that interfere with staying in HIV care and maintaining cART adherence as well.

Forms of trauma commonly reported by cWLHIV include, but are not limited to, child sexual abuse, child physical abuse, sexual assault, physical assault, and intimate partner violence. CWLHIV report higher rates of past and current trauma than do cMLHIV (Brezing et al., 2015), and these rates remain high, with no statistically significant differences across race or class (Whetten et al., 2008; Wyatt et al., 2002). In their meta-analysis of psychological trauma in HIV-positive women, Machtinger, Wilson, Haberer, and Weiss (2012) found and estimated the rate of lifetime sexual abuse at 61%, which is five times the national prevalence for women and estimated the rate of physical abuse at 72%.

One likely reason for these dramatically elevated rates of trauma in cWLHIV is that a history of trauma leads to risk taking that makes people vulnerable to HIV, regardless of gender. For example, Zierler et al. (1991) found that women and men with a history of childhood sexual abuse had a significantly greater risk for contracting HIV due to increased risk behaviors such as sex work, condomless sex, IV drug use, and use of other drugs as a means of self-medication. Wyatt et al. (2002) found similar behavior patterns among cWLHIV and also found that these led to sexually transmitted infections, which also increase HIV risk.

PTSD Prevalence Overall, women with HIV have higher rates of PTSD than do women in the general population. For example, 30% of cWLHIV report recent PTSD (Brezing et al., 2015) in comparison to about 9% for women in the general population (Kilpatrick et al., 2013). Machtinger et al. (2012) found that the rate of recent PTSD for HIV-positive women is 30%, over five times the rate reported nationally, and a rate of 55% for intimate partner violence, which is twice the national rate.

Stigma From the beginning of the epidemic, high levels of stigma toward PLHIV have been reported consistently across many sectors of society (Alonzo & Reynolds, 1995), although the degree and form of stigma can shift based on gender, race, perceived mode of transmission, and age (Berger, 2010; Mahajan et al., 2008). In Goffman's original typology of stigma (Goffman, 2009), he noted that it could take three distinct forms: (1) defects of the body, such as disability or disease; (2) blemishes of character, such as addiction, sexual orientation, or sexual behavior; (3) and "tribal stigma," based on membership in a marginalized group. It can be argued that HIV/AIDS matches all three of Goffman's criteria and that this is why PLHIV are so profoundly stigmatized (Parker & Aggleton, 2003).

To understand the impact of stigma on PLHIV, it is important to distinguish between stigmatizing actions, such as shunning by family members, refusal of medical providers to give treatment, or rejection by friends and internalized stigma, in which a PLHIV feels ashamed, dirty, or embarrassed because of their seropositive status. Internalized stigma may be the direct result of experience of stigmatizing actions or formed solely on individual reaction to receiving an HIV diagnosis. However, in either circumstance the stigma results from societal perception of PLHIV and in both instances, the results are similar (Darlington & Hutson, 2017; Earnshaw et al., 2013).

Much of the literature on HIV stigma indicates that cWLHIV report more severe reactions to stigma than do cMLHIV (Earnshaw et al., 2013; Sandelowski, Lambe, & Barroso, 2004). This difference may be related to the importance of social support and social networks in women's lives: Vyavaharkar et al. (2010) found that women who had a variety of social supports that they found effective also reported significantly lower levels of stigma and depression. However, this difference may also be explained in part by larger, intersecting social forces of racism, sexism, and misogyny; women with HIV face unique kinds of stigma based on their status as women. Indeed, women with HIV face a form of intersectional stigma in which their previous status as "deviant women" by virtue of intravenous drug use, sexual activity, race, and/or class is profoundly compounded by the additional stigma of being HIV positive (Berger, 2010 pp. 3–4).

Trauma, PTSD, Stigma, and cART Adherence PLHIV, who have PTSD and/or report high levels of stigma also demonstrate higher levels of depression, social isolation, anxiety, and hopelessness (Earnshaw et al., 2013; Machtinger et al., 2012; Vanable et al., 2006). Alcohol, nicotine, and other drug use are common among PLHIV (Kalichman et al., 2013; Lillie-Blanton et al., 2010; O'Cleirigh et al., 2015) and are a form of self-medication for psychological distress from stigma and trauma in this population (Mahajan et al., 2008; O'Cleirigh et al., 2015; Valdiserri, 2002; Vanable et al., 2006).

Psychological distress, stigma, and drug use lower cART adherence in complex and sometimes unexpected ways. For example, it has been well documented that for cWLHIV stigma leads to isolation which leads to a lack of social support which leads to depression and that any of these can lead to women becoming lost to care and/or ceasing to take cART regularly (Puskas et al., 2011). However, it is less apparent that for many stigma also drives nonadherence because PLHIV may not want to take cART in the presence of others for fear of their HIV status being discovered (Bottonari, Safren, McQuaid, Hsiao, & Roberts, 2010). Similarly, it is well documented that alcohol and substance use lower adherence simply because intoxication makes it harder to remember to take ARVs (Malta, Strathdee, Magnanini, & Bastos, 2008). However, it may be less obvious that some PLHIV who drink alcohol intentionally skip or stop taking their ARVs as a form of harm reduction because they mistakenly believe that there is a toxic interaction between ARVs and alcohol (Kalichman et al., 2013). Even nicotine, a substance that has no significant mind-altering effects, is correlated with lower cART adherence, engagement in HIV care, and viremia (O'Cleirigh et al., 2015). CWLHIV with any combination of depression, trauma histories, or internalized stigma also characteristically have low self-esteem (Machtinger et al., 2012; Vanable et al., 2006; Vyavaharkar et al., 2010), which has more insidious effects on day-to-day cART adherence: Ongoing, daily self-care is difficult for individuals who do not value themselves. Additional physiological results of these issues include lowered CD4 counts and increased viral load (Mahajan et al., 2008; Vanable et al., 2006) as well as exacerbation of other stress-related health problems (Bottonari et al., 2010; Earnshaw et al., 2013).

Intimate Partner Violence Women with histories of gender-based violence or intimate partner violence are at greater risk for contracting HIV (Campbell et al., 2008; Wyatt et al., 2002), and studies estimate that between 50% and 75% of cWLHIV have also experienced gender-based violence (Schwartz et al., 2014). A growing body of literature also suggests that cWLHIV are more likely to stay in violent relationships with intimate partners (Lopez et al., 2010; Moreno, 2007) and that being in an actively violent relationship lowers cART adherence. This is due in part to the chaos violent relationships create and use of alcohol and other drugs as a method of coping (Lopez et al., 2010). In addition, economic dependence makes women less likely to leave violent relationships, regardless of their HIV status (Anderson & Saunders, 2003).

Paying for Treatment and Medical Care

HIV care and medications are extremely expensive (Schackman et al., 2006). In 2010, the estimated lifetime cost of care was $379,668, and the monthly costs for medication and care were about $23,000 (Centers for Disease Control and Prevention, 2017e). Consequently, middle- and lower-income individuals with HIV tend to eventually be covered by Medicaid due in large part to the costs of their care. However, the cost savings of providing cART versus allowing people with HIV to go untreated are significant and well documented (Schackman et al., 2006; Walensky, Freedberg, Weinstein, & Paltiel, 2007). Currently, HIV care in the USA is funded through a patchwork of federal and state programs, private insurance, pharmaceutical companies, and private charity. The patchwork pattern itself creates tremendous variability in access to care and coverage for care, such that individuals with HIV can become geographically immobile over time because they cannot relocate to a place that would not provide sufficient coverage. Though not well studied, this pattern likely impacts cisgender women as much or more than cisgender men, in part because women with HIV face additional financial vulnerabilities due to income disparity and insurance disparity. We address here several of the types of care most commonly used by cWLHIV.

Public Programs Most cWLHIV are dependent on public insurance for medical care and/or ART (Henry J. Kaiser Family Foundation, 2016). State funding for HIV care at current levels is insufficient to provide HIV care for everyone who needs it (Snider et al., 2014) and would need to be dramatically expanded to fulfill the goal of starting everyone who tests positive on treatment and keep them in treatment. Insufficient public medical coverage demonstrably lowers both access to care and cART adherence (Reif, Whetten, Lowe, & Ostermann, 2006). We describe here some of the forms of public insurance most commonly used by cWLHIV.

Medicaid and Medicaid Expansion Medicaid currently serves more people than any other public health insurance program in the USA and is the single largest source of insurance for PLHIV, providing insurance to about 40% of that population (Henry J. Kaiser Family Foundation, 2016). This program is financed by federal and state governments and administered by states. Consequently, the breadth and depth of coverage varies widely. Prior to the passage of Medicaid expansion under the ACA, eligibility for Medicaid was determined by meeting two federally mandated criteria: poverty thresholds and categorical eligibility based on membership in an eligible population, for example, pregnant women, children, and the disabled. People who did not meet categorical eligibility did not qualify for Medicaid, regardless of income. However, for states that chose to participate in Medicaid expansion under the ACA, categorical eligibility was dropped, with poverty level remaining the sole qualifying criteria. This made impoverished Americans, including many with HIV, Medicaid eligible for the first time. However, most states that are experiencing the greatest increase in new cases of HIV did not participate in Medicaid expansion under the ACA (Reif et al., 2017).

Impact of Medicaid Expansion on the Health of PLHIV The percentage of PLHIV on Medicaid increased from 36% in 2012 to 42% in 2014 as a result of Medicaid expansion with statistically significant drops in the percentage of cWLHIV who were uninsured (Kates & Dawson, 2017). As a part of the Obama Administration's National HIV/AIDS Strategy (White House Office of National AIDS Policy, 2015), reforms to Medicaid and private insurance under the ACA were coordinated with changes to the Ryan White HIV/AIDS program.

Ryan White HIV/AIDS Program The Ryan White Care Act, passed in 1990 is the single largest public program designed to serve the needs of PLHIV. This program is divided into five parts and has traditionally served as a payer of last resort for those with HIV who are uninsured or underinsured. Part A provides grants for medical and support services to areas that are most severely impacted by HIV. Part B provides grants to states and territories, including funding for the AIDS Drug Assistance Program (ADAP). Part C provides grants to community-based AIDS service organizations and Part D provides primary health care services to women, children, and families while Part F includes dental care and several specialized initiatives (Henry J. Kaiser Family Foundation, 2017). ADAP and Part D are our primary focus.

ADAP provides HIV medications to people living with HIV. It is administered at the state level and the quality of ADAP programs varies widely from state to state (McManus, Engelhard, & Dillingham, 2013). The program is financed with federal funds and states may or may not contribute additional subsidies. As a result, while some states providing a formulary of multiple prescription medications beyond cART and/or subsidize or pay private insurance premiums for PLHIV, others have strict cut off points and provide only a limited formulary of HIV medications (National Association of State AIDS Directors, 2017). In the past, waiting lists for ADAP were not uncommon in some states (McManus et al., 2013). With the National HIV/AIDS Strategy and Affordable Care Act, Ryan White Part D is increasingly used to pay insurance premiums for ACA private plans in place of prescription coverage (Kates & Dawson, 2017; National Association of State AIDS Directors, 2017). As a result, the percentage of cWLHIV in Medicaid expansion states receiving private insurance through Ryan White has increased from 23% in 2012 to 46% in 2014. Provision of full insurance is more cost effective than simply dispensing cART and ensures better care and better continuity of care (National Association of State AIDS Directors, 2017).

Ryan White part D was started initially as a demonstration project in response to increasing cases of pediatric AIDS cases. As this demonstration project developed, it took on a more holistic approach, addressing the health needs of children, youth, and women as well as the family system (Health Resources & Services Administration, 2016). It was only when the Ryan White CARE Act was reauthorized in 1996 that Part D became a regular grant program, like the other parts of Ryan White. Currently, this program funds private and public organizations for outreach, prevention, and provision of specialty medical services (Henry J. Kaiser Family Foundation, 2017). It is the only program that addresses the specific needs of cWLHIV and therefore is most tailored to them. However, this program is vulnerable: for the past several years, the President's budget has called for Part D to be ended and collapsed into Part C, but Congress has not acted on this recommendation (Henry J. Kaiser Family Foundation, 2017).

Moving and Staying in Care on Public Insurance Moving to a different city or state creates additional challenges in that it can impact insurance coverage and can reduce services available due to differences in policies and functions of AIDS service organizations.

Although public insurance used by PLHIV is federally mandated, it is administered by states. When a person moves, they must disenroll from Medicaid in the state they are leaving in order to qualify for Medicaid in the state they are arriving to. This process can take considerable coordination across states and involves transfer of prescriptions, medical records, intake appointments, and establishment of new residency prior to transferring Medicaid coverage. These challenges make cART adherence profoundly challenging.

Private Insurance Currently, more PLHIV are covered by private insurance than any previous time. Prior to the passage of the Health Insurance Portability and

Accountability Act (HIPAA) and the ACA, many PLHIV could not get private insurance coverage due to HIV being treated as a preexisting conditions or prohibitively expensive plans. Often those who could afford insurance found that they quickly exhausted coverage after lifetime caps had been met (Henry J. Kaiser Family Foundation, 2017). Often cWLHIV who had some income found themselves ineligible for Ryan White or Medicaid and either excluded from or unable to afford private health insurance, effectively making them uninsurable (Reif et al., 2006).

The ACA effectively eliminated each of these barriers by removing preexisting condition exclusions, providing subsidies for private insurance plans and removing lifetime limits from insurance policies. As a result, private insurance coverage for people with HIV at 100–138% of the federal poverty line has leapt from 45 to 75% and the percentage covered for those at 139–399% of the poverty line has increased by 12 percentage points (Kates & Dawson, 2017). In addition, it has ensured minimum requirements for preventative care, screening, and pharmaceutical coverage. As a result, private insurance coverage for PLHIV has increased.

In recent years, private insurance companies have placed additional cost containment measures as cART becomes increasingly expensive that inadvertently create adherence barriers. Insurance companies have begun to use mail-order pharmacies for PLHIV as well as for people with other chronic medical conditions that require expensive ongoing pharmaceuticals. Mail-order pharmacies offer assurance to private insurers that they can cut costs by better monitoring patient supplies of medications and improving compliance by monthly checks on patients (Thomas & Pollack, 2015). While this innovation is well-received by some PLHIV, others have found that these pharmacies create additional hurdles to remaining cART adherent, including delays in mailing, signature requirements to receive deliveries, risks of medication being left outside and stolen or damaged by extremes in weather which includes normal summer temperatures in much of the country, and increased risk of disclosure of HIV status based on the delivery or its labeling. In recent years, PLHIV have successfully sued several major insurers, on grounds of violation of privacy rights, via the Employee Retirement Income Security Act, and via the Americans with Disabilities Act (Maas, 2013; McAfee, 2015).

Pharmaceutical Company Assistance Programs Currently, the US pharmaceutical companies provide copay assistance programs for patients with private insurance ARV prescription copays. These programs cover the entire cost of monthly copays for most private insurance plans (Poz, 2017). Those with public insurance are ineligible. Additionally, pharmaceutical companies also provide traditional pharmaceutical patient assistance programs to people who do qualify for public insurance programs and are uninsured or underinsured. It is unclear how much patient assistance programs can be utilized as a safety net because eligibility varies widely from company to company and little data exist on how many people have received assistance and how much assistance was given (Choudhry, Lee, Agnew-Blais, Corcoran, & Shrank, 2009).

HIV Criminalization

Communities create policies that unintentionally impede health and health behaviors and therefore lower HIV care engagement and, as result, cART adherence. For example, 33 states have laws designed to criminalize potential HIV exposure (Lehman et al., 2014, p. 997). Many of these laws include behaviors that pose negligible risk for HIV infection, for example, spitting or mutual masturbation. About half of states have notification laws requiring people who know that they have HIV to inform their sexual partners of their HIV status, and some of these states also require that condoms or other barriers be used when engaged in sexual activity (Lehman et al., 2014). People found guilty of violating these laws face felony convictions in most states, prison sentences, and may be required to register as sex offenders (pp. 1000–1001). The majority of these statutes were enacted in the 1980s and 1990s, with the intention of protecting the public health. At that time, there was no effective treatment; so contracting HIV was viewed by many as a death sentence. Hoppe (2017) argues that creation of these laws was an irrational response to a moral panic. In fact, better scientific understanding of HIV transmission and the development of ARVs that make transmission risk negligible render the premise of these statutes obsolete. They also have an unintended consequence of serving as a disincentive for people to get tested for HIV because of the legally precipitous state created by knowledge of a positive test result (Hoppe, 2017). Indeed, in many communities a common catchphrase, "get tested, get arrested," expresses the deep fear of the legal consequences of knowing one's HIV status (Rodriguez, n.d.). For those who do know their status, disclosure may not protect a PLHIV in states that require an affirmative defense (Lehman et al., 2014, p. 1002). Also, implications for cWLHIV in an abusive relationship are even more concerning because revealing their status may put them at risk for intimate partner violence or abandonment (Ahmed, Hanssens, & Kelly, 2009, p. 129).

Implications

As we have summarized above, the constraints on choice and personal agency that cWLHIV experience, and the extent to which these constraints are in part a function of decisions made above the level of the individual, provides a conceptual framework from which to examine policies and practices and informs efforts to improve care and outcomes of care. Moreover, this approach can facilitate the engagement of a range of decision-makers who shape the opportunity of cWLHIV to pursue a healthy life.

Given that the combination of poverty and severe chronic disease becomes insurmountable, existing programs to mitigate the effects of poverty are especially critical for cWLHIV because of their combination of gender- and health-based financial vulnerabilities. Some of the gaps in survival could be mitigated simply through the continuation or even expansion of federal programs that provide housing subsidies, food subsidies, income assistance, and job training. Research on gender, racial/ethnic, and socioeconomic patterns of HIV, AIDS, and survival among PLHIV can also shed light on the extent and nature of disparities.

Strategies for Removing Structural Barriers to Care

From both an individual and population health perspective, the spread of HIV can be reduced and survival increased by eliminating policies that create disincentives for getting tested and seeking care. Perhaps, most critical are those community-level policies that criminalize sexual behaviors. Both criminal penalties and associated stigma become barriers to prevention and treatment, particularly in light of the possibility of prophylaxis to reduce disease transmission. Pre-exposure prophylaxis (PrEP) is now widely used among white men who have sex with men to prevent HIV infection from an HIV-positive sexual partner or one of uncertain HIV status (Grant et al., 2014). It is increasingly being used by women to safely conceive a child with an HIV-positive male partner and is known as PrEPception (Lampe, Smith, Anderson, Edwards, & Nesheim, 2011). Perhaps, the current key issue at the state level is Medicaid expansion and the percentage of the population who are without insurance, or who are unable to obtain sufficient coverage after receiving an HIV diagnosis. Because women are less likely than men to have private insurance, they are particularly vulnerable to gaps in Medicaid and to programs and policies that limit access to women's reproductive health care. These gaps in women's insurance coverage and access to care limit prevention. Given the high rate of gynecological infections that are often among the earliest signs of HIV infection, these gaps can also delay diagnosis and treatment, which in turn contribute to risk of transmission, poorer disease trajectories, and shorter survival.

A combination of state and federal oversight could prevent private insurance companies from employing cost saving strategies, such as mail-order pharmacies, in ways that block cWLHIV from obtaining and taking their medications. Similarly, systematic analysis could be employed to assess the impact of specific programs on patient adherence and on their quality of life. Such work could be done as part of the Agency for Healthcare Research and Quality's Consumer Assessment of Healthcare Providers and Systems (Agency for Healthcare Research and Quality, 2014b). Additional work is needed to develop policies that can improve the adherence and quality of life for cWLHIV, which could include research comparing the impact of policies that differ across states and municipalities and the extent to which they are associated with positive outcomes for cWLHIV as well as cMLHIV.

One of the clearest barriers currently is the combination of differing public insurance programs and coverage and the requirement to disenroll in one state before enrolling in the next. This is quite distinct from the comparatively seamless program of obtaining a driver's license upon moving to a new state. Currently, in an effort to minimize costs, states and mail-order pharmacies work very hard to avoid paying for an additional supply of medications that would be needed to more easily transition into a new system of care. If a federally based public insurance option were made available to all, this would simplify the process of moving and staying in care. For example, the possibility of expanding Medicare beyond its current populations is gaining increasing attention in political and policy circles (Meyer, 2016; Schoen, Buttorff, Andersen, & Davis, 2015). Barring such a change, a coordinated process by which to transfer coverage from one state to another could address significant barriers to care that limit geographic mobility and increase the risk of a period without coverage or medication. Alternatively, reciprocity between state Medicaid systems could be put in place so that people would be able to stay engaged in care as they moved. The groundwork for such a plan is already in place with Medicaid expansion under ACA.

Conclusion

Summary

The expectations regarding behavioral change for newly diagnosed cWLHIV are both high and wide ranging. Although many of these changes can be expected to improve their health trajectories and survival, the societal expectations stem in large part from the possibility that behavioral change, including medication adherence, can and will improve both their health and their quality of life with HIV. Constrained choice theory speaks to the range of decision-makers above the level of the individual who shape an individual's opportunity to choose a healthy life. In other words, policies and practices constrain the range of options from which one can choose the costs or trade-offs that one faces in making such choices, in this case the choices that support behavioral change, including medication adherence.

As we have shown, whereas the benefits of these changes, including medication adherence, are very high for high SES cisgender men and women, who can in many cases retain their middle class or upper middle class lives, the chances of this long-term benefit for many PLHIV are lower, and a disproportionate share of those for whom the barriers are higher and the benefits likely to be less sustainable are cWLHIV. Specifically, cWLHIV face sex-specific biological risks, complications, and disease trajectories that differ from those of cMLHIV and that have been understudied relative to the experiences of cMLHIV. Consequently, medical knowledge is less extensive and complete for cWLHIV, particularly with regard to their responses to treatment, comorbid conditions, and sex-specific complications of HIV.

In addition, the demographic gender differences in income and access to private insurance that cisgender women experience relative to cisgender men are exacerbated among PLHIV. Thus, many of the social forces and practices that contribute to gender differences in cisgender men's and cisgender women's lives are highlighted among PLHIV. These include the constraints on cisgender women's personal agency to engage only in safe sex and limit their risk of infection, and in some cases on their ability to safely communicate about their HIV status to an abusive partner, even if they are required by law to do so. Similarly, cisgender women may be subject to gendered experiences of stigma related to having an STI. For example, the laws that criminalize sexual behaviors, including those that contribute to transmission risk, do not serve to protect cisgender women from transmission but have been used to prosecute cisgender women of color who give birth to a child with HIV.

A range of state and federal policies, particularly health care policy, disproportionately impact cWLHIV in part because cisgender women are less likely than cisgender men to have private health insurance and more likely to have public insurance. Here, we have focused on the lack of a national system of public health insurance or even a system by which to transfer Medicaid coverage from one state to another, the burdens and complexity of transferring between state Medicaid plans, the risks imposed by specialty mail-order pharmacies as the only access to medications, and the issues that arise when payer of last resort programs like ADAP vary widely from state to state. These gaps impact the lives and potentially contribute to the considerably shorter longevity cWLHIV compared to cMLHIV.

Limitations and Strengths

A fundamental limitation of our work here has been a lack of research that is specific to cWLHIV within the existing literature. As a result, we have often been restricted to reporting the experiences of PLHIV generally rather providing information specific to the experiences of cWLHIV.

We acknowledge the importance of intersectionality in understanding HIV/AIDS among cWLHIV and that while we have included element of this paradigm, we have not systematically incorporated it. As the US epidemic moves further into the twenty-first century, it increasingly becomes an epidemic that lays bare a range of societal inequalities. These inequalities are especially apparent for cisgender women, whose HIV risk, disease trajectory, and cART adherence are driven by larger structural forces of socioeconomic, racial/ethnic, and gender inequality. These are best interrogated through an intersectional lens originally developed by Crenshaw (1989) as tool to explain how the discrimination encountered by black women was based in their unique combined statuses based in gender and race and later expanded by Hill-Collins (2002) to address how each individual's social statuses placed them within the axes of oppression and in the context of a matrix of societal domination and how this shaped individual and collective experience. However, public health statistics as well as much of the biomedical literature tend to treat social statuses as discrete categories (Bowleg, 2008, 2012; Watkins-Hayes, 2014) and therefore limited our ability to integrate our ability to an intersectional approach in this chapter. However, where we have incorporated an intersectional approach, it has demonstrated straightforward, measurable disparities in the preexisting health conditions, care engagement, adherence, and viral suppression for cWLHIV and also indicated the need for more research that incorporates intersectional approaches and methodologies.

Although constrained choice is likely applicable to understanding the experiences of transmen and transwomen living with HIV, we have focused exclusively on the experiences of cWLHIV. However, the range and nature of medical issues for transgender women, transgender men, and nonbinary people are more extensive and more diverse than for cisgender women, in part because there are many more variations in anatomy as well as current and lifetime exposure both to hormones and other biological factors and to gendered life experiences.

Future work is needed to consider the utility of constrained choice in examining the experiences of persons living with other diseases and disorders, including those with and without known sex differences, and in identifying potential intervention points to improve prevention, treatment, and outcomes for women and men.

Balancing these limitations are several strengths. First and foremost, cisgender women make up half of all PLHIV worldwide. Moreover, cWLHIV are disproportionately underrepresented in HIV research (Curno et al., 2016; Loutfy et al., 2013). In part, because the HIV epidemic was initially disproportionately male, research and medical care focused on the needs of cMLHIV. However, the social and biological differences between cisgender men and cisgender women create a range of unique risks for cisgender women, as well as sex and gender differences in exposure to factors that constrain choice contribute to different health needs, and complicate medical treatment and adherence.

References

Addo, M. M., & Altfeld, M. (2014). Sex-based differences in HIV type 1 pathogenesis. *The Journal of Infectious Diseases, 209*(suppl_3), S86–S92.

Adimora, A. A., & Auerbach, J. D. (2010). Structural interventions for HIV prevention in the United States. *Journal of Acquired Immune Deficiency Syndromes (1999), 55*(02), S132.

Adimora, A. A., Hughes, J. P., Wang, J., Haley, D. F., Golin, C. E., Magnus, M., … Mannheimer, S. (2014). Characteristics of multiple and concurrent partnerships among women at high risk for HIV infection. *Journal of Acquired Immune Deficiency Syndromes (1999), 65*(1), 99.

Adimora, A. A., Ramirez, C., Schoenbach, V. J., & Cohen, M. S. (2014). Policies and politics that promote HIV infection in the Southern United States. *AIDS, 28*(10), 1393.

Adimora, A. A., Schoenbach, V. J., & Doherty, I. A. (2006). HIV and African Americans in the southern United States: sexual networks and social context. *Sexually Transmitted Diseases, 33*(7), S39–S45.

Agency for Healthcare Research and Quality. (2014a, May). *2013 national healthcare disparities report.* Retrieved from https://archive.ahrq.gov/research/findings/nhqrdr/nhdr13/index.html

Agency for Healthcare Research and Quality. (2014b, April). *CAHPS: Assessing health care quality from the patient's perspective.* AHRQ Pub. No. 14-P004-EF.

Ahmed, A., Hanssens, C., & Kelly, B. (2009). Protecting HIV-positive women's human rights: Recommendations for the United States National HIV/AIDS Strategy. *Reproductive Health Matters, 17*(34), 127–134.

Aidala, A. A., Wilson, M. G., Shubert, V., Gogolishvili, D., Globerman, J., Rueda, S., … Rourke, S. B. (2016). Housing status, medical care, and health outcomes among people living with HIV/AIDS: A systematic review. *American Journal of Public Health, 106*(1), e1–e23.

Alonzo, A. A., & Reynolds, N. R. (1995). Stigma, HIV and AIDS: An exploration and elaboration of a stigma trajectory. *Social Science & Medicine, 41*(3), 303–315.

Andersen, R. M., Davidson, P. L., & Baumeister, S. E. (2014). Improving access to care. In G. F. Kominski (Ed.), *Changing the US health care system: Key issues in health services policy and management* (pp. 33–68). San Francisco, CA: Jossey-Bass.

Anderson, D. K., & Saunders, D. G. (2003). Leaving an abusive partner: An empirical review of predictors, the process of leaving, and psychological well-being. *Trauma, Violence & Abuse, 4*(2), 163–191.

Andrykowski, M. A., Cordova, M. J., Studts, J. L., & Miller, T. W. (1998). Posttraumatic stress disorder after treatment for breast cancer: Prevalence of diagnosis and use of the PTSD Checklist—Civilian Version (PCL—C) as a screening instrument. *Journal of Consulting and Clinical Psychology, 66*(3), 586–590.

Antiretroviral Therapy Cohort Collaboration. (2008). Life expectancy of individuals on combination antiretroviral therapy in high-income countries: A collaborative analysis of 14 cohort studies. *The Lancet, 372*(9635), 293–299.

Ayanian, J. Z., Weissman, J. S., Schneider, E. C., Ginsburg, J. A., & Zaslavsky, A. M. (2000). Unmet health needs of uninsured adults in the United States. *JAMA, 284*(16), 2061–2069.

Bangsberg, D. R., Ragland, K., Monk, A., & Deeks, S. G. (2010). A single tablet regimen is associated with higher adherence and viral suppression than multiple tablet regimens in HIV+ homeless and marginally housed people. *AIDS, 24*(18), 2835–2840.

Baral, S. D., Poteat, T., Strömdahl, S., Wirtz, A. L., Guadamuz, T. E., & Beyrer, C. (2013). Worldwide burden of HIV in transgender women: A systematic review and meta-analysis. *The Lancet Infectious Diseases, 13*(3), 214–222.

Bedimo, A. L., Pinkerton, S. D., Cohen, D. A., Gray, B., & Farley, T. A. (2002). Condom distribution: A cost–utility analysis. *International Journal of STD & AIDS, 13*(6), 384–392.

Berger, M. T. (2010). *Workable sisterhood: The political journey of stigmatized women with HIV/AIDS*. Princeton, NJ: Princeton University Press.

Bird, C. E., & Lang, M. E. (2014). Gender, health, and constrained choice. In W. C. Cockerham, R. Dingwall, & S. R. Quah (Eds.), *The Wiley Blackwell encyclopedia of health, illness, behavior, and society*. Hoboken, NJ: John Wiley & Sons.

Bird, C. E., Lang, M. E., & Rieker, P. P. (2012). Changing gendered patterns of morbidity and mortality. In E. Kuhlmann & E. Annandale (Eds.), *The Palgrave handbook of gender and healthcare* (pp. 145–161). London, England: Palgrave Macmillan.

Bird, C. E., & Rieker, P. P. (2008). Gender and health: The effects of constrained choices and social policies. New York, NY: Cambridge University Press.

Bottonari, K. A., Safren, S. A., McQuaid, J. R., Hsiao, C. B., & Roberts, J. E. (2010). A longitudinal investigation of the impact of life stress on HIV treatment adherence. *Journal of Behavioral Medicine, 33*(6), 486–495.

Bowleg, L. (2008). When Black+ lesbian+ woman≠ Black lesbian woman: The methodological challenges of qualitative and quantitative intersectionality research. *Sex Roles, 59*(5–6), 312–325.

Bowleg, L. (2012). The problem with the phrase women and minorities: Intersectionality—an important theoretical framework for public health. *American Journal of Public Health, 102*(7), 1267–1273.

Bradley, H., Hall, H. I., Wolitski, R. J., Van Handel, M. M., Stone, A. E., LaFlam, M., … Valleroy, L. A. (2014). Vital signs: HIV diagnosis, care, and treatment among persons living with HIV—United States, 2011. *MMWR. Morbidity and Mortality Weekly Report, 63*(47), 1113–1117.

Brezing, C., Ferrara, M., & Freudenreich, O. (2015). The syndemic illness of HIV and trauma: Implications for a trauma-informed model of care. *Psychosomatics, 56*(2), 107–118.

Brown, J. L., Vanable, P. A., Naughton, J. D., & Carey, M. P. (2015). Identifying HIV-Infected women's psychosocial stressors: Findings from a qualitative study. *Journal of HIV/AIDS & Social Services, 14*(2), 188–205.

Campbell, J. C., Baty, M. L., Ghandour, R. M., Stockman, J. K., Francisco, L., & Wagman, J. (2008). The intersection of intimate partner violence against women and HIV/AIDS: A review. *International Journal of Injury Control and Safety Promotion, 15*(4), 221–231.

Carr, R. L., & Gramling, L. F. (2004). Stigma: A health barrier for women with HIV/AIDS. *Journal of the Association of Nurses in AIDS Care, 15*(5), 30–39.
Centers for Disease Control and Prevention. (2010). Racial/ethnic disparities among children with diagnoses of perinatal HIV infection-34 states, 2004–2007. *MMWR. Morbidity and Mortality Weekly Report, 59*(4), 97.
Centers for Disease Control and Prevention. (2016a, November). *HIV in the United States by geographic distribution*. Retrieved from https://www.cdc.gov/hiv/pdf/statistics/cdc-hiv-geographic-distribution.pdf
Centers for Disease Control and Prevention. (2016b, November). *HIV surveillance report, 2015* (Vol. 27). Retrieved from http://www.cdc.gov/hiv/library/reports/hiv-surveillance.html
Centers for Disease Control and Prevention. (2016c, July). *Monitoring selected national HIV prevention and care objectives by using HIV surveillance data United States and 6 dependent areas, 2014*. Retrieved from https://www.cdc.gov/hiv/pdf/library/reports/surveillance/cdc-hiv-surveillance-supplemental-report-vol-21-4.pdf
Centers for Disease Control and Prevention. (2016d, February). *Trends in HIV diagnoses, 2005–2014*. Retrieved from https://www.cdc.gov/nchhstp/newsroom/docs/factsheets/hiv-data-trends-fact-sheet-508.pdf
Centers for Disease Control and Prevention. (2017a, June 9). *HIV among African-Americans*. Retrieved from https://www.cdc.gov/hiv/group/racialethnic/africanamericans/index.html
Centers for Disease Control and Prevention. (2017b, March 9). *HIV among Hispanics/Latinos*. Retrieved from https://www.cdc.gov/hiv/group/racialethnic/hispaniclatinos/index.html
Centers for Disease Control and Prevention. (2017c, March 10). *HIV among pregnant women, infants, and children*. Retrieved from https://www.cdc.gov/hiv/group/gender/pregnantwomen/index.html
Centers for Disease Control and Prevention. (2017d, March 10). *HIV among women*. Retrieved from https://www.cdc.gov/hiv/group/gender/women/index.html
Centers for Disease Control and Prevention. (2017e, March 8). *HIV cost-effectiveness | guidance | program resources | HIV/AIDS | CDC*. Retrieved July 7, 2017, from https://www.cdc.gov/hiv/programresources/guidance/costeffectiveness/index.html
Centers for Disease Control and Prevention. (2017f, June 8). *HIV in the United States: At a glance*. Retrieved from https://www.cdc.gov/hiv/statistics/overview/ataglance.html
Centers for Disease Control and Prevention. (2017g, January 13). *Leading causes of death in females, 2014 (current listing)*. Retrieved from https://www.cdc.gov/women/lcod/2014/black/index.htm
Chesney, M. A. (2006). The elusive gold standard: Future perspectives for HIV adherence assessment and intervention. *JAIDS Journal of Acquired Immune Deficiency Syndromes, 43*, S149–S155.
Choudhry, N. K., Lee, J. L., Agnew-Blais, J., Corcoran, C., & Shrank, W. H. (2009). Drug company–sponsored patient assistance programs: A viable safety net? *Health Affairs, 28*(3), 827–834.
Ciambrone, D. (2003). *Women's experiences with HIV/AIDS: Mending fractured selves*. Binghamton, NY: Haworth Press.
Claborn, K. R., Meier, E., Miller, M. B., & Leffingwell, T. R. (2015). A systematic review of treatment fatigue among HIV-infected patients prescribed antiretroviral therapy. *Psychology, Health & Medicine, 20*(3), 255–265.
Clavel, F., & Hance, A. J. (2004). HIV drug resistance. *New England Journal of Medicine, 350*(10), 1023–1035.
Cohen, M. S., Chen, Y. Q., McCauley, M., Gamble, T., Hosseinipour, M. C., Kumarasamy, N., … Godbole, S. V. (2016). Antiretroviral therapy for the prevention of HIV-1 transmission. *New England Journal of Medicine, 375*(9), 830–839.
Colfax, G. N., Buchbinder, S. P., Cornelisse, P. G., Vittinghoff, E., Mayer, K., & Celum, C. (2002). Sexual risk behaviors and implications for secondary HIV transmission during and after HIV seroconversion. *AIDS, 16*(11), 1529–1535.

Crenshaw, K. (1989). Demarginalizing the intersection of race and sex: A black feminist critique of antidiscrimination doctrine, feminist theory and antiracist politics. *University of Chicago Legal Forum, 1989*(1), 139–167.

Curno, M. J., Rossi, S., Hodges-Mameletzis, I., Johnston, R., Price, M. A., & Heidari, S. (2016). A systematic review of the inclusion (or exclusion) of women in HIV research: From clinical studies of antiretrovirals and vaccines to cure strategies. *JAIDS Journal of Acquired Immune Deficiency Syndromes, 71*(2), 181–188.

Darlington, C. K., & Hutson, S. P. (2017). Understanding HIV-related stigma among women in the Southern United States: A literature review. *AIDS and Behavior, 21*(1), 12–26.

Das, M., Chu, P. L., Santos, G. M., Scheer, S., Vittinghoff, E., McFarland, W., & Colfax, G. N. (2010). Decreases in community viral load are accompanied by reductions in new HIV infections in San Francisco. *PLoS One, 5*(6), 1–9. https://doi.org/10.1371/journal.pone.0011068

Deeks, S. G. (2011). HIV infection, inflammation, immunosenescence, and aging. *Annual Review of Medicine, 62*, 141–155.

Denning, P., & DiNenno, E. (2017, May 17). *Communities in crisis: Is there a generalized HIV epidemic in impoverished urban areas of the United States?* Retrieved from https://www.cdc.gov/hiv/group/poverty.html

Dieffenbach, C. W., & Fauci, A. S. (2009). Universal voluntary testing and treatment for prevention of HIV transmission. *JAMA, 301*(22), 2380–2382.

District of Columbia Department of Health HIV/AIDS, Hepatitis, STD, and TB Administration. (2016). *Annual epidemiology & surveillance report: Surveillance data through December 2015*. Retrieved from https://doh.dc.gov/sites/default/files/dc/sites/doh/publication/attachments/2016%20HAHSTA%20Annual%20Epi%20&%20Surv%20Report%20final.pdf

Dodd, P. J., Garnett, G. P., & Hallett, T. B. (2010). Examining the promise of HIV elimination by 'test and treat' in hyper-endemic settings. *AIDS, 24*(5), 729.

Donnelly, C. A., Bartley, L. M., Ghani, A. C., Le Fevre, A. M., Kwong, G. P., Cowling, B. J., … Anderson, R. M. (2005). Gender difference in HIV-1 RNA viral loads. *HIV Medicine, 6*(3), 170–178.

Earnshaw, V. A., Smith, L. R., Chaudoir, S. R., Amico, K. R., & Copenhaver, M. M. (2013). HIV stigma mechanisms and well-being among PLWH: A test of the HIV stigma framework. *AIDS and Behavior, 17*(5), 1785–1795.

Fleming, D. T., & Wasserheit, J. N. (1999). From epidemiological synergy to public health policy and practice: The contribution of other sexually transmitted diseases to sexual transmission of HIV infection. *Sexually Transmitted Infections, 75*(1), 3–17.

Floridia, M., Giuliano, M., Palmisano, L., & Vella, S. (2008). Gender differences in the treatment of HIV infection. *Pharmacological Research, 58*(3), 173–182.

Gandhi, M., Bacchetti, P., Miotti, P., Quinn, T. C., Veronese, F., & Greenblatt, R. M. (2002). Does patient sex affect human immunodeficiency virus levels? *Clinical Infectious Diseases, 35*(3), 313–322.

Gardner, E. M., McLees, M. P., Steiner, J. F., Del Rio, C., & Burman, W. J. (2011). The spectrum of engagement in HIV care and its relevance to test-and-treat strategies for prevention of HIV infection. *Clinical Infectious Diseases, 52*(6), 793–800.

Gay, C., Portillo, C. J., Kelly, R., Coggins, T., Davis, H., Aouizerat, B. E., … Lee, K. A. (2011). Self-reported medication adherence and symptom experience in adults with HIV. *Journal of the Association of Nurses in AIDS Care, 22*(4), 257–268.

Geronimus, A. T., Hicken, M., Keene, D., & Bound, J. (2006). "Weathering" and age patterns of allostatic load scores among blacks and whites in the United States. *American Journal of Public Health, 96*(5), 826–833.

Goffman, E. (2009). *Stigma: Notes on the management of spoiled identity*. New York, NY: Simon and Schuster.

Granich, R. M., Gilks, C. F., Dye, C., De Cock, K. M., & Williams, B. G. (2009). Universal voluntary HIV testing with immediate antiretroviral therapy as a strategy for elimination of HIV transmission: A mathematical model. *The Lancet, 373*(9657), 48–57.

Grant, R. M., Anderson, P. L., McMahan, V., Liu, A., Amico, K. R., Mehrotra, M., … Buchbinder, S. (2014). Uptake of pre-exposure prophylaxis, sexual practices, and HIV incidence in men and transgender women who have sex with men: A cohort study. *The Lancet Infectious Diseases, 14*(9), 820–829.

Grindley, L. (2014, September 15). *Is undetectable the new safe sex?* Retrieved from https://www.hivplusmag.com/sex-dating/2014/09/15/undetectable-new-safe-sex

Grulich, A. E., van Leeuwen, M. T., Falster, M. O., & Vajdic, C. M. (2007). Incidence of cancers in people with HIV/AIDS compared with immunosuppressed transplant recipients: A meta-analysis. *The Lancet, 370*(9581), 59–67.

Günthard, H. F., Saag, M. S., Benson, C. A., Del Rio, C., Eron, J. J., Gallant, J. E., & Gandhi, R. T. (2016). Antiretroviral drugs for treatment and prevention of HIV infection in adults: 2016 recommendations of the International Antiviral Society—USA panel. *JAMA, 316*(2), 191–210.

Hall, H. I., McDavid, K., Ling, Q., & Sloggett, A. (2006). Determinants of progression to AIDS or death after HIV diagnosis, United States, 1996 to 2001. *Annals of Epidemiology, 16*(11), 824–833.

Health Resources & Services Administration. (2013). *A guide to the clinical care of women with HIV, 2013 edition.* Retrieved from https://hab.hrsa.gov/sites/default/files/hab/clinical-quality-management/womenwithAIDS.pdf

Health Resources & Services Administration. (2014). *Guide for HIV/AIDS clinical care, 2014.* Retrieved from https://hab.hrsa.gov/sites/default/files/hab/clinical-quality-management/2014guide.pdf

Health Resources & Services Administration. (2016, November). *Part D: A living history.* Retrieved from https://hab.hrsa.gov/livinghistory/programs/Part-D.htm

Henry J. Kaiser Family Foundation. (2016, October). *Medicaid and HIV fact sheet.* Retrieved from http://files.kff.org/attachment/Fact-Sheet-Medicaid-and-HIV

Henry J. Kaiser Family Foundation. (2017, February 1). *The Ryan White HIV/AIDS program: The basics.* Retrieved from http://www.kff.org/hivaids/fact-sheet/the-ryan-white-hivaids-program-the-basics/

Hill-Collins, P. (2002). *Black feminist thought: Knowledge, consciousness, and the politics of empowerment.* New York, NY: Routledge.

Hoppe, T. (2017). *Punishing disease: HIV and the criminalization of sickness.* Oakland, CA: University of California Press.

Hull, M. W., Wu, Z., & Montaner, J. S. (2012). Optimizing the engagement of care cascade: A critical step to maximize the impact of HIV treatment as prevention. *Current Opinion in HIV and AIDS, 7*(6), 579–586.

Hunt, P. W. (2012). HIV and inflammation: Mechanisms and consequences. *Current HIV/AIDS Reports, 9*(2), 139–147.

Insight Start Study Group. (2015). Initiation of antiretroviral therapy in early asymptomatic HIV infection. *The New England Journal of Medicine, 373*, 795–807.

Kaiser Family Foundation. (2017). *Women's health insurance coverage* [fact sheet]. Retrieved from https://www.kff.org/womens-health-policy/fact-sheet/womens-health-insurance-coverage-fact-sheet/

Kalichman, S. C., Cherry, C., Amaral, C., White, D., Kalichman, M. O., Pope, H., … Macy, R. (2010). Health and treatment implications of food insufficiency among people living with HIV/AIDS, Atlanta, Georgia. *Journal of Urban Health, 87*(4), 631–641.

Kalichman, S. C., Grebler, T., Amaral, C. M., McNerey, M., White, D., Kalichman, M. O., … Eaton, L. (2013). Intentional non-adherence to medications among HIV positive alcohol drinkers: Prospective study of interactive toxicity beliefs. *Journal of General Internal Medicine, 28*(3), 399–405.

Kalichman, S. C., Williams, E. A., Cherry, C., Belcher, L., & Nachimson, D. (1998). Sexual coercion, domestic violence, and negotiating condom use among low-income African American women. *Journal of Women's Health, 7*(3), 371–378.

Kates, J., & Dawson, L. (2017, February 14). *Insurance coverage changes for people with HIV under the ACA.* Henry J. Kaiser Family Foundation. Retrieved from http://files.kff.org/attachment/Data-Note-Insurance-Coverage-Changes-for-People-with-HIV-Under-the-ACA

Kelly, B., Raphael, B., Judd, F., Perdices, M., Kernutt, G., Burnett, P., … Burrows, G. (1998). Posttraumatic stress disorder in response to HIV infection. *General Hospital Psychiatry, 20*(6), 345–352.

Kempf, M. C., McLeod, J., Boehme, A. K., Walcott, M. W., Wright, L., Seal, P., … Moneyham, L. (2010). A qualitative study of the barriers and facilitators to retention-in-care among HIV-positive women in the rural southeastern United States: Implications for targeted interventions. *AIDS Patient Care and STDs, 24*(8), 515–520.

Kempf, M. C., Pisu, M., Dumcheva, A., Westfall, A. O., Kilby, J. M., & Saag, M. S. (2009). Gender differences in discontinuation of antiretroviral treatment regimens. *Journal of Acquired Immune Deficiency Syndromes (1999), 52*(3), 336–341.

Kilpatrick, D. G., Resnick, H. S., Milanak, M. E., Miller, M. W., Keyes, K. M., & Friedman, M. J. (2013). National estimates of exposure to traumatic events and PTSD prevalence using DSM-IV and DSM-5 criteria. *Journal of Traumatic Stress, 26*(5), 537–547.

King, M. S. (2016). *Five reasons 'HIV undetectable' must equal 'untransmittable'*. Retrieved from http://marksking.com/my-fabulous-disease/five-reasons-hiv-undetectable-must-equal-untransmittable/

Kirby, D. (2002). The impact of schools and school programs upon adolescent sexual behavior. *Journal of Sex Research, 39*(1), 27–33.

Krawczyk, C. S., Funkhouser, E., Kilby, J. M., & Vermund, S. H. (2006). Delayed access to HIV diagnosis and care: Special concerns for the Southern United States. *AIDS Care, 18*(S1), 35–44.

Krieger, N. (2001). Theories for social epidemiology in the 21st century: An ecosocial perspective. *International Journal of Epidemiology, 30*(4), 668–677.

Lampe, M. A., Smith, D. K., Anderson, G. J., Edwards, A. E., & Nesheim, S. R. (2011). Achieving safe conception in HIV-discordant couples: The potential role of oral preexposure prophylaxis (PrEP) in the United States. *American Journal of Obstetrics and Gynecology, 204*(6), 488. e1–8.

Lehman, J. S., Carr, M. H., Nichol, A. J., Ruisanchez, A., Knight, D. W., Langford, A. E., … Mermin, J. H. (2014). Prevalence and public health implications of state laws that criminalize potential HIV exposure in the United States. *AIDS and Behavior, 18*(6), 997–1006.

Leserman, J. (2008). Role of depression, stress, and trauma in HIV disease progression. *Psychosomatic Medicine, 70*(5), 539–545.

Lillie-Blanton, M., Stone, V. E., Snow Jones, A., Levi, J., Golub, E. T., Cohen, M. H., … Wilson, T. E. (2010). Association of race, substance abuse, and health insurance coverage with use of highly active antiretroviral therapy among HIV-infected women, 2005. *American Journal of Public Health, 100*(8), 1493–1499.

Lopez, E. J., Jones, D. L., Villar-Loubet, O. M., Arheart, K. L., & Weiss, S. M. (2010). Violence, coping, and consistent medication adherence in HIV-positive couples. *AIDS Education and Prevention, 22*(1), 61–68.

Loutfy, M. R., Sherr, L., Sonnenberg-Schwan, U., Walmsley, S. L., Johnson, M., & Monforte, A. D. A. (2013). Caring for women living with HIV: Gaps in the evidence. *Journal of the International AIDS Society, 16*(1), 1–14. https://doi.org/10.7448/IAS.16.1.18509

Maas, A. (2013, June). *Anthem settles suit over mandatory mail order for HIV/AIDS drugs*. AIS Health. Retrieved from https://aishealth.com/archive/nspn0613-06

Machtinger, E. L., Wilson, T. C., Haberer, J. E., & Weiss, D. S. (2012). Psychological trauma and PTSD in HIV-positive women: A meta-analysis. *AIDS and Behavior, 16*(8), 2091–2100.

Magnus, M., Herwehe, J., Murtaza-Rossini, M., Reine, P., Cuffie, D., Gruber, D., & Kaiser, M. (2013). Linking and retaining HIV patients in care: The importance of provider attitudes and behaviors. *AIDS Patient Care and STDs, 27*(5), 297–303.

Mahajan, A. P., Sayles, J. N., Patel, V. A., Remien, R. H., Ortiz, D., Szekeres, G., & Coates, T. J. (2008). Stigma in the HIV/AIDS epidemic: A review of the literature and recommendations for the way forward. *AIDS, 22*(Suppl 2), S67–S79.

Malta, M., Strathdee, S. A., Magnanini, M. M., & Bastos, F. I. (2008). Adherence to antiretroviral therapy for human immunodeficiency virus/acquired immune deficiency syndrome among drug users: A systematic review. *Addiction, 103*(8), 1242–1257.

Marks, G., Gardner, L. I., Craw, J., & Crepaz, N. (2010). Entry and retention in medical care among HIV-diagnosed persons: A meta-analysis. *AIDS, 24*(17), 2665–2678.
Marmot, M. (2005). Social determinants of health inequalities. *The Lancet, 365*(9464), 1099–1104.
Martin, L., & Kagee, A. (2011). Lifetime and HIV-related PTSD among persons recently diagnosed with HIV. *AIDS and Behavior, 15*(1), 125–131.
McAfee, D. (2015, March 30). *United, HIV/AIDS patients settle mail-order drug dispute law 360.* Ret1rieved from https://www.law360.com/articles/520419/united-hiv-AIDS-patients-settle-mail-order-drug-dispute
McEwen, B. S. (1998). Stress, adaptation, and disease: Allostasis and allostatic load. *Annals of the New York Academy of Sciences, 840*(1), 33–44.
McFall, A. M., Dowdy, D. W., Zelaya, C. E., Murphy, K., Wilson, T. E., Young, M. A., … Althoff, K. N. (2013). Understanding the disparity: Predictors of virologic failure in women using highly active antiretroviral therapy vary by race and/or ethnicity. *Journal of Acquired Immune Deficiency Syndromes (1999), 64*(3), 289–298.
McManus, K. A., Engelhard, C. L., & Dillingham, R. (2013). Current challenges to the United States' AIDS drug assistance program and possible implications of the Affordable Care Act. *AIDS Research and Treatment, 2013*, 1–7. https://doi.org/10.1155/2013/350169
Merenstein, D., Schneider, M. F., Cox, C., Schwartz, R., Weber, K., Robison, E., … Plankey, M. W. (2009). Association of child care burden and household composition with adherence to highly active antiretroviral therapy in the women's interagency HIV study. *AIDS Patient Care and STDs, 23*(4), 289–296.
Messer, L. C., Quinlivan, E. B., Parnell, H., Roytburd, K., Adimora, A. A., Bowditch, N., & DeSousa, N. (2013). Barriers and facilitators to testing, treatment entry, and engagement in care by HIV-positive women of color. *AIDS Patient Care and STDs, 27*(7), 398–407.
Meyer, H. (2016). Clinton's Medicare buy-in concept revives debate on public option. *Modern Healthcare, 46*(20), 10–11.
Mojola, S. A. (2014). *Love, money, and HIV: Becoming a modern African woman in the age of AIDS*. Oakland, CA: University of California Press.
Montaner, J. S., Lima, V. D., Harrigan, P. R., Lourenço, L., Yip, B., Nosyk, B., … Hogg, R. S. (2014). Expansion of HAART coverage is associated with sustained decreases in HIV/AIDS morbidity, mortality and HIV transmission: The "HIV Treatment as Prevention" experience in a Canadian setting. *PLoS One, 9*(2), 1–10. https://doi.org/10.1371/journal.pone.0087872
Montessori, V., Press, N., Harris, M., Akagi, L., & Montaner, J. S. (2004). Adverse effects of antiretroviral therapy for HIV infection. *Canadian Medical Association Journal, 170*(2), 229–238.
Moreno, C. L. (2007). The relationship between culture, gender, structural factors, trauma, and HIV/AIDS for Latinas. *Qualitative Health Research, 17*(3), 340–352.
Mugavero, M. J., Lin, H. Y., Willig, J. H., Westfall, A. O., Ulett, K. B., Routman, J. S., … Allison, J. J. (2009). Missed visits and mortality among patients establishing initial outpatient HIV treatment. *Clinical Infectious Diseases, 48*(2), 248–256.
National Association of State AIDS Directors. (2017). *National ADAP monitoring: 2017 annual report.* Retrieved from https://www.nastad.org/sites/default/files/nas001_report_v4_spreads-new3.pdf
Nguyen, V. K., Bajos, N., Dubois-Arber, F., O'Malley, J., & Pirkle, C. M. (2011). Remedicalizing an epidemic: From HIV treatment as prevention to HIV treatment is prevention. *AIDS, 25*(3), 291–293.
O'Cleirigh, C., Valentine, S. E., Pinkston, M., Herman, D., Bedoya, C. A., Gordon, J. R., & Safren, S. A. (2015). The unique challenges facing HIV-positive patients who smoke cigarettes: HIV viremia, ART adherence, engagement in HIV care, and concurrent substance use. *AIDS and Behavior, 19*(1), 178–185.
Operario, D., & Nemoto, T. (2010). HIV in transgender communities: Syndemic dynamics and a need for multicomponent interventions. *Journal of Acquired Immune Deficiency Syndromes (1999), 55*(Suppl 2), S91–S93.
Parker, R., & Aggleton, P. (2003). HIV and AIDS-related stigma and discrimination: A conceptual framework and implications for action. *Social Science & Medicine, 57*(1), 13–24.

Poizot-Martin, I., Solas, C., Allemand, J., Obry-Roguet, V., Pradel, V., Bregigeon, S., … Lacarelle, B. (2013). Renal impairment in patients receiving a tenofovir-cART regimen: Impact of tenofovir trough concentration. *Journal of Acquired Immune Deficiency Syndromes, 62*(4), 375–380.

Pomerantz, R. J., de la Monte, S. M., Donegan, S. P., Rota, T. R., Vogt, M. W., Craven, D. E., & Hirsch, M. S. (1988). Human immunodeficiency virus (HIV) infection of the uterine cervix. *Annals of Internal Medicine, 108*(3), 321–327.

Poteat, T., Wirtz, A. L., Radix, A., Borquez, A., Silva-Santisteban, A., Deutsch, M. B., … Operario, D. (2015). HIV risk and preventive interventions in transgender women sex workers. *The Lancet, 385*(9964), 274–286.

Poz. (2017, May 31). *HIV drug assistance programs*. Retrieved from https://www.poz.com/basics/hiv-basics/drug-assistance-programs

Prevention Access Campaign. (2017, July 6). *Consensus statement*. Retrieved from https://www.preventionaccess.org/consensus

Pulerwitz, J., Amaro, H., Jong, W. D., Gortmaker, S. L., & Rudd, R. (2002). Relationship power, condom use and HIV risk among women in the USA. *AIDS Care, 14*(6), 789–800.

Puskas, C. M., Forrest, J. I., Parashar, S., Salters, K. A., Cescon, A. M., Kaida, A., … Hogg, R. S. (2011). Women and vulnerability to HAART non-adherence: A literature review of treatment adherence by gender from 2000 to 2011. *Current HIV/AIDS Reports, 8*(4), 277.

Raymond, A., Hill, A., & Pozniak, A. (2013). Large disparities in HIV treatment cascades between eight European and high-income countries-analysis of break points. *Journal of the International AIDS Society, 17*(4 Suppl 3), 1–2. https://doi.org/10.7448/IAS.17.4.19507

Raz, L., & Miller, V. M. (2013). Considerations of sex and gender differences in preclinical and clinical trials. In V. Regitz-Zagrosek (Ed.), *Sex and gender differences in pharmacology* (pp. 127–147). New York, NY: Springer.

Reif, S., Safley, D., McAllaster, C., Wilson, E., & Whetten, K. (2017). State of HIV in the US deep South. *Journal of Community Health, 47*(1), 1–10.

Reif, S., Whetten, K., Lowe, K., & Ostermann, J. (2006). Association of unmet needs for support services with medication use and adherence among HIV-infected individuals in the southeastern United States. *AIDS Care, 18*(4), 277–283.

Reisner, S. L., Poteat, T., Keatley, J., Cabral, M., Mothopeng, T., Dunham, E., … Baral, S. D. (2016). Global health burden and needs of transgender populations: A review. *The Lancet, 388*(10042), 412–436.

Reskin, B. F., & Roos, P. A. (2009). *Job queues, gender queues: Explaining women's inroads into male occupations*. Philadelphia, PA: Temple University Press.

Ridgeway, C. L. (2011). *Framed by gender: How gender inequality persists in the modern world.* New York, NY: Oxford University Press.

Riley, E. D., Gandhi, M., Hare, C. B., Cohen, J., & Hwang, S. W. (2007). Poverty, unstable housing, and HIV infection among women living in the United States. *Current HIV/AIDS Reports, 4*(4), 181–186.

Rocheleau, G., Brumme, C. J., Shoveller, J., Lima, V. D., & Harrigan, P. R. (2018). Longitudinal trends of HIV drug resistance in a large Canadian cohort, 1996–2016. *Clinical Microbiology and Infection, 24*(2), 185–191.

Rodger, A. J., Cambiano, V., Bruun, T., Vernazza, P., Collins, S., Van Lunzen, J., … Asboe, D. (2016). Sexual activity without condoms and risk of HIV transmission in serodifferent couples when the HIV-positive partner is using suppressive antiretroviral therapy. *JAMA, 316*(2), 171–181.

Rodriguez, C. (n.d.). *Living with HIV: The choices and consequences of disclosure*. The Center for HIV Law and Policy. Retrieved from https://www.hivlawandpolicy.org/fine-print-blog/living-hiv-choices-and-consequences-disclosure

Royce, R. A., Seña, A., Cates, W., Jr., & Cohen, M. S. (1997). Sexual transmission of HIV. *New England Journal of Medicine, 336*(15), 1072–1078.

Samji, H., Cescon, A., Hogg, R. S., Modur, S. P., Althoff, K. N., Buchacz, K., … Justice, A. (2013). Closing the gap: Increases in life expectancy among treated HIV-positive individuals in the United States and Canada. *PLoS One, 8*(12), 1–8. https://doi.org/10.1371/journal.pone.0081355

Sandelowski, M., Lambe, C., & Barroso, J. (2004). Stigma in HIV-positive women. *Journal of Nursing Scholarship, 36*(2), 122–128.
Schackman, B. R., Gebo, K. A., Walensky, R. P., Losina, E., Muccio, T., Sax, P. E., … Freedbeerg, K. A. (2006). The lifetime cost of current human immunodeficiency virus care in the United States. *Medical Care, 44*(11), 990–997.
Scherzer, R., Estrella, M., Yongmei, L. I., Deeks, S. G., Grunfeld, C., & Shlipak, M. G. (2012). Association of tenofovir exposure with kidney disease risk in HIV infection. *AIDS, 26*(7), 867–875.
Schoen, C., Buttorff, C., Andersen, M., & Davis, K. (2015). Policy options to expand Medicare's low-income provisions to improve access and affordability. *Health Affairs, 34*(12), 2086–2094.
Schwartz, R. M., Weber, K. M., Schechter, G. E., Connors, N. C., Gousse, Y., Young, M. A., & Cohen, M. H. (2014). Psychosocial correlates of gender-based violence among HIV-infected and HIV-uninfected women in three US cities. *AIDS Patient Care and STDs, 28*(5), 260–267.
Siddiqi, A. E., Hall, H. I., Hu, X., & Song, R. (2016). Population-based estimates of life expectancy after HIV diagnosis: United States 2008–2011. *Journal of Acquired Immune Deficiency Syndromes, 72*(2), 230–236.
Snider, J. T., Juday, T., Romley, J. A., Seekins, D., Rosenblatt, L., Sanchez, Y., & Goldman, D. P. (2014). Nearly 60,000 uninsured and low-income people with HIV/AIDS live in states that are not expanding Medicaid. *Health Affairs, 33*(3), 386–393.
Swan, H., & O'Connell, D. J. (2012). The impact of intimate partner violence on women's condom negotiation efficacy. *Journal of Interpersonal Violence, 27*(4), 775–792.
Taylor, A. W., Nesheim, S. R., Zhang, X., Song, R., FitzHarris, L. F., Lampe, M. A., … Sweeney, P. (2017). Estimated perinatal HIV infection among infants born in the United States, 2002–2013. *JAMA Pediatrics, 171*(5), 435–442.
Thomas, K., & Pollack, A. (2015, July 15). Specialty pharmacies proliferate, along with questions. *New York Times*. Retrieved from https://www.nytimes.com/2015/07/16/business/specialty-pharmacies-proliferate-along-with-questions.html
Townsend, C. L., Byrne, L., Cortina-Borja, M., Thorne, C., de Ruiter, A., Lyall, H., … Tookey, P. A. (2014). Earlier initiation of ART and further decline in mother-to-child HIV transmission rates, 2000–2011. *AIDS, 28*(7), 1049–1057.
UNAIDS. (2016). *2015 Progress report on the global plan towards the elimination of new HIV infections among children and keeping their mothers alive*. Retrieved from http://www.unAIDS.org/sites/default/files/media_asset/JC2774_2015ProgressReport_GlobalPlan_en.pdf
Valdiserri, R. O. (2002). HIV/AIDS stigma: An impediment to public health. *American Journal of Public Health, 92*(3), 341–342.
Vanable, P. A., Carey, M. P., Blair, D. C., & Littlewood, R. A. (2006). Impact of HIV-related stigma on health behaviors and psychological adjustment among HIV-positive men and women. *AIDS and Behavior, 10*(5), 473–482.
Vyavaharkar, M., Moneyham, L., Corwin, S., Saunders, R., Annang, L., & Tavakoli, A. (2010). Relationships between stigma, social support, and depression in HIV-infected African American women living in the rural Southeastern United States. *Journal of the Association of Nurses in AIDS Care, 21*(2), 144–152.
Walensky, R. P., Freedberg, K. A., Weinstein, M. C., & Paltiel, A. D. (2007). Cost-effectiveness of HIV testing and treatment in the United States. *Clinical Infectious Diseases, 45*(Suppl 4), S248–S254.
Watkins-Hayes, C. (2014). Intersectionality and the sociology of HIV/AIDS: Past, present, and future research directions. *Annual Review of Sociology, 40*, 431–457.
Weiser, S. D., Young, S. L., Cohen, C. R., Kushel, M. B., Tsai, A. C., Tien, P. C., … Bangsberg, D. R. (2011). Conceptual framework for understanding the bidirectional links between food insecurity and HIV/AIDS. *The American Journal of Clinical Nutrition, 94*(6), 1729S–1739S.
Whetten, K., Reif, S., Whetten, R., & Murphy-McMillan, L. K. (2008). Trauma, mental health, distrust, and stigma among HIV-positive persons: Implications for effective care. *Psychosomatic Medicine, 70*(5), 531–538.

White House Office of National AIDS Policy. (2015, July). *National HIV/AIDS strategy for the United States: Updated to 2020*. Retrieved from https://www.hiv.gov/sites/default/files/nhas-update.pdf

Whiteside, A. (2016). *HIV & AIDS: A very short introduction*. Oxford, England: Oxford University Press.

Wilper, A. P., Woolhandler, S., Lasser, K. E., McCormick, D., Bor, D. H., & Himmelstein, D. U. (2009). Health insurance and mortality in US adults. *American Journal of Public Health, 99*(12), 2289–2295.

World Health Organization. (2013, June). *Consolidated guidelines on the use of antiretroviral drugs for treating and preventing HIV infection*. Retrieved from http://www.who.int/hiv/pub/guidelines/arv2013/intro/keyterms/en/

Wyatt, G. E., Myers, H. F., Williams, J. K., Kitchen, C. R., Loeb, T., Carmona, J. V., … Presley, N. (2002). Does a history of trauma contribute to HIV risk for women of color? Implications for prevention and policy. *American Journal of Public Health, 92*(4), 660–665.

Yin, M. T., Zhang, C. A., McMahon, D. J., Ferris, D. C., Irani, D., Colon, I., … Shane, E. (2011). Higher rates of bone loss in postmenopausal HIV-infected women: A longitudinal study. *The Journal of Clinical Endocrinology & Metabolism, 97*(2), 554–562.

Zierler, S., Feingold, L., Laufer, D., Velentgas, P., Kantrowitz-Gordon, I., & Mayer, K. (1991). Adult survivors of childhood sexual abuse and subsequent risk of HIV infection. *American Journal of Public Health, 81*(5), 572–575.

Chapter 6
Strategic Communication Research to Illuminate and Promote Public Engagement with Climate Change

Connie Roser-Renouf and Edward Wile Maibach

Part I: Rationale, Mission, and Approach

Introduction

In this chapter, we offer readers a nontraditional research narrative that is in varying degrees theoretical, empirical, practical, and autobiographical. In a limited sense, the story we tell is ours—because we are the two scientists who founded the communication research team in question, that recently celebrated its tenth anniversary—but in a fuller sense it is the story of the many faculty members and students at our university and other universities, with whom we have been fortunate to collaborate; our use of a plural pronoun to tell this story is meant to convey all of these people's contributions to it. And, while our narrative focuses primarily on our research, we recognize that we stand on the shoulders of the giants who preceded us in the social sciences, and on the shoulders of investigators who are working concurrently with us in universities around the world; they deserve a full measure of credit for any progress we are making.

Our story also requires an upfront disclosure. We accept as true that harmful, human-caused climate change is happening, because—based on the evidence—nearly all of the world's climate scientists, and all of the world's legitimate science societies, are convinced this is so. As social scientists with deep roots in the public health community, we feel an obligation to forewarn and forearm humanity so that

C. Roser-Renouf (✉)
Center for Climate Change Communication, George Mason University, Fairfax, VA, USA
e-mail: croserre@gmu.edu

E. W. Maibach
Department of Communication, Center for Climate Change Communication, George Mason University, Fairfax, VA, USA
e-mail: emaibach@gmu.edu

D. A. Hope, R. A. Bevins (eds.), *Change and Maintaining Change*, Nebraska Symposium on Motivation 65, https://doi.org/10.1007/978-3-319-96920-6_6

people and society can understand the risks they face and make the best possible decisions regarding how to manage those risks. We see this as akin to warning people and society about the health risks of tobacco use, and informing them of the range of potential options to manage those risks. In short, it is fair to say that we have an agenda: to promote comprehension of climate change risks and thoughtful deliberation and decision-making about how best to respond to them, or stated more briefly, to promote public engagement in climate change. Some critics claim that having an agenda inherently biases scientists and renders them advocates rather than honest brokers. We disagree; advocating for informed decision-making, based on the best available information, is a valuable approach to being an honest broker.

Communication Science in the Public's Interest

Social scientists have long studied the processes by which communication influences public knowledge, attitudes, and behavior on a range of important societal issues. Much of that research has focused on understanding the potential negative impacts of mass communication on society by fostering, for example, aggression, social mistrust, and negative stereotypes through television content. Another large body of research has focused on the potential of strategic (or purposive) communication to enhance public well-being, with an emphasis on health and health behaviors, such as smoking prevention and cessation, drunk driving prevention, and seat belts, condoms, and physical activity promotion. The bulk of this work has focused on changing the behaviors of at-risk individuals, although some has focused on building public support for policy changes that protect the public, such as banning smoking from public places.

Much can be learned about how to build public engagement with climate change from the extant research focusing on other societal challenges. However, in many ways, climate change poses different and potentially more difficult challenges for those who seek to promote public engagement in it.

- Most Americans hold serious misperceptions about climate change, viewing the threat as small and distant in space (not here), time (not yet), and species (not us).
- Many politically conservative Americans flat out reject its reality (in response to what they have been told by their political leaders and by fossil fuel industry sponsored denial campaigns), and they are passionately and ideologically opposed to most proposed solutions.
- The most important solutions—i.e., greatly accelerating the transition to clean energy (so as to leave fossil fuels in the ground), and turning the tide on global deforestation and soil degradation—are neither well-understood nor directly influenced by ordinary citizens.
- The problem is global, having worldwide causes, and requiring worldwide solutions, which creates myriad challenges to mounting effective responses beyond those normally inherent in individual, local, and national problems.

- The need for large-scale global solutions is urgent because the earth's climate system could reach one or more "tipping points" in the very near future, which would cause dramatic harm to humanity and to the ecosystems on which humans depend. Recent research finds that if carbon emissions continue to rise after 2020, the temperature goals set in the Paris climate accord are likely to become unattainable (Figueres et al., 2017).

Thus, we face an urgent threat that is poorly understood by large segments of the public. Threat reduction will require widespread collective action, which is unlikely in the current highly polarized political context. These are the challenges we are working to address.

Health Threats Posed by Climate Change

Climate change has a long list of impacts that are harmful to humans, including more extreme weather, heat, drought, flooding, sea level rise, increased ranges for vector-borne illnesses, longer allergy seasons, and increases in water and foodborne illnesses. Drought and sea level rise increase competition for scarce resources in the developing nations, fostering conflicts and migration. The Third National Climate Assessment by the US Global Change Research Program—a collaboration of 13 federal agencies, including NASA and NOAA—tells us that these are not impacts expected in the future—they are happening now (Walsh et al., 2014).

Figure 6.1 was developed by the US Centers for Disease Control and Prevention (CDC) (2016) to illustrate the connections between climate change and the harm it causes to humans, with changes to the climate illustrated in the innermost circle. As CO_2 levels increase, temperatures rise, causing more extreme weather and sea level rise. These changes lead to increases in the risk factors shown in the middle circle, and ultimately, to the impacts on people shown in the outer circle. Increases in extreme heat, for example, entail longer lasting heat waves and less cooling overnight, which increase heat-related illnesses and cardiovascular failure. Insects and animals that carry deadly diseases, such as malaria and Lyme disease, are expanding their ranges, moving northward as higher temperatures increase the range within which they can survive. Environmental degradation in the form of droughts and flooding make once productive agricultural land less capable of supporting the people who live upon it. Increased competition in the developing nations for scarce resources like potable water fosters civil conflict and forces people to migrate from their homes (Centers for Disease Control and Prevention (CDC), 2016; Luber et al., 2014)

Clearly, climate change is not simply a danger to polar bears. Recognition of its massive threat to human's well-being prompted creation of the Center for Climate Change Communication at George Mason University in the fall of 2007.

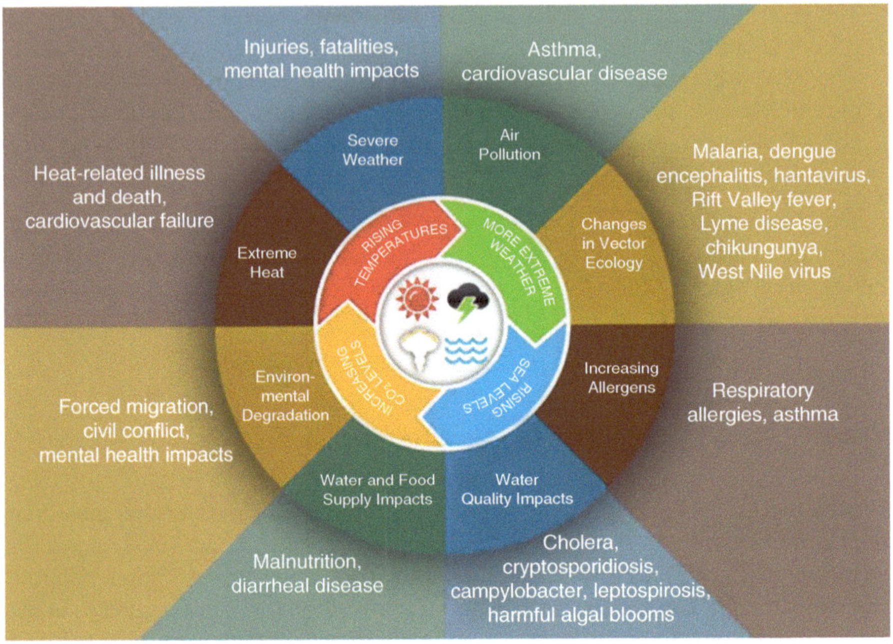

Fig. 6.1 Impacts of climate change on human health (Source: Centers for Disease Control and Prevention (CDC), 2016: https://www.cdc.gov/climateandhealth/effects/default.htm)

Strategic Communication Research in Service of Earth's Climate

We created the Center for Climate Change Communication (4C) in 2007 to promote public engagement in climate change through audience research, message testing, and the application of theories in science and risk communication. Specifically, the Center's stated mission is to "develop and apply social science insights to help society make informed decisions that will stabilize earth's life-sustaining climate and prevent further harm from climate change."

Our work is guided by several premises. First, "issue engagement" has cognitive, affective, and behavioral components (Ockwell, Whitmarsh, & O'Neill, 2009), all of which we consider in our research. Second, while communication is not a magic bullet, most successful strategic communication campaigns are "big messy programs" (Hornik, 2002) that convey simple, clear messages, repeated often, through multiple trusted sources (Maibach, in press). With these in mind, we have focused on the methods of increasing knowledge, and changing attitudes and behavior with a range of trusted sources working in diverse communication settings, both mediated and interpersonal.

Our four primary activities are:

1. Survey research and interviews to illuminate the processes by which public understanding, concern, and skepticism about climate change are created;
2. Experimental research to identify effective messages in controlled settings;
3. Audience segmentation to identify motivationally coherent segments that may be effectively targeted with content specific to their needs and interests;
4. Outreach to increase public engagement including: field experiments and demonstration projects that test and/or scale up promising approaches to public engagement; and trainings and briefings to help communication practitioners and policy-makers improve their communication effectiveness through application of research findings.

Our program is grounded in the recognition that successful messaging begins with understanding the audience, and that a combination of surveys, interviews, and experiments are the best foundation for building this understanding. Surveys and interviews can identify correlational relationships; experiments can then test whether the relationships are causal. For example, our research with cross-sectional survey data showed that awareness of the scientific consensus on climate change predicted mitigation policy support through several mediating key beliefs—that climate change is real, human-caused, harmful, and solvable—and that this model was a better fit to the data than alternative models using the same variables but alternative paths of influence (Ding, Maibach, Zhao, Roser-Renouf, & Leiserowitz, 2011). Through multiple message experiments, we have assessed the impact of the scientific consensus message, confirming that the relationship originally identified with cross-sectional data is causal, and extending the findings by comparing different forms of the message (Myers, Maibach, Peters, & Leiserowitz, 2015; van der Linden, Leiserowitz, Feinberg, & Maibach, 2014; van der Linden, Leiserowitz, Rosenthal, & Maibach, 2017).

Survey data can also identify promising approaches for climate change messaging when combined with experimental data. For example, in one experiment we found that messages framing climate change as a health issue were positively received across opinion groups (Myers, Nisbet, Maibach, & Leiserowitz, 2012). We subsequently assessed public understanding of the health threats of climate change in a survey, finding that few people were aware of the threats (Leiserowitz, Maibach, et al., 2014; Maibach, Leiserowitz, et al., 2015; Roser-Renouf, Stenhouse, Rolfe-Redding, Maibach, & Leiserowitz, 2014), which suggested that health would be a promising framing for information campaigns.

With this framework in mind, we began a program of research to identify effective methods of increasing the American public's issue engagement, mitigation policy support, sustainable behavior, and climate change activism. While our primary objective has been applied—i.e., to build public engagement with climate change, our work has also entailed contributions to the academic literature on climate change communication, and the training of young scholars to help build what is still a small research community into a larger, robust field. This more basic research feeds not only our own public engagement initiatives but also provides insights useful to the fields of environmental communication and environmental psychology overall.

Part II: Theoretical Grounding—Theories of Change

The People and Places Framework

Much of our research is grounded in cognitive and social psychology. Theories of individual behavior, however, are not sufficient to understand individuals, social networks, or society as a whole. Social-ecological models such as the People and Places Framework (Maibach, Roser-Renouf, & Leiserowitz, 2008) remind us that actions are shaped not only by individual factors like risk perceptions, but also by social factors, like norms and social networks, as well as the physical and the policy environment (see Fig. 6.2). Volumes have been written on each of the theoretical perspectives encompassed by the People and Places Framework; below, we provide the briefest of summaries of those that most strongly guide our research.

Attributes of Place

Social-ecological models make it clear that sustainable behavior is not possible if the local environment does not support it—if there is, for example, no mass transit in a community and housing is distant from work places, people will be forced to drive, regardless of their feelings about climate change. Research testing the ABC model of Guagnano, Stern, and Dietz (1995) shows that the relationship between A (attitudes) and B (behavior) is contingent on C (conditions): Most people engage in

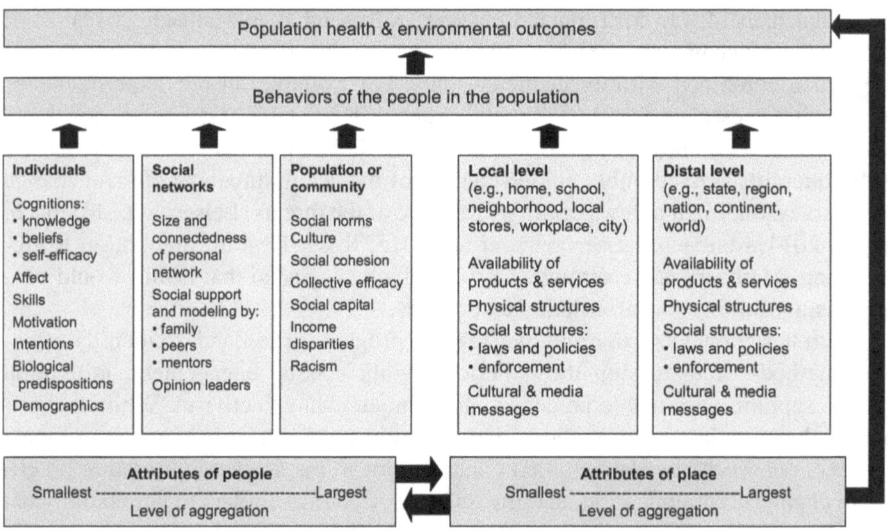

Fig. 6.2 The people and places framework (Source: Maibach et al., 2009)

very easy behaviors, such as curbside recycling, regardless of their attitudes, while few engage in very difficult behaviors, such as cycling long distances to work. Only actions of moderate difficulty are strongly related to attitudes. This points to the importance of place-based changes: sustainability will not be achieved by persuading people to change their behavior if the context does not support that behavior.

Our studies have shown that climate change attitudes are only weakly predictive of conservation behaviors in the USA. Home energy use is more strongly related to demographic factors like home-ownership, age, and income, and is more strongly motivated by economics than the environment (Maibach, Roser-Renouf, Akerlof, Leiserowitz, & Nisbet, 2010). Boucher (2016) used data from one of our nationally representative surveys and found that climate change beliefs influence the size of people's "carbon footprint" only at the highest level of issue engagement. Thus, the data support the insights provided by the model on the importance of place in determining behavior.

For people to live sustainably, policies and regulations are needed that change place-based characteristics in ways that encourage sustainable behavior, e.g., zoning that reduces the distances between work sites and housing, a carbon tax, and government rebates on purchases of solar panels and electric cars. These changes are less likely to be enacted in the absence of community pressure, however, which is why some researchers argue that climate change activism is the most important action citizens can take (Ockwell et al., 2009). Thus, although our work to-date has drawn primarily on theories from the "people" side of the figure, the "places" side has been central to the selection of our dependent variables: We have focused most heavily on dependent variables that can lead to the largest reductions in carbon emissions, i.e., support for policies to mitigate climate change, and citizen activism in support of these policies.

Audience Perspectives

Our research is grounded strongly in *Social Cognitive Theory* (Bandura, 2001), which posits that people's behavior is influenced by their expectations about the likelihood and desirability of outcomes associated with behaviors, and by their perceptions of their own ability to perform the actions that lead to positive outcomes, i.e., their self-efficacy. In the case of climate change, collective efficacy and proxy efficacy are also relevant, i.e., the ability of one's group to accomplish a shared task with a desirable outcome (e.g., influencing legislators), and the ability of those who represent one's group (in this case, policy-makers), to take actions that will lead to positive outcomes (e.g., enacting effective mitigation policies; Bandura, 2000).

Theories that focus specifically on risk assessment and response can be considered in the context of social cognitive theory in that they examine outcome expectations and efficacy beliefs with a specific focus on perceived outcomes of threats.[1] We draw heavily on the *Extended Parallel Process Model* (Maloney, Lapinski, & Witte, 2011; Witte, 1992), which posits that in response to a perceived threat, people first consider two dimensions of a threat's outcomes—its severity and their vulnerability to it. If perceived severity and vulnerability are high, they next assess the effectiveness and feasibility of methods of threat reduction. If the threat is perceived as high, but the methods of responding to it are perceived as ineffective or infeasible (i.e., people hold low response- and self-efficacy perceptions), they may engage in defensive avoidance; if, however, they perceive responses to be effective and feasible, they are likely to take action.

We also draw heavily on *Dual-Processing Theories* that examine the ways that different types of information processing affect responses to messages. For our purposes, Tversky's and Kahneman's contrast between effortful and automatic processing is most relevant, i.e., some information is processed immediately, effortlessly, and automatically, while other content requires cognitive effort and thoughtful attention (Kahneman, 2003). The less effortful a message is, the wider its reception is likely to be (which is not the same as persuasion, but a necessary first step, in the view of most researchers).

A second dual-processing approach, the *Elaboration Likelihood Model* (ELM) developed by Petty and Cacioppo (1986), is also relevant in its exploration of the role of issue involvement as a predictor of the depth of message processing and responsiveness to peripheral message cues, such as the credibility of the source, as compared to the strength of the arguments presented. These theories suggest guidelines on the design of messages: Effortful content is only appropriate for audiences who are motivated to expend the necessary cognitive effort to process it, and the more easily and automatically a message can be processed, the wider the audience who will understand it.

Motivation may shape not only the depth of processing, but also the cognitive strategies employed: When people are motivated to reach a particular conclusion, they often do so, applying differing standards for evidence to arguments that are congruent and incongruent with their desired conclusion (Kunda, 1990). "Solution aversion"—a dislike for proposed policy solutions to climate change—has been shown to motivate much of conservatives' rejection of climate science (Campbell & Kay, 2014).

A third audience perspective we have drawn on is *Construal Level Theory* (Trope & Liberman, 2011). When people consider distant attitude objects, their thoughts tend to be abstract and global, while their thinking about closer objects will be more concrete. Distance is defined here along multiple dimensions, including time, space, and social similarity. This perspective informs our efforts to focus climate change communications on local impacts that are happening now: On most—but not all—dimensions of psychological distance, greater distance is associated with lower issue engagement (Spence, Poortinga, & Pidgeon, 2012).

[1] They differ from Social-Cognitive Theory in the emphasis some place on emotions—specifically, fear—as drivers of behavior.

Social System Perspectives

At the level of social systems, our work has been most heavily influenced by research on the diffusion of innovations (Rogers, 2010), the two-step flow of information, and opinion leadership (Katz, 1957; Valente, 2012). Innovations in technology, ideas, and behaviors spread through social systems following an S-shaped curve, adopted first by a few innovators, who typically learn of the innovation from mediated sources. They are followed by early adopters, who are often opinion leaders. These opinion leaders play a pivotal role in promoting adoption by a larger proportion of the public: People are more readily persuaded by friends and family—and especially by the opinion leaders in their social network—than by mass media. Thus, information flows in at least two steps, and in many cases, multiple steps, from media through the interpersonal channels of opinion leaders to a broader audience. This perspective has particularly influenced our strategic objectives for the segment of the public who is highly concerned about climate change (the Alarmed; see Part IV), as we seek ways to activate them as opinion leaders, who will share their knowledge and concern with their friends and family.

Theories About Media Effects

There are multiple theories that shed light on the ways that mediated content is received, used, and responded to. We draw heavily on two types.

Framing Theory: Message frames can provide receivers with heuristics, or cognitive shortcuts, shaping the way they form opinions, and frames that align with individuals' values and predispositions can be particularly influential in shaping opinions. Focusing people's attention on an issue's personally important dimensions through message framing can increase message acceptance (Chong & Druckman, 2007). Of particular import for climate change communication is research demonstrating that political polarization on the issue can be reduced by messages that are framed in terms of conservative values (Feinberg & Willer, 2013; Feygina, Jost, & Goldsmith, 2010; Wolsko, Ariceaga, & Seiden, 2016).

Selective Exposure and Reinforcing Spirals: People tend to selectively expose themselves to media content that reflects their existing views, as conflicting information may arouse feelings of dissonance and discomfort (Sears & Freedman, 1967). Selectivity protects people from experiencing the discomfort of hearing that their opinions and beliefs may be wrong, and is facilitated by the current fragmented media landscape (Bennett & Iyengar, 2008). Widespread use of internet news sources with varying degrees of accuracy and objectivity facilitates selective exposure and may be exacerbating the polarized state of public opinion in the USA (Tewksbury, 2005).

Media content helps audiences to form opinions but thereafter tends to have a reinforcing effect, as people choose to expose themselves to information that is consistent with their beliefs, which strengthens these beliefs and fosters future selective exposure in a "reinforcing spiral" (Slater, 2007).

Social Marketing Approach

Although not a theory, the practice of social marketing—initiatives focused on helping populations of people change their behavior in ways that are beneficial to them and to society—brings an important practical perspective to our translational research. Social marketing initiatives seek to promote beneficial behaviors not by changing people, but rather by changing the behavior being promoted. Specifically, to increase the likelihood that people will adapt a new behavior, social marketers endeavor to make the behavior easy to perform, rich in benefits that have perceived value to the adopters, and perceived to be socially normative. By (1) identifying and reducing barriers that impede people's performance of a beneficial behavior; (2) identifying and offering benefits that people value; and (3) demonstrating that the behavior is normative or is becoming more normative, social marketers, in essence, make the behavior "easy, fun, and popular." This approach, for example, directly shaped our *Climate Matters* program, which has enabled hundreds of American TV weathercasters to begin reporting on the local impacts of climate change in their community (Maibach et al., 2016).

Part III: Research

Research Collaborations and Climate Change in the American Mind

In 2008, we began a research collaboration with Yale's newly formed Program on Climate Change Communication titled *Climate Change in the American Mind* (*CCAM*). The *CCAM* collaboration entails biannual nationally representative surveys, which provide data on a wide range of variables, including Americans' understanding of climate change, their perceptions of its threat, support for mitigation policies, climate-relevant behaviors, values, interpersonal communication, media use, and perceptions of the credibility of information sources.

To date, we have conducted 19 *CCAM* surveys, two of which were recontacts of prior respondents, yielding panel data, and two of which included samples of adolescent–parent dyads, which allowed us to examine family dynamics around climate change. One of these surveys included an over-sample of Republicans, to examine their beliefs in greater depth; and another used a split-half design to compare responses when questions ask about "climate change," rather than "global warming," which is our standard term.[2]

The surveys serve multiple purposes, both applied and theoretical. Topline data are reported in research monographs and polling reports, and academic papers are written examining the dynamics at play in the formation of climate change opinions and the drivers of climate-relevant behavior. The surveys are the foundation for the Yale Climate Opinion Maps, which downscale to the state, county, and media market levels many of the variables we have tracked on climate change beliefs and attitudes (Howe, Mildenberger, Marlon, & Leiserowitz, 2015).

The survey data are also our most used resource for briefing communication practitioners and policy-makers. These poll findings—which typically show strong public support for climate action and clean energy—are widely cited in the news media, and are of great interest to policy-makers who support, or are considering supporting, climate action policies. An article in the National Journal, a political newspaper, reported White House sources as saying that our polling reports helped convince President Obama to make climate action a bigger priority in his second term, because they demonstrated that the public would support this move (Davenport, 2013). More recently (but less successfully), we have released polling reports showing strong public disapproval for the prospect of the US withdrawal from the Paris Climate Accord.

Media Effects on Perceptions and Issue Engagement

Just over a third of Americans believe that they have personally experienced climate change (36% in May 2017; Leiserowitz, Maibach, Roser-Renouf, Rosenthal, & Cutler, 2017), while the remaining two-thirds are relying on other sources of information to form their beliefs about the reality and harmfulness of climate change. When personal experience with a phenomenon is absent, media effects on beliefs and attitudes are likely to be greater (Ball-Rokeach & DeFleur, 1976). Thus, understanding the roles that the news media are playing in shaping public beliefs has been an important focus for our research. Some of this work has examined direct effects of exposure on beliefs, but a larger portion has analyzed the ways that individual attitudes and beliefs shape the ways that people use, process, and respond to mass media. From this work, we understand more clearly the role media play in the attitudinal polarization and skepticism surrounding climate change in the USA.

Political polarization on climate change in the USA can be dated back to the late 1990s, when the attitudes of Republicans and Democrats began to diverge (Krosnick, Holbrook, & Visser, 2000), eventually reaching a point where skepticism became something of a litmus test for Republicans (Dunlap & McCright, 2011). Major contributors to the polarization include disinformation campaigns funded by the fossil

[2]While the climate science community prefers the term "climate change," we continue using "global warming" in our surveys because it is still the most commonly used term among Americans (Leiserowitz, Feinberg, et al., 2014).

fuel industry, and media coverage of the issue, which for many years presented a "false balance" in coverage of the issue, fostering beliefs in the audience that the science is contested (Boykoff, 2007; Somerville & Hassol, 2011). A fragmented media environment, selective exposure to compatible news sources, and motivated reasoning within the audience (Campbell & Kay, 2014; Kunda, 1990) have all contributed to sustaining the polarization.

In 2011, we assessed differences in the impacts of attention to political news on climate change, as compared to scientific and environmental news. Political news has typically focused on controversy and has given voice to climate skeptics among Republican political elites, while scientific and environmental news have typically conveyed science-based information. We found that attention to science and environmental news is associated with beliefs more consistent with the global warming science, and with higher risk perceptions, and that the opposite is true of attention to political news: After controlling for attention to science and environmental news exposure, attention to political news has significant negative relationships with understanding that climate change is real, human-caused, and harmful, and that scientists agree on the issue (Zhao, Leiserowitz, Maibach, & Roser-Renouf, 2011; see Fig. 6.3).

Within categories of news, particular news sources are significant contributors to the polarization. Content analyses show that conservative news media, such as Fox News and The Wall Street Journal, carry more articles and opinion pieces that cast doubt on the scientific consensus than liberal and middle-of-the-road sources, such as MSNBC, CNN, The New York Times, and The Washington Post (Feldman, Maibach, Roser-Renouf, & Leiserowitz, 2012; Theel, Greenberg, & Robbins, 2013).

An analysis of 2008 *CCAM* data found a negative association between Fox News viewership and acceptance of global warming, even after controlling for numerous potential confounding factors. Conversely, viewing CNN and MSNBC was associated with greater acceptance of global warming. Further analyses revealed that the views of Republicans were strongly linked with the news outlet they watched, regardless of how well that outlet aligned with their political predispositions.

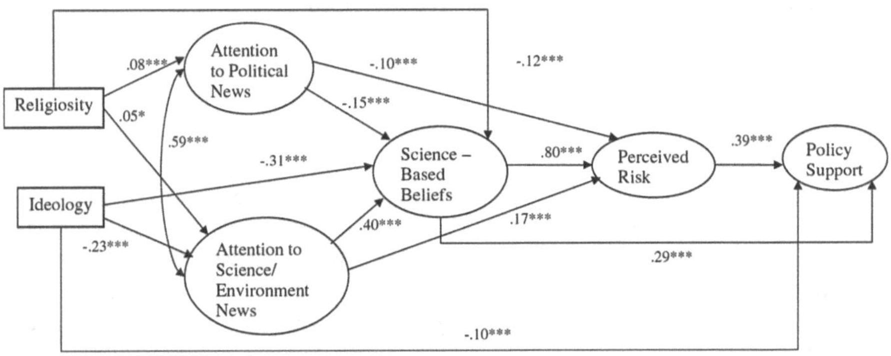

Fig. 6.3 Differential effects of attention to political and science/environmental news (Source: Zhao et al., 2011)

In contrast, Democrats did not vary much in their beliefs as a function of cable news use. This asymmetry suggests that Republicans are less skeptical when they are exposed to information on the reality and urgency of climate change (Feldman et al., 2012).

Selective exposure to conservative news sources inhibits change, however, and can act over time to reinforce and strengthen climate skepticism—a process demonstrated in an analysis of *CCAM* panel data. Selectivity combined with media effects created a reinforcing spiral: Consuming conservative or nonconservative media at Wave 1 made people more likely to consume those same media at Wave 2, partly as an indirect result of the media's effects on global warming belief certainty and policy preferences. Wave 2 media use, in turn, further strengthened audiences' global warming belief certainty and policy preferences (Feldman, Myers, Hmielowski, & Leiserowitz, 2014; see Fig. 6.4). The data further demonstrated that conservative media use decreased trust in scientists which, in turn, decreased certainty that global warming is happening. By contrast, use of nonconservative media increased trust in

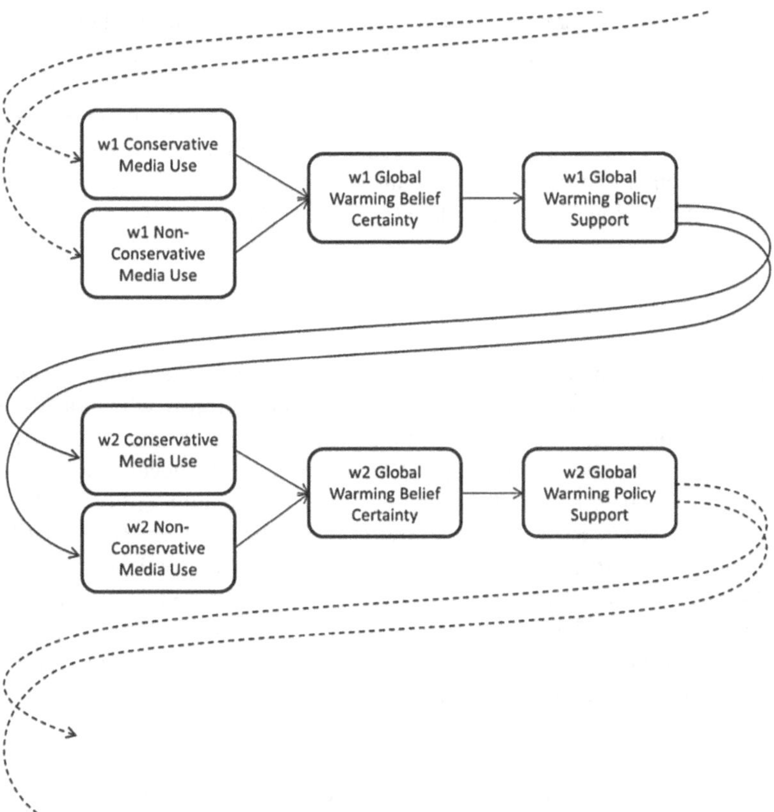

Fig. 6.4 Reinforcing spirals model (Source: Feldman et al., 2014)

scientists, which, in turn, increased certainty that global warming is happening (Hmielowski, Feldman, Myers, Leiserowitz, & Maibach, 2013).

Together, slanted news coverage, selective exposure, and motivated reasoning can result in diametrically different interpretations of the same news. For example, 60% of the Republicans who were aware of Climategate[3] said they lost trust in scientists as a result, while three-quarters of Democrats said their trust in scientists was not affected (Leiserowitz, Maibach, Roser-Renouf, Smith, & Dawson, 2012).

Cognitive Drivers of Issue Engagement

Despite the fact that climate skepticism is higher among Republicans than Democrats in the USA, two-thirds of moderate and liberal Republicans now recognize that climate change is real (65%), as do 45% of conservative Republicans (Leiserowitz et al., 2017). Feldman et al. (2012) found that Republicans were less skeptical if they viewed CNN or MSNBC suggests that accurate information changes people's minds, even if tribal commitments do play a major role in determining beliefs (Kahan, Jenkins-Smith, & Braman, 2011). Moreover, experiments by Ranney and his colleagues (e.g., Ranney & Clark, 2016) demonstrate that information can and does change minds, and that these effects endure over time. Thus, an important focus of our research has been to identify the specific and essential information that builds issue engagement and mitigation policy support, and that changes behavior. The key beliefs described below form a template for climate change communication.

Four Key Beliefs

Support for climate change mitigation policies and both political and consumer climate change activism are significantly higher among those who hold four key beliefs: They are certain that climate change is (1) real, (2) human-caused, and (3) harmful, and (4) they believe that collectively humans can successfully reduce climate change (i.e., they have collective efficacy; Roser-Renouf, Atkinson, Maibach, & Leiserowitz, 2016; Roser-Renouf, Maibach, Leiserowitz, & Zhao, 2014). Our analyses of *CCAM* data show that people who hold these four beliefs are more likely to be affectively involved with the issue, i.e., they worry more and view the issue as personally important. They are more likely to act as opinion leaders on the issue by discussing it with their family and friends; to have contacted legislators in support of mitigation policies; and to make consumer choices with the objective of influencing others' consumption and changing corporate practices.

---

[3] In November, 2009, over 1000 stolen emails between climate scientists were publically released, along with claims that they were evidence of scientific misconduct to mislead the public about climate change. Dubbed "Climategate," the event drew widespread media attention. Multiple university investigations showed the charges against the scientists to be unfounded, and cleared them of all charges.

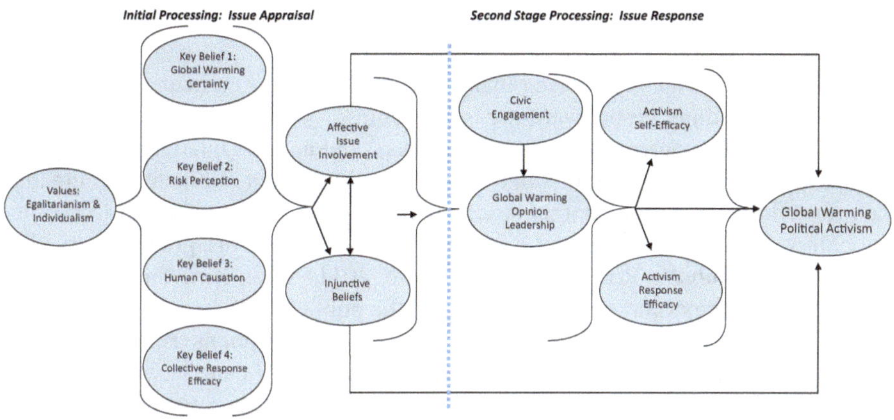

Fig. 6.5 Two-stage information processing model of climate change activism (Source: Roser-Renouf, Maibach, Leiserowitz, & Zhao, 2014)

We modeled climate change political activism with the Two-Stage Information-Processing Model (see Fig. 6.5), which is grounded in Social Cognitive Theory. It operationalizes climate change outcome expectations with two beliefs—climate change is real and harmful—and efficacy beliefs with two additional beliefs—humans are capable of reducing climate change and humans are causing it.[4] These beliefs are strongly predictive of affective issue involvement and injunctive beliefs (i.e., beliefs that government, corporations, and citizens should take action to reduce the threat), which, in turn, predict opinion leadership, political efficacy perceptions, and activism (Roser-Renouf, Maibach, Leiserowitz, Feinberg, et al., 2014).

A Fifth Key Belief: The Scientific Consensus

In light of our research showing that recognition of the scientific consensus increases each of the original four beliefs, we have added a fifth key belief to the four listed above. This simple, clear message—"97% of climate scientists are convinced that human-caused climate change is happening"—is a useful and effective heuristic for shallow information-processors: People who are either unable or unwilling to learn more about the science demonstrating that human-caused climate change is occurring can easily understand that experts agree on these facts. Moreover, the consensus message directly addresses one of the primary tactics used by disinformation campaigns, i.e., asserting that the science is not settled and scientists disagree on the issue. Published papers have quantified the high scientific consensus dating back to a paper published by Naomi Oreskes in 2004 (Oreskes, 2004), and replicated multiple times using multiple methods: The "consensus on consensus" is that 97%

[4] Humans are capable of reducing climate change *because* humans are causing it; hence, human causation is a logical foundation for efficacy.

of climate scientists concur on the reality of anthropogenic climate change (Cook et al., 2016).

Our initial 2008 survey showed that fewer than half of Americans thought that "most scientists think global warming is happening" (46%), while a third believed "there is a lot of disagreement among scientists," and another quarter said they did not know. By June of 2010, following the release of the stolen "Climategate" emails, the proportion recognizing that most scientists are in agreement fell by 14 percentage points to 33%, and the proportion who thought scientists disagree grew to 39% (Leiserowitz, Maibach, Roser-Renouf, & Smith, 2011). Correcting this misperception seemed an important avenue to engaging the public.

Our efforts to assess the importance of consensus perceptions as a predictor of other beliefs and attitudes began with an analysis of *CCAM* data, in which consensus perceptions were predicted to both directly increase policy support and injunctive beliefs (i.e., beliefs that societal actors—government, corporations, and citizens—should take action on climate change), and to indirectly increase these dependent variables through the four key beliefs (see Fig. 6.6). The analysis strongly supported the hypotheses, and in comparisons to alternative models, only the hypothesized model fit the data well (Ding et al., 2011).

In light of these survey results, we began testing the relationships experimentally and examining ways that the consensus could most effectively be communicated. A comparison of metaphors, descriptive text, and a pie chart to communicate the consensus found that all three were effective, but that the pie chart and descriptive text had greater recall and were most effective across political party lines (van der Linden et al., 2014).

A second experiment showed that numeric estimates of the consensus were more effective than non-numeric estimates in increasing consensus recognition (Myers et al., 2015); and a third experiment found that asking participants to estimate the level of consensus prior to revealing the actual level led to higher consensus estimates than simply the information alone, indicating that an "estimation-and-reveal" technique in public communication about the scientific consensus can be effective (Myers et al., 2015). All three experiments found consensus messaging to be effective across party lines.

An experimental replication and extension of the Ding and colleagues findings tested a "gateway belief model," showing that increasing public perceptions of the

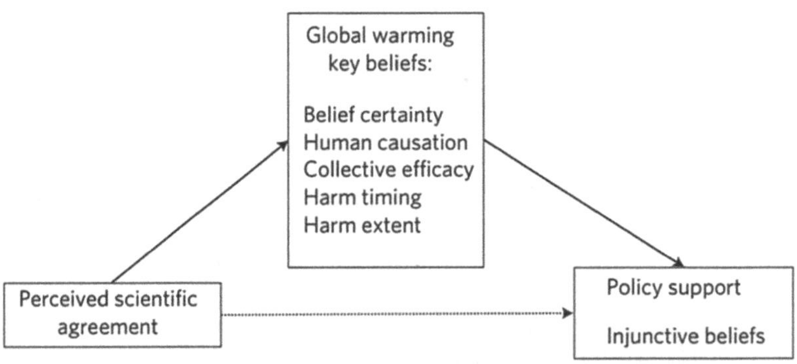

Fig. 6.6 Conceptual model of the relationships among consensus perceptions, key beliefs and support for mitigation (Source: Ding et al., 2011)

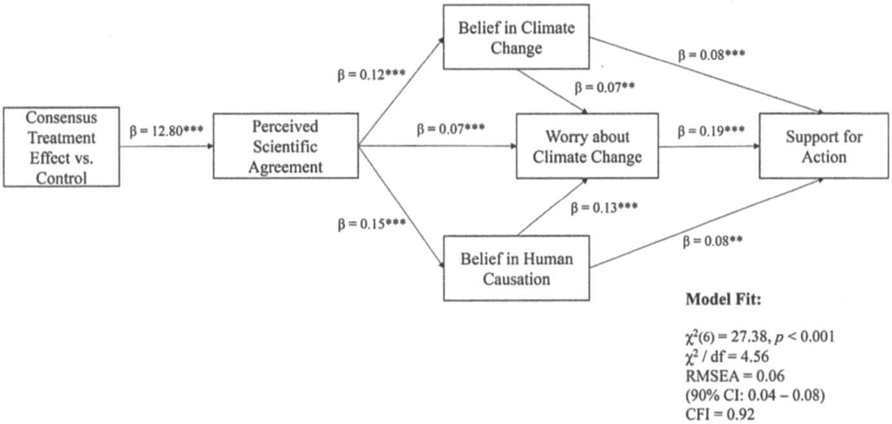

Fig. 6.7 The gateway belief model. $*p < 0.05$, $**p < 0.01$, $***p < 0.001$. $N = 1104$. Coefficients are unstandardized and adjusted for covariates; gender, age, education and political party (Source: van der Linden, Leiserowitz, et al., 2015)

scientific consensus is significantly and causally associated with an increase in the belief that climate change is happening, human-caused, and a worrisome threat. In turn, changes in these key beliefs are predictive of increased support for public action (see Fig. 6.7; van der Linden, Leiserowitz, Feinberg, & Maibach, 2015).

While these studies indicate that the consensus message can be effective, they may have limited external validity because outside the lab setting people are exposed to both information and disinformation. To begin to address this issue, we tested whether people can be "inoculated" against misinformation by providing not only the correct information, but also by explaining the biased motivations and factual errors of disinformation campaigns. The study found that not only is inoculation effective, it also works across the political spectrum (van der Linden et al., 2017).

In sum, these studies show that five key beliefs—climate change is real, harmful, human-caused, and solvable, and that scientists agree on its reality, human-causation, and harmfulness—are powerful drivers of mitigation policy support and climate change activism. In the next section, we describe studies that have examined drivers of affective involvement with climate change, focusing on perceptions of its harmfulness and personal relevance.

Affective Drivers of Issue Engagement

Extreme Weather and Experiential Learning

Even among Americans who accept that climate change is real, many continue to see it as a distant threat—distant in space (i.e., not here), time (i.e., not yet), and species (i.e., not us). Many think that it is a threat to polar bears, future generations, and people in the developing nations, but not to them, their families, or their communities (Leiserowitz, 2006). This is, perhaps, the most challenging of the barriers we face, as the impacts of climate change are not yet readily apparent to most people,[5] and in their absence, it is challenging to build issue engagement when many other threats appear to be more immediate and pressing. Humans have a "limited pool of worry" (Weber, 2006), and climate change can easily fall to the bottom of the list.

Weber's aptly subtitled 2006 paper, "Why global warming doesn't scare us (yet)" made the point that affect is a stronger driver of risk perceptions than cognitions, and that people need personal experience with global warming to become truly involved with the issue. In response to increases in extreme weather in the USA (and Hurricane Sandy in particular), we focused our spring 2013 *CCAM* survey on Americans' experience of extreme weather events, and their perceptions of the link between weather and climate change. We found that two-thirds of Americans (64%) believed that weather in the USA has become worse over the past several years, and over half (58%) agreed with the statement that "Global warming is affecting weather in the United States." Many believed that global warming increased the severity of extreme weather events such as Superstorm Sandy (46%) and record high temperatures (50%) (Leiserowitz, Maibach, Roser-Renouf, Feinberg, & Howe, 2013).

Subsequent research on the accuracy of self-reported weather experiences revealed that reported experiences correspond well with recorded event impacts, both in the USA (Howe, Boudet, Leiserowitz, & Maibach, 2014) and in India (Howe, Thaker, & Leiserowitz, 2014). Belief that extreme weather is becoming more frequent is associated with higher concern about climate change, and is higher among those who watch television weather forecasts—a finding that points to the influence of weathercasters (Bloodhart, Maibach, Myers, & Zhao, 2015).

Together, these results suggested that extreme weather events can serve as "teachable moments" that help people to recognize the reality of climate change (Somerville & Hassol, 2011). Analyses of panel *CCAM* data indicate that this holds true for people who are uncertain about the reality of climate change: For those who are highly engaged and strongly convinced of the reality/non-reality of climate change, weather conditions are used to bolster their existing beliefs—an example of motivated reasoning—but among those who less are engaged and unsure of their global warming beliefs, personal experience is associated with increased certainty in the reality of climate change (Myers, Maibach, Roser-Renouf, Akerlof, & Leiserowitz, 2013; see Fig. 6.8[6]).

Thus, the evidence suggests that extreme weather can help the majority of Americans who are still at least somewhat uncertain about the reality of climate change to learn that climate change is real and is affecting the USA. Further, these findings suggest that television weather forecasts can help people to make the link

---

[5] The 2017 hurricane season may change this. At this writing, however, it is too early to say.

[6] Figure 6.8 shows only a small piece of the model-testing. The analysis assessed six different models, including models with both synchronous and lagged effects of belief certainty and personal experience at T1 and T2, as well as all relevant controls, for both the highly and less engaged groups. Only two variables are shown here for simplicity. See the full paper for complete results.

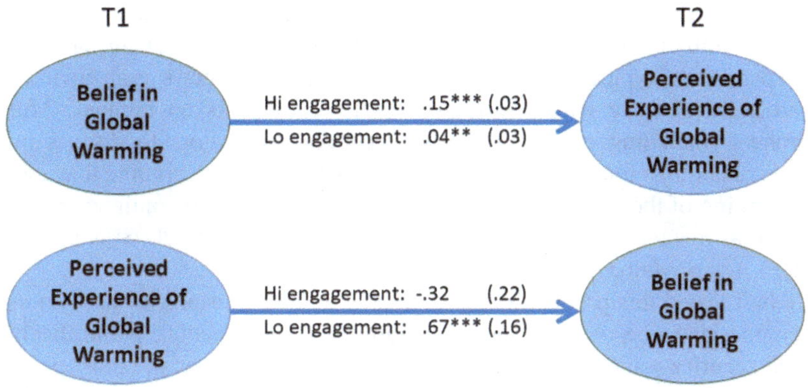

Fig. 6.8 Responses to personal experience of climate change: motivated reasoning and experiential learning. Note: Figure shows standardized βs with standardized error in parentheses; full models are not shown. $^{**}p < 0.01$; $^{***}p < 0.001$ (Source: Adapted from Myers et al., 2013)

between weather and climate change by highlighting the ways in which current weather anomalies are exemplars of the changes associated with climate change. These findings laid the foundation for our work with TV weathercasters, which is described in Part V.

Health Harms

A primary motivation for the establishment of our research center was our recognition of the serious impacts climate change has on humans' health and well-being—a recognition increasingly shared by the public health and medical communities. Interviews we conducted with directors of city and county public health department in 2008 found that roughly 60% agreed that one or more serious public health problems would occur in their jurisdiction over the coming two decades due to climate change (Balbus et al., 2008). Only 11% strongly agreed, however, and 4 years later, the proportion that strongly agreed with the statement had more than doubled to 29% (Roser-Renouf, Maibach, & Li, 2016).

More recently, our surveys of medical societies have revealed that physicians are now seeing impacts of climate change in their patient populations. This includes doctors who treat pulmonary diseases, allergies, asthma, and those whose practices include a high proportion of African-American patients, i.e., populations we expect to experience greater health impacts of climate change (Sarfaty et al., 2015, 2016; Sarfaty, Kreslake, Casale, & Maibach, 2015; Sarfaty, Mitchell, Bloodhart, & Maibach, 2014). For example, a 2014 survey of members of the National Medical Association—an organization of doctors who treat and/or are African-American—found that 61% say climate change is now affecting the health of their patients a great deal or a moderate amount (Sarfaty et al., 2014).

While public health and medical professionals are aware of the health threats associated with climate change, most of the public has been unaware. This may be due, in part, to the typical framing of global warming in the news as an environmental and political issue with few references to its impacts on humans. Multiple researchers (including our team) have urged communicators to discuss human impacts, rather than impacts on iconic species like polar bears, arguing that a greater understanding of the health impacts could engage people who continue to perceive the threat as distant and personally irrelevant (Maibach et al., 2008; Nisbet, 2009; van der Linden, Maibach, & Leiserowitz, 2015).

We first tested this proposition by assessing audience responses to short essays that emphasized one of three message frames—environmental, public health, or national security—and found that the public health frame was the most positively received of the three, and that this held true regardless of the respondents' prior beliefs about climate change (i.e., even climate skeptics responded positively; Myers et al., 2012).

In light of this finding, we assessed public understanding of the health impacts of climate change in a *CCAM* survey in 2014. Close to two-thirds of Americans had given little to no thought to the impacts of global warming on people's health (61%), and only a quarter could accurately name any type of climate change-related health harm in an open-ended question (27%; Leiserowitz, Maibach, et al., 2014; Maibach, Leiserowitz, et al., 2015). Accurate knowledge of the types of climate change harm was almost exclusively restricted to respondents who were highly concerned about climate change (i.e., the Alarmed, who are described in Part IV; they comprised 13% of the population at that time), and even among the most highly engaged, understanding was low with only a third able to name the most familiar climate-related health threat (lung diseases; Roser-Renouf, Maibach, Leiserowitz, Feinberg, Rosenthal & Kreslake, 2014).

The ideal source for health impacts messaging is, naturally, a physician. In *CCAM* questions regarding trusted sources, respondents said their primary care physician is their most trusted source of information on the health harms of climate change; many also trust the Centers for Disease Control and Prevention, the World Health Organization, and their local public health department (Maibach, Kreslake, et al., 2015). Together, these findings show that: (1) the public knows little about the health impacts of climate change; (2) health framing is positively received across opinion groups; and (3) physicians are trusted sources of information on this topic. Hence, we have been working with medical societies to recruit physicians to act as spokespeople on the issue. This work is described in Part V.

Moral Dimensions

While risk perceptions are important drivers of affective involvement, another possible approach to engaging Americans is through their religious values. As a nation, we are unique among developed countries in our high religiosity. Over half of

Americans (54%) say religion plays a very important role in their lives, as compared, for example, to 24% of Canadians and 21% of Australians (Pew Research Center, 2015). Many climate skeptics are high in religiosity, and our baseline survey suggested that many Americans could be responsive to a moral framing of climate change. When asked to name the most important outcome of action to reduce global warming, one in five said it would "protect God's creation." Few, however, recognized other moral outcomes of mitigation: 4% said the most important reason to mitigate would be to "save many people around the world from poverty and starvation," and only 1% said the most important reason was to "protect the world's poorest people from environmental harm caused by the world's richest people" (Maibach, Roser-Renouf, & Leiserowitz, 2009).

Pope Francis' release of an encyclical on climate change in 2015 addressed these latter points directly. His emphasis on the moral imperative of mitigation to protect the vulnerable poor worldwide was a framing most Americans had not previously heard, and given the high level of religiosity among Americans, the moral framing had high potential: In the spring of 2015, only 35% of Americans said global warming is a moral issue, in contrast to the proportions that said it is an environmental (76%), scientific (71%), or political (54%) issue (Leiserowitz, Maibach, Roser-Renouf, Feinberg, & Rosenthal, 2015b).

The pope was also a new voice on the issue, speaking from outside the politically polarized arena. He spoke with the moral authority of his position leading the second largest religious denomination in the USA,[7] and when the pope stated that climate change is a moral issue that people of faith are called to address, he may have reached an audience that other sources have struggled to engage, i.e., the segments of the public that regard climate change as an issue that politicians debate and scientists study, but that has little personal relevance (Roser-Renouf, Stenhouse, et al., 2014).

To assess the pope's impact, we conducted three *CCAM* surveys focusing on exposure to and acceptance of his message. The initial survey was conducted in the spring of 2015, prior to release of the encyclical at a time when few Americans (5%) were aware of it (Maibach, Leiserowitz, et al., 2015). The second and third surveys were conducted in the fall, following the pope's visit to the USA; one of these surveys was a new independent cross-section, and the other was a recontact of our spring respondents.

Both of the fall surveys showed that perceptions that global warming is a moral issue increased significantly between the spring and fall (see Table 6.1). Americans also became more certain that climate change harms the poor and people in the developing nations, and the proportions that said the issue is personally important and worrisome increased (Leiserowitz, Maibach, Roser-Renouf, Feinberg, & Rosenthal, 2015a; Maibach, Leiserowitz, et al., 2015; previously unpublished *CCAM* data).

[7] Twenty-one percent of Americans are Catholic, second only to Evangelical Protestants, who make up a quarter of the population (Pew Research Center, 2013).

Table 6.1 Changes in perceptions of global warming, March–October 2015

	Panel[a]		Cross-sections[b]	
	March	Oct.	March	Oct.
GW is a moral issue (%)	32	38	35	41
Certain GW is happening	34	40	37	40
Issue is very/moderately important personally	19	26	21	26
Very/extremely worried	51	56	52	57
GW will harm world's poor a great deal/moderate amount	49	61	53	61
GW will harm developing nations a great deal/moderate amount	48	63	52	61

[a]All panel comparisons significant, $p < 0.001$. Unweighted $n = 905$ (Sources: Maibach, Leiserowitz, et al., 2015; previously unpublished CCAM data)
[b]Moral issue, $p < 0.05$; certainty GW is happening, n.s.; personal importance and worry, $p < 0.01$; gw will harm poor and developing nations, $p < 0.001$. March unweighted $n = 1263$; Oct. unweighted $n = 1344$ (Sources: Leiserowitz et al., 2015a; previously unpublished CCAM data)

Further, exposure activated people who were already concerned about climate change prior to the pope's encyclical. They engaged in more consumer activism, and expressed greater willingness to join a campaign to convince government officials to act on climate; that is, people became more likely to act on their beliefs (see Fig. 6.9; Myers, Roser-Renouf, Maibach, & Leiserowitz, 2017). The least common (and probably most difficult) behavior we assessed—contacting government officials in support of mitigation policies—was unaffected by exposure to the pope, but both boycotting and buycotting, based on companies' climate change-related practices, increased as a function of exposure to the pope's climate change message.

We found that by the fall of 2016, when the pope's views on climate change were no longer prominent in the news, perceptions that climate change is a moral issue had reverted to their spring 2015 levels (Leiserowitz et al., 2017). This drop may reflect the absence of message repetition: Without the reinforcement provided by hearing the moral message repeated, the changes witnessed in 2015 faded. Nonetheless, given its at least temporary effects on issue engagement, we view the moral climate message as a potentially effective means of engaging faith communities.

Efficacy and Solvability Perceptions

If people come to recognize the threat of climate change without also believing there is something they can do to avert the threat, "fear control," becomes more likely: Defensive avoidance, denial, and distortion are response strategies people may employ in the face of an unavoidable threat (Witte, 1992). Hence, it is counterproductive to frighten people with information on the harmfulness of climate change without simultaneously providing them with images of a positive future and the actions they personally can take to move society toward that future.

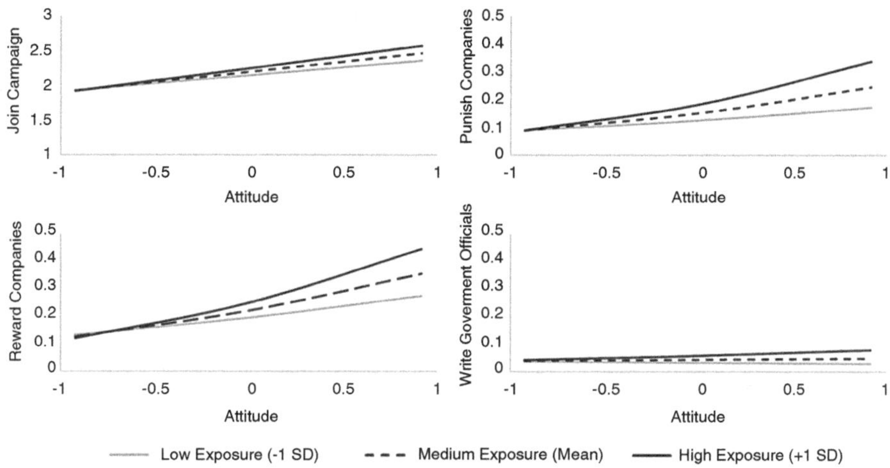

Fig. 6.9 Relationships between climate change attitudes and four activist behaviors, as a function of exposure to the Pope's climate change message. Relationships between attitudes and four behaviors at Time 2, as moderated by exposure to the Pope's message about global warming, controlling for likeliness of doing the behavior at Time 1. Note: The interactions between exposure to the Pope's message and attitude were significant for willingness to join a campaign, punishing companies by boycotting their products, and rewarding companies that are taking action to reduce global warming, but was not significant for contacting government officials. The non-significant interaction is shown for reference. The figures for punishing companies, rewarding companies and writing government officials show the conditional probabilities of performing those behaviors on the *y*-axis across levels of attitude and exposure, while the figure for joining a campaign to convince elected officials to take action to reduce global warming is on the measured scale for that variable, ranging from 1 = "I definitely would not do it," to 5 = "I am participating in a campaign like this now" (Source: Myers et al., 2017)

Efficacy beliefs are currently lacking in the USA: 42% of Americans agree with the statement, "The actions of a single individual won't make any different in global warming," and few are confident that we can and will reduce global warming. While 7% believe we will successfully reduce climate change, 44% believe we will not—either because people are not willing to change their behavior, humans are not capable of reducing climate change, or climate change is not happening. A plurality (49%) say it is unclear what will happen (see Table 6.2; Leiserowitz et al., 2017).

Low efficacy perceptions reduce the motivation to act (Bandura, 2001), and they represent a significant barrier to public engagement. Climate change is a collective problem that requires collective action. Unlike health threats—e.g., smoking–most individual actions to reduce climate change appear to have minimal impact: If I quit smoking, my health immediately begins to improve; if I quit driving, no reduction in climate change is apparent. However, this perspective fails to account for the significant contagion effects of individual action (Christakis & Fowler, 2013). Unfortunately, most people are unaware of the power of social influence (Nolan, Schultz, Cialdini, Goldstein, & Griskevicius, 2008).

Our research on political activism has highlighted the implications of efficacy perceptions for individual action: Among respondents who were certain climate

Table 6.2 Global warming solvability and collective efficacy perceptions

Humans can reduce global warming, and we are going to do so successfully	7%
Humans could reduce global warming, but it's unclear at this point whether we will do what's needed	49%
Humans could reduce global warming, but people aren't willing to change their behavior, so we're not going to	24%
Humans can't reduce global warming, even if it is happening	12%
Global warming isn't happening	8%

Unweighted $n = 1266$ (Source: Leiserowitz et al., 2017)

change is real, and who had high-risk perceptions (two of key beliefs), 3% had contacted a legislator in support of mitigation over the prior year. Among those who held these beliefs, but who also understood that humans cause and therefore can reduce climate change (two additional key beliefs that encompass efficacy), 40% had contacted a legislator (Roser-Renouf, Maibach, Leiserowitz, Feinberg, et al., 2014). The belief that activism is effective and a high sense of personal efficacy to engage in it were both significant predictors of political activism on climate.

In our examination of consumer activism, we found that the belief that consumer activism can influence the practices of companies (i.e., high perceived effectiveness) strongly predicted the goal of influencing other consumers and companies with one's purchase decisions, which in turn predicted both opinion leadership and green consumption choices. The perceived effectiveness of consumer activism was quite low, however: 72% of respondents said their actions influenced companies "not at all" or "only a little" (Roser-Renouf, Maibach, Leiserowitz, Feinberg, & Rosenthal, 2016).[8]

Best Practices for Climate Change Communications

In light of the research described above, together with other related research on science and risk communication, we published an overview of best practices for communicators and policy-makers (van der Linden, Leiserowitz, et al., 2015). In brief, we suggest that communicators:

- Localize the threat, emphasizing that it is hurting people in the audience's own community here and now. Distant peoples and species are less engaging.
- Rely less on messaging that requires analytical thought and cognitive effort. Messages should, instead, be easily and automatically understood, with an emphasis on concrete experiences that audience members can relate to their own lives.

[8] This is a misperception. Boycotts that receive at least some national media attention have about a one-in-four success rate in influencing corporate practices (Friedman, 1985; King, 2008; Roser-Renouf, Atkinson, Maibach & Leiserowitzl, 2016); and for those that include public protests or demonstrations, the success rate jumps to about half (Friedman, 1985).

- Leverage both descriptive and injunctive norms by highlighting the effective actions others are taking and the power of collective action; and by avoiding communications that imply negative attitudes and harmful behaviors are widespread.
- Emphasize the current benefits of mitigation actions, i.e., the co-benefits to our health and safety. Because humans are averse to losses, messages that suggest we sacrifice now for gains in the future are more likely to fall on deaf ears.
- Appeal to people's deeply held values concerning environmental protection and concerning the well-being of others.

Part IV: Audience Segmentation

Global Warming's Six Americas

The five best practices described above apply to messaging a broad audience. It is also true, however, that one size does not fit all. Audiences are diverse in their beliefs, informational needs, values, and interests, and within each of the best practices there are a range of communication options. Some audiences are willing to expend cognitive effort to learn more about an issue they care about. Some are already frightened and need less information on threats and more on solutions. And, some are open to making high-effort behavior changes, while others are only willing to change small, simple behaviors. Campaigns to increase engagement must therefore work at multiple levels, contingent on characteristics of the audiences they are attempting to reach.

To distinguish target audiences for strategic communications, we used our first *CCAM* survey data (2008) to segment the American adult public into six audiences: *Global Warming's Six Americas* (Maibach et al., 2009; Maibach, Leiserowitz, Roser-Renouf, & Mertz, 2011). The segmentation distinguishes among these audiences using 36 questions assessing four sets of characteristics: beliefs and attitudes; issue involvement; climate-relevant behaviors; and preferred societal responses. These segmentation findings and a screening instrument we developed for use by other researchers have become some of our most widely used applications, as they provide an in-depth analysis of groups that are both internally consistent, and distinct from one other.

The Six Americas range across a spectrum of concern and issue engagement, with segments that accept and reject climate science at the ends of a continuum, and those that are less certain and less engaged in the middle (see Fig. 6.10). At one end of the spectrum are the *Alarmed*, who are very concerned about the issue, accept that climate change is real, human-caused, and harmful, and who support aggressive action to reduce it. At the other end are the Dismissive, who are unlikely to believe that climate change is real or a problem, and are likely to believe it is a scientific hoax. Between these two extremes are four groups—the *Concerned, Cautious,*

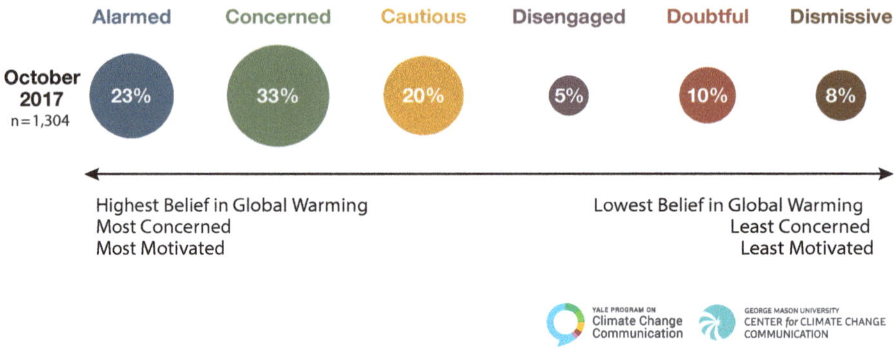

Fig. 6.10 Global Warming's Six Americas, October 2017

Disengaged, and Doubtful—with lower certainty and issue engagement. A selection of the measures used to identify the segments is shown in Table 6.3, illustrating differences among the groups.[9]

Unsurprisingly, the Dismissive and Doubtful are more likely to be conservative Republicans, while the Alarmed and Concerned are more likely to be liberal Democrats (Maibach et al., 2009). On scales of cultural values (Wildavsky & Dake, 1990), the Dismissive end of the spectrum favors individualism over egalitarianism, while the reverse is true of the segments at the Alarmed end. People at the Dismissive end of the spectrum are more likely to be evangelical Christians, to reject evolution, and to be biblical literalists. Conversely, the Alarmed are more likely than other segments to be atheists, and they are more likely to accept evolution and reject literal interpretations of the Bible (see Maibach et al., 2009; Roser-Renouf, Maibach, Leiserowitz, Feinberg, & Rosenthal, 2016).

The segments are not strongly distinguished by demographics, although there is some tendency for the Dismissive to be older, white males. Hispanics tend to be in the Alarmed and Concerned segments; and people with lower socioeconomic status tend to be in the Disengaged segment. None of these differences are as strong as the differences in attitudes and beliefs, however (Maibach et al., 2011).

Applications and Extensions

We have tracked the Six Americas since 2008 and worked with many organizations to apply the results, including federal agencies, park rangers, science museums, faith-based environmental groups, public health departments, water utilities, and transportation agencies. The segmentation has been used to profile specific subpopulations, including American zoo and aquarium visitors (Kelly et al., 2014), agricultural extension agents (Bowers, Monroe, & Adams, 2016), visitors to national

[9] The full segmentation screener with all 36 items, a 15-item abbreviated screening instrument, and the methodology used in the segmentation can be found in Maibach et al. (2011).

Table 6.3 Selected segmentation measures by Six Americas segment

Categories of questions	Survey questions	Segments						F or χ^2
		Alarmed	Concerned	Cautious	Disengaged	Doubtful	Dismissive	
Global warming beliefs	Certainty global warming is happening[a]	8.66	7.84	6.57	6.07	4.80	2.87	451
	Human causation[b]	94%	77%	50%	47%	19%	5%	438.63
	Most scientists agree gw is happening[c]	87%	69%	33%	22%	22%	12%	363.7
	Personal risk[d]	3.30	2.78	2.19	2.23	1.44	1.07	247.54
	Risk to future generations[d]	3.98	3.9	3.1	1	2.21	1.12	936.04
	Collective efficacy/solvability[e]	3.93	3.76	3.59	3.40	2.43	1.55	254.62
Issue involvement	Affective rating of global warming[f]	5.82	5.38	4.17	4.29	3.67	3.11	172.66
	Worry about global warming[g]	3.7	3.05	2.3	2.25	1.59	1.14	599.79
	Personal importance of issue[h]	4.31	3.22	2.54	2.40	1.69	1.31	474.46
	"I could easily change my mind about global warming."[i]	1.31	1.97	2.61	2.77	2.10	1.52	112.55
	How often thought about global warming[j]	3.60	2.65	2.08	1.80	1.99	2.18	142.62
Behavior	Contacted govt. official in support of mitigation[k]	41%	9%	8%	0	1%	0	222.69
	Rewarded companies that reduced emissions by buying their products[k]	73%	33%	23%	8%	11%	2%	297.63
	Stage of change for using mass transit/car pool instead of driving[l]	3.92	3.40	3.12	2.61	2.33	2.48	14.90
Preferred societal response	Priority of global warming for president and Congress[m]	3.76	3.1	2.22	2.45	1.45	1.03	425.67
	Citizens should do more/less to reduce warming[n]	4.66	4.22	3.61	3.82	3.05	2.31	205.09

All comparisons $p < 0.001$; unweighted $n = 1266$ (Source: Leiserowitz et al., 2017; previously unpublished CCAM data)

[a]1 = certain global warming not happening; 5 = don't know; 9 = certain global warming is happening

[b]Percent who say that assuming global warming is happening, it is primarily human-caused

[c]Percent who say that most scientists agree that global warming is happening

[d]1 = low harm; 4 = a great deal of harm; note: this analysis treats "don't know" responses as missing. In the analyses to create the segmentation, these variables are treated as dummy variables and "don't know" is included in the analysis. See Maibach et al. (2011) for details

(continued)

Table 6.3 (continued)

[e]1 = global warming isn't happening; 2 = even if global warming is happening, humans can't reduce it; 3 = humans could reduce global warming, but humans aren't willing to change our behavior, so we're not going to; 4 = humans could reduce global warming, but it's not clear at this point whether we'll do what's necessary; 5 = humans can and will successfully reduce global warming
[f]1 = very good; 6 = very bad
[g]1 = not at all worried; 4 = very worried
[h]1 = not at all important; 5 = extremely important
[i]1 = strongly disagree; 4 = strongly agree
[j]1 = not at all; 4 = a great deal
[k]Percent who have performed action at least once over the past year
[l]1 = never do this and don't plan to in the future; 10 = always do this and plan to do so more often in the future
[m]1 = low; 4 = very high
[n]1 = much less; 5 = much more

parks (Schweizer, Davis, & Thompson, 2013), museum visitors (Leiserowitz & Smith, 2011; Phipps, 2011), and adolescents (Flora & Roser-Renouf, 2014). It has been used to study specific audience segments, for example, the Alarmed (Doherty & Webler, 2016), and as an outcome measure to assess the impact of climate change educational interventions (Flora et al., 2014). Experimental research has used the segmentation as an independent variable to identify differences in the segments' responses to different message frames (Myers et al., 2012) and their responses to personal experiences with climate change (Myers et al., 2013).

The segmentation has been replicated in Australia (Morrison, Duncan, Sherley, & Parton, 2013), Germany (Metag, Füchslin, & Schäfer, 2015), India (Leiserowitz, Thaker, Feinberg, & Cooper, 2013), and Singapore (Detenber, Rosenthal, Liao, & Ho, 2016). The segments identified in Australia and Germany closely resemble those in the USA, with the important difference that Germany has no Dismissive segment. In India, the segments are quite different, with the largest segment of the population unfamiliar with the term "climate change," but once it has been explained, they readily agree that it is occurring. And, in Singapore, only three segments were identified, with varying levels of concern and issue engagement, but little evidence of climate skepticism. To date, the results suggest that the segments are similar across developed nations, but that in developing nations, attitudes are structured differently.

In an important recent development, we have developed a reliable, much shorter, four-item Six Americas screening instrument (Chryst et al., in press). This shorter instrument will make the segmentation tool practical for many additional research and communication planning purposes.

Theoretical Underpinnings of the Six Americas and Their Implications for Communication Campaigns

Two theoretical dimensions underlie the Six Americas—*attitudinal valence* and *cognitive issue involvement* (see Fig. 6.11; Roser-Renouf, Maibach, Leiserowitz, & Zhao, 2014). These dimensions link the segmentation to the literatures on information processing, risk communication, and opinion leadership cited in the section on Theories of Change, and suggest a wealth of communication strategies for reaching and influencing the six groups.

Attitudinal valence is defined here as *the inclination to accept or reject the science of climate change*, as reflected in acceptance of the key climate change beliefs: Climate change is happening; harmful; human-caused; solvable; and scientists agree on its reality and human causes.

Issue involvement refers to *cognitive issue involvement*[10] as reflected in the amount of thought devoted to the issue and attitudinal certainty. Both the *Alarmed*

[10] This pattern does not describe affective involvement, as reflected in worry, concern, or personal importance. These characteristics follow the same pattern as attitudinal valence.

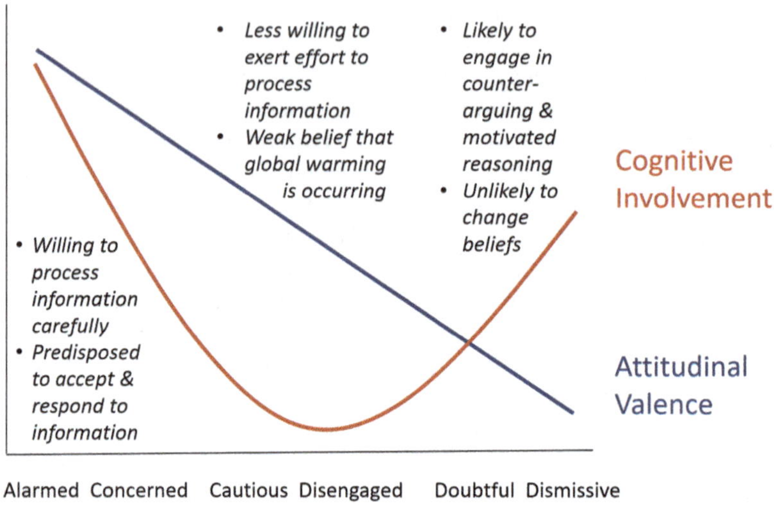

Fig. 6.11 Information-processing propensities among the Six Americas (Source: Roser-Renouf, Stenhouse, et al., 2014)

and *Dismissive* think about the issue and are certain of their opinions, but the *Alarmed* are likely to accept all the key beliefs and are predisposed to accept messages that are consistent with the science, while the *Dismissive* reject the key beliefs and are predisposed to reject and counterargue these same messages. The segments between the two end points devote less thought to the issue and are less certain of their views. The curvilinear relationship shown in Fig. 6.11 is apparent in the segment means for thought and attitudinal certainty shown in Table 6.3, with thought following the pattern in the figure, and willingness to change one's mind, a mirror image of this pattern.

The interaction of attitudes and involvement is strongly predictive of the level of attention people pay to information on global warming, their willingness to attend closely to information and process it deeply, and their inclination to accept information or to counterargue and reject it.

Informational Needs and Interests

Communicators reduce their effectiveness if they focus on the information they want the audience to understand, while ignoring the information the audience is interested in hearing. When asked what information they would be most interested in receiving from a climate scientist (Fig. 6.12; Roser-Renouf, Stenhouse, et al., 2014), clear patterns are apparent among the Six Americas: The Alarmed overwhelmingly are interested in hearing about solutions to climate change—the actions they can personally take, as well as the actions that the USA can take.

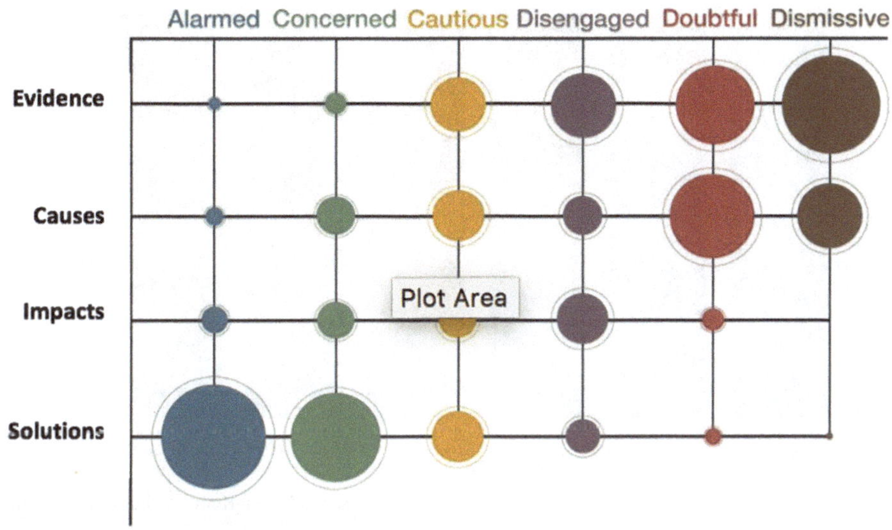

Fig. 6.12 Nature of the one question the Six Americans would most like to pose to a climate scientist. The Six Americas are interested in learning different types of information about global warming, with the skeptical segments on the right most interested in information about the evidence for and causes of global warming, the concerned segments on the left interested in information about action to mitigate climate change, and the less involved segments in the middle varying widely in their questions. Unweighted $N = 1010$ (Source: Roser-Renouf, Stenhouse, et al., 2014; figure edited from original by Ian Barin)

They also want to hear whether it is too late. The Concerned are also most interested in solutions information, although some express interest in causes and impacts.

The Dismissive and Doubtful are most interested in information about the reality and causes of global warming. However, because both groups tend to be skeptical of the science, it is highly likely that many of them will engage in counterarguing and motivated reasoning if presented with this information, so other ways of communicating with them are sometimes wiser. An initial focus on solutions that are consistent with conservative values may be a better starting point, both to avoid triggering identity protection ("This is a 'liberal' issue, and I'm a conservative"), and to address the fact that people are less likely to accept the problem as valid if they believe that the solutions are unacceptable, i.e., "solution aversion" increases motivated skepticism about climate change (Campbell & Kay, 2014).

Patterns are less clear among the Cautious and Disengaged—their responses are distributed across all four types of information. Because these groups have given the issue very little thought, it is likely that many do not actually have actual questions, and have simply picked a random response on the survey. In light of this, we would mostly like them to learn that climate change is happening now in the USA and is

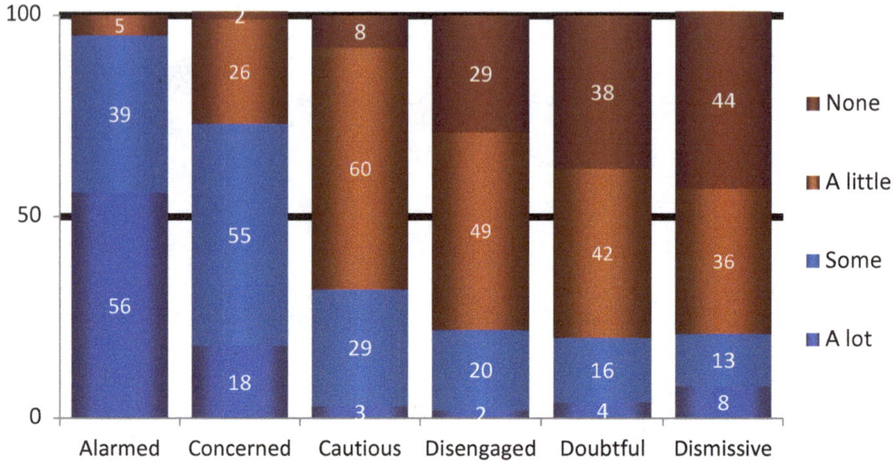

Fig. 6.13 Attention paid to global warming information (Source: Roser-Renouf, Stenhouse, et al., 2014)

harming people here; this follows from risk communication models, such as the Extended Parallel Process Model (Witte, 1992): People begin to search for information on solutions to a problem after they realize that it is harmful and that they are vulnerable.

The challenge is to gain the middle segments' attention long enough to communicate this information: They pay little attention to global warming information (Fig. 6.13). This holds true of the Doubtful and Dismissive as well, although we also know that a fraction of the Dismissive are paying close attention to information on the issue, as they are actively engaged in attempts to undermine the science.[11] Low-information seekers are the people we seek to reach with messages that require minimal cognitive effort, and for whom the five best practices most strongly apply. The heuristics and cues that audiences with low-issue involvement rely on, as identified in the Elaboration Likelihood Model (Petty & Cacioppo, 1986), are essential in reaching these groups with both the information that will interest them and draw them into the issue, as well as the information we believe they need.

In reaching them, simple, clear messages that trigger automatic processing are essential: Three-quarters of the Disengaged say they have difficulty understanding news reports on global warming, and majorities of the Disengaged, Doubtful, and Dismissive say they do not want to hear about the subject (See Table 6.4;

[11] This is readily apparent in the comments sections accompanying online news reports about climate change, which typically contain large numbers of comments disputing climate science.

Table 6.4 Ability and motivational barriers to climate change communication

	Alarmed (%)	Concerned (%)	Cautious (%)	Disengaged (%)	Doubtful (%)	Dismissive (%)
"I have difficulty understanding news reports about global warming"	23	39	44	77	35	19
"In general, I don't like to read or hear anything about global warming"	10	28	37	59	57	72

Note: Cells show the proportions in each segment who agreed with the statements (Source: Roser-Renouf, Stenhouse, et al., 2014)

Roser-Renouf, Stenhouse et al., 2014). Even among the Alarmed, close a quarter report they have difficulty understanding global warming news.

Communication Objectives and Strategies

Based on our understanding of the segments' beliefs, their issue involvement, information needs, interests, and their willingness and ability to attend to information on global warming, we have developed general objectives and communication strategy recommendations for audiences who are very concerned about climate change (the Alarmed and many of the Concerned); the skeptics (the Dismissive and many of the Doubtful); and the uncertain, uninvolved middle segments (the Cautious and Disengaged, and some of the Concerned and Doubtful). A full application of the segmentation would entail six different sets of recommendations, but space in this chapter, as well as the challenges of putting such a complex campaign into place, make it more practical to distinguish between three approaches instead of six.

The Middle Segments

The best practices apply to communicating across segments, but are most relevant for the uncertain middle segments, as they are unlikely to attend to effortful content, such as reading textual material or interpreting graphs and figures. Communicators should attempt to engage the middle segments with easily processed messages that illustrate local, concrete impacts, as well as the co-benefits of actions that will mitigate the threat. Invoking norms constructively is also likely to be beneficial. Use of peripheral cues—likable and authoritative sources, humor, and narratives of people they can identify with—can help as well. Essentially, the two core social marketing recommendations we have mentioned several times apply most strongly to the middle segments; that is, (1) simple, clear messages, repeated often, by a variety of trusted sources, and (2) recommended behaviors should be presented as easy, fun, and popular. Messages should communicate the key beliefs—particularly the scientific consensus message—and behaviors should be simple, while still being effective at reducing emissions.

An excellent example of a campaign that employed these techniques is the "Wicked Smaht" campaign in Boston, which effectively applied the research described in this chapter. The campaign communicated the key beliefs—climate change is real, harmful, human-caused, and solvable, and scientists agree—over the course of a year on subways and buses (Sciencetogo.org, 2017). A dozen posters were designed, and a new one appeared each month (see Fig. 6.14 for examples). The first poster adapted the "estimate and reveal" technique tested by Myers et al. (2015): It engaged people with a question about the scientific consensus, which would not be answered until the second month, when the message described the 97% consensus among climate scientists that human-caused climate change is happening. For 4 months, each poster addressed a different impact of climate change on Boston: sea level rise, extreme storms, heat waves, and the spread of vector-borne diseases. The final 5 months addressed solutions by describing local organizations, individuals, and groups that were working to reduce their emissions—an approach

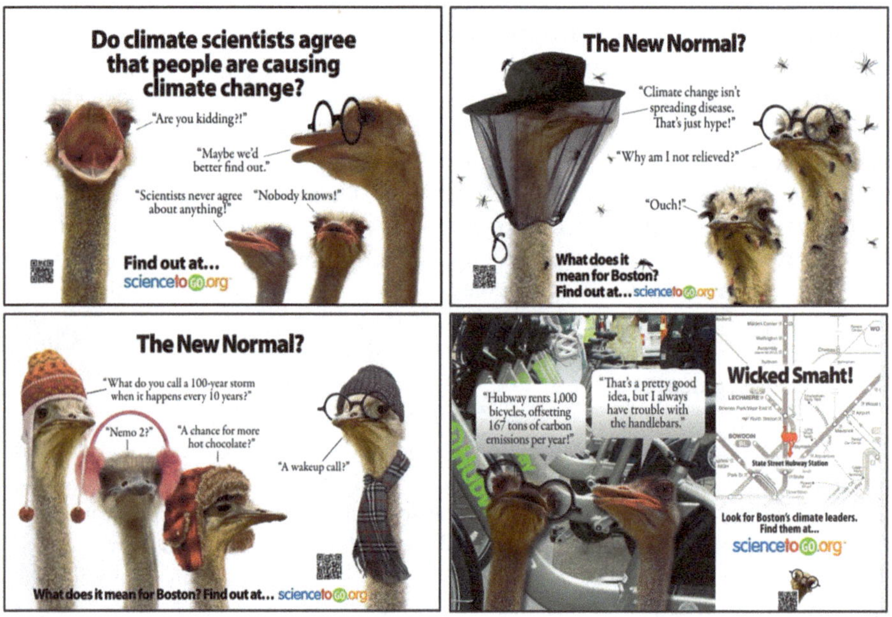
Do climate scientists agree that people are causing climate change?
"Are you kidding?!"
"Maybe we'd better find out."
"Scientists never agree about anything!"
"Nobody knows!"
Find out at...
sciencetoGO.org
The New Normal?
"Climate change isn't spreading disease. That's just hype!"
"Why am I not relieved?"
"Ouch!"
What does it mean for Boston?
Find out at... sciencetoGO.org
The New Normal?
"What do you call a 100-year storm when it happens every 10 years?"
"Nemo 2?"
"A chance for more hot chocolate?"
"A wakeup call?"
What does it mean for Boston? Find out at... sciencetoGO.org
"Hubway rents 1,000 bicycles, offsetting 167 tons of carbon emissions per year!"
"That's a pretty good idea, but I always have trouble with the handlebars."
Wicked Smaht!
State Street Hubway Station
Look for Boston's climate leaders. Find them at...
sciencetoGO.org

Fig. 6.14 "Wicked Smaht" campaign posters (Source: sciencetogo.org; designs by Tom Bowman, Bowman Change, Inc.; Robert J Gould, One Degree Strategies, LLC; and Ed Hackley, Ed Hackley Design; used by permission)

intended to activate social norms by presenting sustainable behaviors as "popular," as well as building collective efficacy, hope, and perceptions that climate change is solvable. The use of one clever ostrich in glasses with several less-clever ostriches who often voiced climate skeptic arguments allowed for humor and a light touch, avoiding any gloom-and-doom or guilt messaging.

The Alarmed (and to Some Extent, the Concerned)

Unlike the middle segments, the Alarmed and many of the Concerned are willing to extend the time and cognitive effort necessary to learn more detailed information about climate change. They are also looking for ways they personally can help reduce the threat. Hence, rather than trying to change their attitudes on the issue and engage them, we aim to enlist them as opinion leaders, social role models, and climate activists.

The Alarmed and Concerned are likely to comprise the largest proportion of adult visitors to online sources of information on climate change, such as the National Climate Assessment, NASA's and NOAA's online climate change resources, AAAS's "What We Know" site, and Skeptical Science—all excellent sources of climate change information.[12] Close to 90% of visitors to NASA's climate change website, for example, belong to these two segments (59% Alarmed and 29% Concerned; Myers, Rolfe-Redding, Roser-Renouf, & Maibach, 2014). The same is true of visitors to science and technology museums (74%, Leiserowitz & Smith, 2011), and zoos and aquaria (64%; Kelly et al., 2014).

Information obtained from these and similar sources is likely to be shared with others: 85% of the Alarmed say they discuss global warming often or occasionally with family and friends (Leiserowitz et al., 2017). Moreover, people trust their family and friends as information sources on global warming as strongly as they trust climate scientists (i.e., 69% trust their family and friends and 70% trust scientists; Leiserowitz et al., 2015b). Hence, providing them with some of the facts that support the key beliefs can equip them to convince those around them. Information on risks should always be paired with efficacy-building hopeful messages, as despair and a sense that it is too late can foster issue avoidance, rather than heightening engagement.

Advocacy organizations seeking to recruit new members should note that only 8% of the Alarmed say they are currently participating in a campaign to convince government officials to reduce global warming, but another two-thirds say they would be willing to join such a campaign (68%). Moreover, more than half say they have never been contacted by an environmental organization that works on global warming (55%; Leiserowitz et al., 2017). One of the strongest predictors of political

[12] See: nca2014.globalchange.gov/; climate.nasa.gov; noaa.gov/climate; whatweknow.aaas.org/; and skepticalscience.com/.

participation is being asked (Brady, Verba, & Schlozman, 1995), and in recruiting the Alarmed, activist groups should stress that their participation can make a difference, as this is a strong predictor of joining a social movement (Burstein, Einwohner, & Hollander, 1995). The social marketing admonition that recommended behaviors should appear easy, fun, and popular applies here as well: Many people join advocacy groups for the social benefits of group membership (Van Zomeren, Postmes, & Spears, 2008).

The Dismissive (and to Some Extent, the Doubtful)

While we might like to overcome the skepticism in these segments regarding the reality and human causes of climate change, changing people's minds when they are firmly convinced of their opinions is difficult and rare. A more promising objective may be to build their support for a swift transition to clean energy by focusing on its co-benefits and through discussing policies that are consistent with conservative values.

Half of the Dismissive and Doubtful identify as Republicans, and the vast majority of these say they are conservative Republicans. With strong individualistic values, they dislike the policy options for reducing climate change that have been promoted by liberals. Further, the climate skepticism among Republican party's political elites has been a particularly powerful contributor to the issue's polarization. A longitudinal study comparing factors that contributed to decline in climate change beliefs and concern between 2002 and 2010 found that statements by political elites had by far the greatest impact on conservatives' expressed concern about climate change—greater than weather extremes, advocacy campaigns, scientific news, media coverage, or extreme weather[13] (Brulle, Carmichael, & Jenkins, 2012).

Some experimental work has identified promising messages for reaching and influencing Republicans and conservatives, e.g., explanations of the science (Ranney & Clark, 2016) and the scientific consensus message (van der Linden et al., 2017). Conservatives and Republicans have also been found to respond well to environmental messages that use conservative value frames—loyalty, purity, authority, and patriotism (Feinberg & Willer, 2013; Feygina et al., 2010; Wolsko et al., 2016).

Segment and party identification are not synonymous, however: Close to half of Republicans belong to the Doubtful and Dismissive groups (48%), but one in five Republicans belong to Alarmed and Cautious segments (21%), and close to a third belong to the Cautious and Disengaged (31%; previously unpublished *CCAM* data, May 2017). Hence, research demonstrating that Republicans have been influenced by particular messages or message frames does not necessarily generalize to the Doubtful and Dismissive.

One study we conducted to test the impact of various message frames on the Six Americas was highly instructive. We expected a national security framing of climate change to be positively received by the Doubtful and Dismissive; instead, it elicited anger.

[13] The authors note that although weather did not affect opinions during the years they analyzed, it could in the future.

The most positively received message across all segments was a public health framing of climate change that emphasized the health co-benefits of redesigning urban areas to encourage walking and biking and reducing the need to drive (Myers et al., 2012).

In light of this study, as well as Brulle et al.'s (2012) evidence of the influence of political elites, our primary recommendation for communicating with the Dismissives and Doubtful is to reach out through conservative sources they trust who are proposing conservative responses to climate change they can accept. When acceptable solutions are available to them, the motivated reasoning and solution aversion that have promoted climate skepticism (Campbell & Kay, 2014) may be reduced. We will return to this approach in Part V, when we describe the activities of *RepublicEn*, our outreach program to conservatives led by Bob Inglis, a former Republican Congressman from South Carolina who advocates for free-market responses to climate change.

Part V: Outreach

The research described in Part II identified three sources who were particularly likely to be influential with audiences, i.e., television meteorologists, medical professionals, and Republican elites. We have major outreach programs with each of these, and—in light of the importance of journalists in shaping audience perceptions of the issue—we are about to extend our work with meteorologists into television newsrooms.

We also advise a wide range of other climate change communicators, as we work to instantiate a "big messy program" with many credible messengers delivering the same simple, clear messages through multiple channels. These other communicators include federal and state agencies, park rangers, public health departments, science and natural history museums, aquaria, zoos, college campus leaders, and faith communities.

Demonstration Project: Climate Matters

Our most significant outreach program has been to TV weathercasters, through *Climate Matters,* a demonstration project that trains and supports TV weathercasters to report on the local impacts of climate change in their media market. The NSF-funded program has gradually expanded over the past 8 years from a pilot project with one weathercaster in Columbia, South Carolina to nationwide operation with over 500 weathercasters in over half the nation's media markets. In September 2017, in partnership with five journalism professional societies (Radio & Television Digital News Association, National Association of Black Journalists, National Association of Hispanic Journalists, Society of Environmental Journalists, and the Kneeland Project), the program began expanding beyond weathercaster into television, radio, newspaper, and digital newsrooms.

Rationale for Communicating Climate Change Through TV Weather Forecasts

For a variety of reasons, TV weathercasters are potentially effective climate change communicators. Their audience is large, and diverse in age, income, education, and racial demographics. Our *CCAM* surveys have shown them to be a highly trusted source of global warming information, and 70% of the public say they watch the local weather forecast closely (e.g., Maibach et al., 2009). Further, they are highly skilled science communication professionals.

The local weather forecast has the potential to help viewers link climate issues with their personal lives. People learn complex information most quickly when it is offered in the form of concrete examples and narratives that are easily applied to their experience. The more times they encounter information presented this way, the stronger the lesson will be. When weathercasters are able to present information about climate change in conjunction with related local weather events, it can help people understand that they are personally experiencing the effects of climate change, fostering the understanding that it is a serious issue. Severe weather events offer particularly strong climate change learning opportunities, as many of these events are becoming more common and more severe as a result of global warming.

Weathercasters' Climate Change Beliefs, Attitudes, and On-Air Reporting

Climate Matters was initiated at a time when few television newscasts were actually reporting about climate change on the air. In 2010, more than half of television news directors said their newscasts discussed climate change less than once a month (Maibach, Wilson, & Witte, 2010a); and 80% of weathercasters said they discussed climate change less than once a month during their forecasts (Maibach, Wilson, & Witte, 2010b).

In 2009, immediately prior to the launch of the pilot test in South Carolina, we used snowball sampling to identify TV weathercasters who were actively reporting on climate change but were able to identify only 16 weathercasters of this type anywhere in the USA (Rowan et al., in press).

In a 2010 survey we conducted with weathercasters nationwide, we learned that 94% of weathercasters said they are the only people in their newsroom trained in science or the environment (Maibach, Wilson, & Witte, 2010b). While all have had extensive experience as science communicators, and many have had scientific training, at that time only slightly more than half believed that climate change is happening, and only a third believed that it is human-caused (54% and 31%, respectively;

Maibach, Wilson, & Witte, 2010c).[14] Many weathercasters said they would like to report on climate change, but most cited a range of barriers that impede them from doing so including: lack of time on air; lack of time to produce stories; lack of access to broadcast quality climate change graphics; lack of access to climate scientists; and the belief that it is inappropriate to discuss climate change on air.

The Launch and National Scale-Up of Climate Matters

In 2010, we launched *Climate Matters* as a 1-year pilot test at WLTX-TV, the CBS affiliate in Columbia, South Carolina, in partnership with their chief meteorologist Jim Gandy, his news director Marybeth Jacoby, and Climate Central (a science communication nonprofit organization). A team of broadcast meteorologists, climate scientists, communication scientists, writers, and graphic designers developed scripts and graphical materials for 12 short segments on climate change, which Gandy presented on air throughout the year, when time permitted and conditions were appropriate. These video segments were also displayed on the station's website, along with additional print content developed by Gandy throughout the year. The segment topics were selected based on foreseeable local weather events (see Table 6.5). Each 90-s segment was designed to be a self-contained short lesson on climate change, focusing on one or two major points selected to be as connected as possible to the experiences of the viewer. For example, a segment on poison ivy explained how certain plant pests thrive under increasing carbon dioxide levels and are likely to become more prevalent without intervention. The team's goal was to show viewers that climate change is an issue that already impacts their everyday lives, thus helping to correct the misperception that climate change is a distant problem.

The effects of the Climate Matters pilot test were assessed with surveys conducted before the program's launch, and at the end of the year; both cross-sectional and panel data were collected. These surveys revealed that, in comparison to viewers of other stations in Columbia, WLTX viewers became significantly more likely to report that climate change was happening and harmful, regardless of whether or not they specifically remembered seeing the segments. Those who were able to recall specific Climate Matters segments were also more likely to attribute climate change to human causes (Zhao et al., 2014).

[14] Over the past 7 years, we have made consistent efforts to educate members of this community about climate change, primarily through presentations and workshops at their annual professional meetings. In our 2017 survey of weathercasters, we found that 95% now say climate change is happening, an increase of 41 percentage points. Understanding of human causation has also changed, though less dramatically: 49% now say it is mostly or entirely human-caused, an increase of 18 percentage points, and another 21% say it is equally caused by human activity and natural events (Maibach et al., 2017).

Table 6.5 Climate Matters design

Date	Activity	
11 May–15 July 2010	Baseline survey of panel sample	
2 Aug. 2010	Campaign began	
	Segment name	**Description (length)**
2 Aug. 2010 (again 8 Sept. 2010)	High temperatures	Increasing number of >95° F days as GHG emissions increase—separate segment for each summer month (1:18)
12 Aug. 2010	Extreme heat	Increasing likelihood of >101° F days for today, 2040s, and 2070s (1:16)
25 Aug. 2010	Climate	Baseball statistics analogy explains difference between weather and climate (1:54)
16 Sept. 2010	Hurricanes	Climate change may make hurricanes less frequent but more intense (1:30)
1 Oct. 2010	Intense storms	Climate change may be making intense rainfall more intense in the U.S. (1:55)
12 Nov. 2010	Sea level rise	Rate of sea level rise along South Carolina coast may triple (1:54)
9 Mar. 2011	Poison ivy	More CO_2 may make some plant pests like poison ivy grow better (1:31)
22 Apr. 2011	Human cause	How we know greenhouse gas increase is due to people (1:20)
12 May 2011	Air quality	Connection between warmer temperature and code red smog days (1:07)
31 May 2011	Heat and human health	Heat is already the top weather-related killer in the U.S., and GHGs will likely increase the heat index in the Southeast (1:23)
9 June 2011	Drought	Drought outlook to explain risk for increased drought in a warmer world (2:23)
12 June 2011	Global weirding	Global warming can cause opposite weather extremes (1:26)
10 July–30 Aug. 2011	Follow-up survey of panel sample; survey of new cross-sectional sample	

In 2012, Climate Matters was expanded to ten TV stations in ten different media markets, with all participating weathercasters receiving localized climate change content, including high-resolution graphics ready for on-air use. Starting in 2013, participation in Climate Matters grew rapidly (supported by a combination of NSF and philanthropic funding). By the beginning of 2014, for example, over 100 weathercasters were participating. Currently (in Feb. 2018), we have over 500 weathercasters participating in the project (including 31 who broadcast in Spanish), broadcasting from 262 stations in 136 of America's 210 media markets, including 24 of the top 25 media markets. Moreover, on-air reporting about climate change by weathercasters increased over 1200% in the 4-year span from 2013 to 2016.

In short, the program—now a partnership involving our university, Climate Central, NOAA (National Oceanic and Atmospheric Association), NASA, and the

American Meteorological Society—has blossomed into a resource for informal climate education nationwide. Every week, a team of meteorologists, research scientists, data analysts, journalists, and creative designers put together a comprehensive package of content about various current climate change topics. Each package includes TV-ready visuals, detailed descriptions of the latest science behind the week's topic, current climate change information from NASA, NOAA, and other sources of climate change data, and a roundup of new climate research findings. The packages are designed to be current and relevant, and to dramatically reduce the production burden for weathercasters interested in including climate change education as part of their segments. *Climate Matters* has also expanded beyond the short TV weather segment to support weathercasters in climate change education across a variety of mediums. To engage with growing digital content consumption, *Climate Matters* offers interactive media and tweetable facts that can be easily embedded in station websites or social media. They provide a range of resources that are suitable for the local community outreach presentations that many weathercasters give. *Climate Matters* also provides video and production support to meteorologists who are interested in developing and producing their own original climate change stories and specials.

An impact evaluation of the national scale-up of Climate Matters is currently underway. Multilevel modeling is being used to analyze *CCAM* data on audience beliefs within media markets, using a quasi-experimental, dose–response, nonequivalent group design with multiple time points.

Climate Matters Expands into Newsrooms

In September of 2017, *Climate Matters* began offering resources to non-weather journalists to extend the reach of local climate reporting and education. In partnership with a range of journalism associations (including Society of Environmental Journalists, Radio & TV Digital News Association, National Association of Black Journalists, National Association of Hispanic Journalists, and The Kneeland Project), we are now offering *Climate Matters* reporting resources to journalists around the nation. We have high hopes that extending *Climate Matters* deeper into the newsroom (i.e., beyond TV weathercasters) will help end the dearth of local climate reporting, and thereby help Americans better understand the local relevance of the problem, and local solutions.

Additional Outreach Efforts

Program on Climate and Health

Our Program on Climate and Health was started in 2013 under the directorship of a physician—Mona Sarfaty, MD—in recognition of the severe impacts climate change has on human health. The program has several objectives: to illuminate public and health professionals' understanding of the health harms associated with climate change and the health benefits created by climate solutions; to increase public and health professional awareness of the climate change and health connections; and to encourage life-saving preventive and protective action.

Over the past several years, we have surveyed physicians in multiple medical societies, focusing on specialties that are most likely to include patients vulnerable to climate change (including the National Medical Association, which serves African-American physicians and patients; the American Academy of Allergies, Asthma and Immunology; and the American Thoracic Society); and we have used our *CCAM* surveys to further explore public understanding of the climate–health nexus. Three important findings have emerged from this research thus far: (1) Most Americans are largely unaware of the health harms associated with climate change (and who is mostly likely to be harmed); (2) Conversely, most physicians are aware of the health harms, and many are convinced that climate change is already harming some of their patients; and (3) People trust their physicians most as a source of information about climate and health. These findings strongly suggest an important role for America's physicians in educating the public and policy-makers about the human health aspects of climate change.

The Medical Society Consortium on Climate and Health

In the spring of 2017, we launched an important new initiative—*The Medical Society Consortium on Climate and Health*—with the aim of activating the American medical community to teach the public and policy-makers about the human health relevance of climate change. Specifically, the mission of the Consortium is to inform the public and policy-makers about the harmful effects of climate change on Americans, and about the immediate and long-term health benefits associated with decreasing greenhouse gas emissions and other preventive and protective measures. Initially composed of nine major medical societies (which collectively represent half of America's doctors), the Consortium recently released its first report entitled: "*Medical Alert! Climate Change is Harming our Health*" (Medical Society Consortium on Climate and Health, 2017).

Since the spring of 2017, membership in the Consortium has grown to 13 medical societies, and 19 other health and climate science organizations have joined as "affiliates." In addition, several hundred physicians have volunteered to help the Consortium by serving as climate and health advocates in their community—to speak with community groups, the media, and local policy-makers.

The trusted voices of these 13 medical societies and hundreds of volunteer physicians are seeking to convey five simple messages: (1) There is a scientific consensus about human-caused climate change, therefore doctors have a responsibility to take action so that people are not needlessly hurt. (2) In communities across America, climate change is already harming people's health. (3) The health of any American can be harmed by climate change, but some people face greater risks than others (e.g., children, pregnant women, elder, people with chronic illness and allergies, and the poor). (4) Unless we take concerted action, the harms to our health are going to worsen. (5) The most important action we can take to protect our health is to reduce heat-trapping pollution by reducing energy waste and accelerating the transition to clean, renewable energy.

Engaging Conservatives: *RepublicEn*

RepublicEn was started in 2012 by Bob Inglis, a former six-term Republican Congressman from South Carolina, who serves as the group's executive director. Inglis lost his seat in Congress in 2010 in large part due to his acceptance of the science of climate change and his advocacy for free-market solutions to mitigate the threat. Through *RepublicEn*, he is seeking to catalyze a new narrative on climate change among conservatives based in free-market thinking, with the objective of generating support for climate solutions and the political will needed to press for an aggressive response.

Through media interviews, community events, and a rapidly growing online community, the *RepublicEn* team educates Republicans on climate science, public opinion and—perhaps most importantly, in light of what we understand about solution aversion—tax reform. They call for the repeal of all subsidies for fuel production, and for a revenue-neutral carbon tax on companies for the greenhouse gases they emit (see Fig. 6.15).

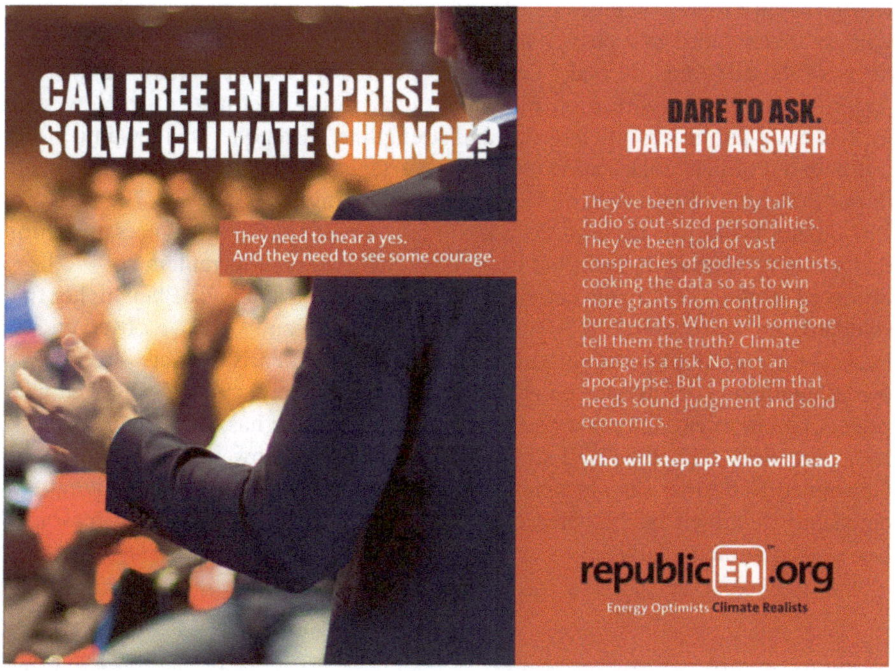
CAN FREE ENTERPRISE SOLVE CLIMATE CHANGE?
They need to hear a yes.
And they need to see some courage.
DARE TO ASK.
DARE TO ANSWER
They've been driven by talk radio's out-sized personalities. They've been told of vast conspiracies of godless scientists, cooking the data so as to win more grants from controlling bureaucrats. When will someone tell them the truth? Climate change is a risk. No, not an apocalypse. But a problem that needs sound judgment and solid economics.
Who will step up? Who will lead?
republicEn.org
Energy Optimists Climate Realists

Fig. 6.15 *RepublicEn* Facebook post (Source: https://www.facebook.com/republicen/photos/a.210244879118841.55519.114226275387369/1051156848360969/?type=3&theater)

In 2015, Inglis was awarded the *John F. Kennedy Profile in Courage* Award by the John F. Kennedy Library Foundation. On September 12, 2016, Inglis and *RepublicEn* advisor Katharine Hayhoe—a climate scientist at Texas Tech University—were named on the Politico 50 list for their work on what Politico called articulating "the conservative case for fighting climate change." Politico's top 50 ranking is described as a "guide to the thinkers, doers and visionaries transforming American politics in 2016" (Politico Magazine, 2016).

Ironically, given the inexplicable anti-climate science views being expressed by President Trump and his administration, the past year may prove to be a watershed moment for Republican embrace of climate solutions. A growing list of prominent Republicans have come out in support of a revenue-neutral carbon tax to address climate change and strengthen our economy, 29 Republican members of Congress have joined the Climate Solutions Caucus, and our *RepublicEn* team is more energized than ever. Inglis recently summarized his feelings about the opportunity at hand: "We're making progress. Conservatives are going to come around on climate. We're going to realize that we're all in this together, and the world is going to celebrate American leadership. This is our generation's moon shot" (RepublicEn, 2017).

Part VI: Conclusions

Our research center continues to expand both its outreach and research activities with as much speed and energy as we can muster. Although we have addressed many of the questions we had a decade ago, as many or more remain. And, while Americans increasingly recognize the reality and threat of climate change, we still lack an issue-public of sufficient size and strength to push policy-makers into effective action. Political polarization remains a barrier to progress on climate, and much of our thinking is focused on methods of de-polarizing the issue.

Looking back over the past decade's work, we can say with some satisfaction that we have been both busy and productive, and we plan to remain so. We have observed progress on climate action in the USA—the Clean Power Plan, higher fuel standards for automobiles, the Paris Climate Accord—and we have observed setbacks—the current plans to withdraw the USA from the Paris Climate Accord, and the appointments of climate change skeptics to head federal agencies charged with protecting our environment and resources. Public opinion has been trending in the right direction, with over half of the American public now in the Alarmed and Concerned Six Americas segments, but the 3-year window to start reducing our emissions identified by Figueres et al. (2017) is closing. There is still reason to hope, but no time to dally.

References

Balbus, J., Ebi, K., Finzer, L., Malina, C., Chadwick, A., McBride, D., … Maibach, E. (2008). *Are we ready? Preparing for the public health challenges of climate change*. Retrieved from National Association of County and City Health Officials website: http://www.naccho.org/uploads/downloadable-resources/Are-we-ready_14_view.pdf

Ball-Rokeach, S. J., & DeFleur, M. L. (1976). A dependency model of mass-media effects. *Communication Research, 3*, 3–21. https://doi.org/10.1177/009365027600300101

Bandura, A. (2000). Exercise of human agency through collective efficacy. *Current Directions in Psychological Science, 9*, 75–78. https://doi.org/10.1111/1467-8721.00064

Bandura, A. (2001). Social cognitive theory: An agentic perspective. *Annual Review of Psychology, 52*, 1–26. https://doi.org/10.1146/annurev.psych.52.1.1

Bennett, W. L., & Iyengar, S. (2008). A new era of minimal effects? The changing foundations of political communication. *Journal of Communication, 58*, 707–731. https://doi.org/10.1111/j.1460-2466.2008.00410.x

Bloodhart, B., Maibach, E., Myers, T., & Zhao, X. (2015). Local climate experts: The influence of local TV weather information on climate change perceptions. *PLoS One, 10*, e0141526. https://doi.org/10.1371/journal.pone.0141526

Boucher, J. L. (2016). Culture, carbon, and climate change: A class analysis of climate change belief, lifestyle lock-in, and personal carbon footprint. *Social Ecology: Journal for Environmental Thought and Sociological Research, 25*, 53–80. https://doi.org/10.17234/SocEkol.25.1.3

Bowers, A. W., Monroe, M. C., & Adams, D. C. (2016). Climate change communication insights from cooperative extension professionals in the US southern states: Finding common ground. *Environmental Communication, 10*, 656–670. https://doi.org/10.1080/17524032.2016.1176947

Boykoff, M. T. (2007). Flogging a dead norm? Newspaper coverage of anthropogenic climate change in the United States and United Kingdom from 2003 to 2006. *Area, 39*, 470–481. https://doi.org/10.1111/j.1475-4762.2007.00769.x

Brady, H. E., Verba, S., & Schlozman, K. L. (1995). Beyond SES: A resource model of political participation. *American Political Science Review, 89*(2), 271–294. https://doi.org/10.2307/2082425

Brulle, R. J., Carmichael, J., & Jenkins, J. C. (2012). Shifting public opinion on climate change: An empirical assessment of factors influencing concern over climate change in the US, 2002–2010. *Climatic Change, 114*(2), 169–188. https://doi.org/10.1007/s10584-012-0403-y

Burstein, P., Einwohner, R., & Hollander, J. (1995). The success of political movements: A bargaining perspective. In J. Jenkins & B. Klandermans (Eds.), *Politics of social protest: Comparative perspectives on states and social movements* (pp. 275–295). Minneapolis, MN: University of Minnesota Press.

Campbell, T. H., & Kay, A. C. (2014). Solution aversion: On the relation between ideology and motivated disbelief. *Journal of Personality and Social Psychology, 107*, 809. https://doi.org/10.1037/a0037963

Centers for Disease Control and Prevention (CDC). (2016). *Climate effects on health*. Retrieved from CDC website: https://www.cdc.gov/climateandhealth/effects/

Chong, D., & Druckman, J. N. (2007). Framing theory. *Annual Review of Political Science, 10*, 103–126. https://doi.org/10.1146/annurev.polisci.10.072805.103054

Christakis, N. A., & Fowler, J. H. (2013). Social contagion theory: Examining dynamic social networks and human behavior. *Statistics in Medicine, 32*, 556–577. https://doi.org/10.1002/sim.5408

Chryst, B., Marlon, J., van der Linden, S., Leiserowitz, A., Maibach, E., & Roser-Renouf, C. (in press). Six Americas short survey. *Environmental Communication*.

Cook, J., Oreskes, N., Doran, P. T., Anderegg, W. R., Verheggen, B., Maibach, E. W., … Nuccitelli, D. (2016). Consensus on consensus: A synthesis of consensus estimates on human-caused global warming. *Environmental Research Letters, 11*(4). https://doi.org/10.1088/1748-9326/11/4/048002

Davenport, C. (2013, July 25). Why it finally makes sense to talk about climate change. *National Journal.*
Detenber, B., Rosenthal, S., Liao, Y., & Ho, S. S. (2016). Audience segmentation for campaign design: Addressing climate change in Singapore. *International Journal of Communication, 10*, 4736–4758 Retrieved from http://hdl.handle.net/10220/41984
Ding, D., Maibach, E., Zhao, X., Roser-Renouf, C., & Leiserowitz, A. (2011). Support for climate policy and societal action are linked to perceptions about scientific agreement. *Nature Climate Change, 1*, 462–466. https://doi.org/10.1038/NCLIMATE1295
Doherty, K. L., & Webler, T. N. (2016). Social norms and efficacy beliefs drive the alarmed segment's public-sphere climate actions. *Nature Climate Change, 6*, 879–884. https://doi.org/10.1038/nclimate3025
Dunlap, R. E., & McCright, A. M. (2011). Organized climate change denial. In J. Dryzek, R. Norgaard, & D. Schlosberg (Eds.), *The Oxford handbook of climate change and society* (pp. 144–160). New York, NY: Oxford University Press.
Feinberg, M., & Willer, R. (2013). The moral roots of environmental attitudes. *Psychological Science, 24*, 56–62. https://doi.org/10.1177/0956797612449177
Feldman, L. M., Maibach, E., Roser-Renouf, C., & Leiserowitz, A. (2012). Climate on cable: The nature and impact of global warming coverage on Fox News, CNN, and MSNBC. *International Journal of Press/Politics, 17*, 3–31. https://doi.org/10.1177/1940161211425410
Feldman, L. M., Myers, T. A., Hmielowski, J. D., & Leiserowitz, A. A. (2014). The mutual reinforcement of media selectivity and effects: Testing the reinforcing spirals framework in the context of global warming. *Journal of Communication, 64*, 590–611. https://doi.org/10.1111/jcom.12108
Feygina, I., Jost, J. T., & Goldsmith, R. E. (2010). System justification, the denial of global warming, and the possibility of "system-sanctioned change". *Personality and Social Psychology Bulletin, 36*, 326–338. https://doi.org/10.1177/0146167209351435
Figueres, C., Schellnhuber, H. J., Whiteman, G., Rockström, J., Hobley, A., & Rahmstorf, S. (2017). Three years to safeguard our climate. *Nature, 546*, 593–595. https://doi.org/10.1038/546593a
Flora, J., & Roser-Renouf, C. (2014). Climate change activism and youth. In UNICEF (Ed.), *The challenges of climate change: Children on the front line* (pp. 86–91). Retrieved from https://s3.amazonaws.com/academia.edu.documents/34335801/Challenges_of_Climate_Change-Children_on_the_Front_Line.pdf?AWSAccessKeyId=AKIAIWOWYYGZ2Y53UL3A&Expires=1506619508&Signature=ntciaZCcEDuQVqs0z1mIVhC0YaA%3D&response-content-disposition=inline%3B%20filename%3DInequality_climate_change_and_children_s.pdf
Flora, J. A., Saphir, M., Lappé, M., Roser-Renouf, C., Maibach, E. W., & Leiserowitz, A. A. (2014). Evaluation of a national high school entertainment education program: The Alliance for Climate Education. *Climatic Change, 127*, 419–434. https://doi.org/10.1007/s10584-014-1274-1
Friedman, M. (1985). Consumer boycotts in the United States, 1970–1980: Contemporary events in historical perspective. *Journal of Consumer Affairs, 19*, 96–117. https://doi.org/10.1111/j.1745-6606.1985.tb00346.x
Guagnano, G. A., Stern, P. C., & Dietz, T. (1995). Influences on attitude-behavior relationships: A natural experiment with curbside recycling. *Environment and Behavior, 27*, 699–718. https://doi.org/10.1177/0013916595275005
Hmielowski, J. D., Feldman, L. M., Myers, T. A., Leiserowitz, A. A. & Maibach, E.W. (2013). An attack on science?: Media use, trust in scientists, and perceptions of global warming. *Public Understanding of Science, 23*, 866–883. https://doi.org/10.1177/0963662513480091
Hornik, R. (2002). *Public health communication: Evidence for behavior change*. Mahwah, NJ: Lawrence Erlbaum.
Howe, P. D., Boudet, H., Leiserowitz, A., & Maibach, E. W. (2014). Mapping the shadow of experience of extreme weather events. *Climatic Change, 127*, 381–389. https://doi.org/10.1007/s10584-014-1253-6
Howe, P. D., Mildenberger, M., Marlon, J. R., & Leiserowitz, A. (2015). Geographic variation in opinions on climate change at state and local scales in the USA. *Nature Climate Change, 5*(6), 596. https://doi.org/10.1038/NCLIMATE2583

Howe, P. D., Thaker, J., & Leiserowitz, A. (2014). Perceptions of changes in rainfall and extreme events among the Indian public. *Climatic Change, 127*, 211–225. https://doi.org/10.1007/s10584-014-1245-6

Kahan, D. M., Jenkins-Smith, H., & Braman, D. (2011). Cultural cognition of scientific consensus. *Journal of Risk Research, 14*, 147–174. https://doi.org/10.1080/13669877.2010.511246

Kahneman, D. (2003). A perspective on judgment and choice: Mapping bounded rationality. *American Psychologist, 58*, 697–720. https://doi.org/10.1037/0003-066X.58.9.697

Katz, E. (1957). The two-step flow of communication: An up-to-date report on an hypothesis. *Public Opinion Quarterly, 21*, 61–78. https://doi.org/10.1086/266687

Kelly, L. A. D., Luebke, J. F., Clayton, S., Saunders, C. D., Matiasek, J., & Grajal, A. (2014). Climate change attitudes of zoo and aquarium visitors: Implications for climate literacy education. *Journal of Geoscience Education, 62*, 502–510. https://doi.org/10.5408/13-078.1

King, B. G. (2008). A political mediation model of corporate response to social movement activism. *Administrative Science Quarterly, 53*, 395–421. https://doi.org/10.2189/asqu.53.3.395

Krosnick, J. A., Holbrook, A. L., & Visser, P. S. (2000). The impact of the fall 1997 debate about global warming on American public opinion. *Public Understanding of Science, 9*, 239–260. https://doi.org/10.1088/0963-6625/9/3/303

Kunda, Z. (1990). The case for motivated reasoning. *Psychological Bulletin, 108*, 480. https://doi.org/10.1037/0033-2909.108.3.480

Leiserowitz, A. (2006). Climate change risk perception and policy preferences: The role of affect, imagery, and values. *Climatic Change, 77*, 45–72. https://doi.org/10.1007/s10584-006-9059-9

Leiserowitz, A., Feinberg, G., Rosenthal, S., Smith, N., Anderson A., Roser-Renouf, C., & Maibach, E. (2014, May). *What's in a name? Global warming vs. climate change*. Retrieved from George Mason Center for Climate Change Communication website: https://www.climatechangecommunication.org/?s=+Global+Warming+vs.+Climate+Change

Leiserowitz, A., Maibach, E., Roser-Renouf, C., Feinberg, G., & Howe, P. (2013, April). *Extreme weather and climate change in the American mind, April 2013*. Retrieved from George Mason Center for Climate Change Communication website: https://www.climatechangecommunication.org/?s=Extreme+Weather+and+Climate+Change+in+the+American+Mind%2C+April+2013

Leiserowitz, A., Maibach, E., Roser-Renouf, C., Feinberg, G., & Rosenthal, S. (2015a, October). *Climate change in the American mind: October, 2015*. Retrieved from George Mason Center for Climate Change Communication website: https://www.climatechangecommunication.org/?s=Climate+change+in+the+American+mind%3A+October%2C+2015

Leiserowitz, A., Maibach, E., Roser-Renouf, C., Feinberg, G., & Rosenthal, S. (2015b, March). *Climate change in the American Christian mind: March, 2015*. Retrieved from George Mason Center for Climate Change Communication website: https://www.climatechangecommunication.org/?s=Climate+change+in+the+American+Christian+mind%3A+March%2C+2015

Leiserowitz, A., Maibach, E., Roser-Renouf, C., Feinberg, G., Rosenthal, S., & Marlon, J. (2014, October). *Public perceptions of the health consequences of global warming: October, 2014*. Retrieved from George Mason Center for Climate Change Communication website: https://www.climatechangecommunication.org/?s=Public+Perceptions+of+the+Health+Consequences+of+Global+Warming

Leiserowitz, A., Maibach, E., Roser-Renouf, C., Rosenthal, S., & Cutler, M. (2017). *Climate change in the American mind: May 2017*. Retrieved from George Mason Center for Climate Change Communication website: https://www.climatechangecommunication.org/all/may2017ccam/

Leiserowitz, A., Maibach, E., Roser-Renouf, C., & Smith, N. (2011, May). *Climate change in the American mind: Americans' global warming beliefs and attitudes in May 2011*. Retrieved from George Mason Center for Climate Change Communication website: https://www.climatechangecommunication.org/all/the-climate-change-in-the-american-mind-series-may-2011-2/

Leiserowitz, A., Maibach, E., Roser-Renouf, C., Smith, N., & Dawson, Y. E. (2012). Climategate, public opinion, and the loss of trust. *American Behavioral Scientist, 57*, 818–837. https://doi.org/10.1177/0002764212458272

Leiserowitz, A., & Smith, N. (2011). *Knowledge of climate change among visitors to Science & Technology Museums*. Retrieved from Yale Program on Climate Change Communication website: http://environment.yale.edu/climate/files/MuseumReport.pdf

Leiserowitz, A., Thaker, J., Feinberg, G., & Cooper, D. (2013) *Global warming's six Indias*. Yale University. Retrieved from Yale Program on Climate Change Communication website: http://climatecommunication.yale.edu/wp-content/uploads/2016/02/2013_05_Global-Warming%E2%80%99s-Six-Indias.pdf

Luber, G., Knowlton, K., Balbus, J., Frumkin, H., Hayden, M., Hess, J., & Ziska, L. (2014). Human health. Climate change impacts in the United States: The third national climate assessment. In J. M. Melillo, Terese (T. C.) Richmond, and G. W. Yohe (Eds.), *Third national climate assessment* (pp. 220–256). https://doi.org/10.7930/J0PN93H5. Retrieved from http://nca2014.globalchange.gov/report/sectors/human-health

Maibach, E. (in press). Increasing public awareness and facilitating behavior change: Two guiding heuristics. In L. Hannah & T. Lovejoy (Eds.), *Climate change and biodiversity* (2nd ed.). New Haven, CT: Yale University Press.

Maibach, E., Cullen, H., Placky, B., Witte, J., Seitter, K., Gardiner, N., … Sublette, S. (2016). TV meteorologists as local climate educators. In *Oxford research encyclopedia of climate science*. https://doi.org/10.1093/acrefore/9780190228620.013.505

Maibach, E., Kreslake, J., Roser-Renouf, C., Rosenthal, S., Feinberg, G., & Leiserowitz, A. (2015). Do Americans understand that global warming is harmful to human health? Evidence from a national survey. *Annals of Global Health, 81*, 396–409. https://doi.org/10.1016/j.aogh.2015.08.010

Maibach, E., Leiserowitz, A., Roser-Renouf, C., & Mertz, C. K. (2011). Identifying like-minded audiences for global warming public engagement campaigns: An audience segmentation analysis and tool development. *PLoS One, 6*, e17571. https://doi.org/10.1371/journal.pone.0017571

Maibach, E., Leiserowitz, A., Roser-Renouf, C., Myers, T., Rosenthal, S., & Feinberg, G. (2015). *The Francis effect: How Pope Francis changed the conversation about global warming*. Retrieved from George Mason Center for Climate Change Communication website: https://www.climatechangecommunication.org/?s=The+Francis+Effect%3A+How+Pope+Francis+Changed+the+Conversation+about+Global+Warming

Maibach, E., Perkins, D., Timm, K., Myers, T., Placky, B., Sublette, S., … Seitter, K. (2017). *A 2017 national survey of broadcast meteorologists: Initial findings*. Retrieved from George Mason Center for Climate Change Communication website: https://www.climatechangecommunication.org/tag/2017+tv-weathercasters/

Maibach, E., Roser-Renouf, C., Akerlof, K., Leiserowitz, A., & Nisbet, M. (2010). Saving energy is a value shared by all Americans: Results of a global warming audience segmentation analysis. In K. Erhardt-Martinez & J. Laitner (Eds.), *People-centered initiatives for increasing energy savings* (pp. 99–112). Retrieved from http://www.aceee.org/sites/default/files/publications/ebook/eb01.pdf

Maibach, E., Roser-Renouf, C., & Leiserowitz, A. (2008). Communication and marketing as climate change intervention assets: A public health perspective. *American Journal of Preventive Medicine, 35*, 488–500. https://doi.org/10.1016/j.amepre.2008.08.016

Maibach, E., Roser-Renouf, C., & Leiserowitz, A. (2009). *Global Warming's Six Americas 2009: An audience segmentation analysis*. Retrieved from George Mason Center for Climate Change Communication website: https://www.climatechangecommunication.org/all/climate-change-in-the-american-mind-global-warmings-six-americas/

Maibach, E., Wilson, K., & Witte, J. (2010a). *A national survey of news directors about climate change: Preliminary findings*. Retrieved from George Mason Center for Climate Change Communication website: https://www.climatechangecommunication.org/?s=A+National+Survey+of+News+Directors+about+Climate+Change

Maibach, E., Wilson, K., & Witte, J. (2010b). *A national survey of television meteorologists about climate change: Preliminary findings*. Fairfax, VA: George Mason University, Center for Climate Change Communication Retrieved from George Mason Center for Climate Change Communication website: https://www.climatechangecommunication.org/tag/2010+tv-weathercasters/

Maloney, E. K., Lapinski, M. K., & Witte, K. (2011). Fear appeals and persuasion: A review and update of the extended parallel process model. *Social and Personality Psychology Compass, 5*, 206–219. https://doi.org/10.1111/j.1751-9004.2011.00341.x

Medical Society Consortium on Climate and Health. (2017). *Medical alert! Climate change is harming our health*. Retrieved from George Mason Center for Climate Change Communication website: https://www.climatechangecommunication.org/all/medical-alert-climate-change-is-harming-our-health/

Metag, J., Füchslin, T., & Schäfer, M. S. (2015). Global warming's five Germanys: A typology of Germans' views on climate change and patterns of media use and information. *Public Understanding of Science, 26*, 434–451. https://doi.org/10.1177/0963662515592558

Morrison, M., Duncan, R., Sherley, C., & Parton, K. (2013). A comparison between attitudes to climate change in Australia and the United States. *Australasian Journal of Environmental Management, 20*, 87–100. https://doi.org/10.1080/14486563.2012.762946

Myers, T., Rolfe-Redding, J., Roser-Renouf, C., & Maibach, E. (2014). *Visitors' experiences with NASA's earth observatory and global climate change resources*. Fairfax, VA: George Mason University, Center for Climate Change Communication.

Myers, T. A., Maibach, E., Peters, E., & Leiserowitz, A. (2015). Simple messages help set the record straight about scientific agreement on human-caused climate change: The results of two experiments. *PLoS One, 10*, e0120985. https://doi.org/10.1371/journal.pone.0120985

Myers, T. A., Maibach, E. W., Roser-Renouf, C., Akerlof, K., & Leiserowitz, A. A. (2013). The relationship between personal experience and belief in the reality of global warming. *Nature Climate Change, 3*, 343–347. https://doi.org/10.1038/nclimate1754

Myers, T. A., Nisbet, M. C., Maibach, E. W., & Leiserowitz, A. A. (2012). A public health frame arouses hopeful emotions about climate change: A letter. *Climatic Change, 13*, 1105–1112. https://doi.org/10.1007/s10584-012-0513-6

Myers, T. A., Roser-Renouf, C., Maibach, E., & Leiserowitz, A. (2017). Exposure to the Pope's climate change message activated convinced Americans to take certain activism actions. *Global Challenges, 1*, 1–8. https://doi.org/10.1002/gch2.201600019

Nisbet, M. C. (2009). Communicating climate change: Why frames matter for public engagement. *Environment: Science and Policy for Sustainable Development, 51*, 12–23. https://doi.org/10.3200/ENVT.51.2.12-23

Nolan, J. M., Schultz, P. W., Cialdini, R. B., Goldstein, N. J., & Griskevicius, V. (2008). Normative social influence is underdetected. *Personality and Social Psychology Bulletin, 34*(7), 913–923. https://doi.org/10.1177/0146167208316691

Ockwell, D., Whitmarsh, L., & O'Neill, S. (2009). Reorienting climate change communication for effective mitigation: Forcing people to be green or fostering grass-roots engagement? *Science Communication, 30*, 305–327. https://doi.org/10.1177/1075547008328969

Oreskes, N. (2004). The scientific consensus on climate change. *Science, 306*(5702), 1686–1686. https://doi.org/10.1126/science.1103618

Petty, R. E., & Cacioppo, J. T. (1986). The elaboration likelihood model of persuasion. *Advances in Experimental Social Psychology, 19*, 123–205. https://doi.org/10.1016/S0065-2601(08)60214-2

Pew Research Center. (2013). *Question search*. Retrieved from http://www.pewglobal.org/question-search/?qid=408&cntIDs=&stdIDs=

Pew Research Center. (2015). *How do Americans stand out from the rest of the world?* Retrieved from http://www.pewresearch.org/fact-tank/2015/03/12/how-do-americans-stand-out-from-the-rest-of-the-world/

Phipps, M. (2011). *Global Warming's Six Americas: A science museum of Minnesota audience segmentation analysis*. Retrieved from http://www.informalscience.org/sites/default/files/6Americas_with2011data.pdf

Politico Magazine. (2016). *Politico 50: Our guide to the thinkers, doers and visionaries transforming American politics in 2016*. Retrieved from http://www.politico.com/magazine/politico50/2016

Ranney, M. A., & Clark, D. (2016). Climate change conceptual change: Scientific information can transform attitudes. *Topics in Cognitive Science, 8*, 49–75. https://doi.org/10.1111/tops.12187

RepublicEn. (2017). *RepublicEn: Engaging conservatives*. Retrieved from George Mason Center for Climate Change Communication website: https://www.climatechangecommunication.org/republicen/

Rogers, E. M. (2010). *Diffusion of innovations*. New York, NY: Simon and Schuster.

Roser-Renouf, C., Atkinson, L., Maibach, E., & Leiserowitz, A. (2016). The consumer as climate activist. *International Journal of Communication, 10*, 4759–4783 Retrieved from http://ijoc.org/index.php/ijoc/article/view/4702

Roser-Renouf, C., Maibach, E., Leiserowitz, A., Feinberg, G., & Rosenthal, S (2016). *Faith, morality and the environment: Portraits of Global Warming's Six Americas*. Retrieved from George Mason Center for Climate Change Communication website: https://www.climatechangecommunication.org/all/faith-morality-and-the-environment-2016/

Roser-Renouf, C., Maibach, E., Leiserowitz, A., Feinberg, G., Rosenthal, S., & Kreslake, J. (2014). *Global Warming's Six Americas: Perceptions of the health consequences of global warming and update on key beliefs*. Retrieved from George Mason Center for Climate Change Communication website: https://www.climatechangecommunication.org/all/global-warmings-six-americas-in-october-2014-perceptions-of-the-health-consequences-of-global-warming-and-update-on-key-beliefs-2/

Roser-Renouf, C., Maibach, E., Leiserowitz, A., & Rosenthal, S. (2016). *Takin' it to the mall: Consumer activism on global warming*. Retrieved from George Mason Center for Climate Change Communication website: https://www.climatechangecommunication.org/all/takin-it-to-the-mall-consumer-activism-on-global-warming/

Roser-Renouf, C., Maibach, E., Leiserowitz, A., & Zhao, X. (2014). The genesis of climate change activism: From key beliefs to political action. *Climatic Change, 125*, 163–178. https://doi.org/10.1007/s10584-014-1173-5

Roser-Renouf, C., Maibach, E. W., & Li, J. (2016). Adapting to the changing climate: An assessment of local health department preparations for climate change-related health threats, 2008-2012. *PLoS One, 11*, e0151558. https://doi.org/10.1371/journal.pone.0151558

Roser-Renouf, C., Stenhouse, N., Rolfe-Redding, J., Maibach, E., & Leiserowitz, A. (2014). Engaging diverse audiences with climate change: Message strategies for Global Warming's Six Americas. In A. Hansen & R. Cox (Eds.), *Handbook of environment and communication* (pp. 368–386). New York, NY: Routledge.

Rowan, K., Kotcher, J., Walsh-Thomas, J., Baldwin, P., Trowbridge, J., Thaker, J., … Maibach, E. (in press). Best practices of "innovator" TV meteorologists who act as climate change educators. In D. O'Hair (Ed.), *Risk and health communication in an evolving media environment*. London, England: Routledge.

Sarfaty, M., Kreslake, J., Bloodhart, B., Price, K., Casale, T., Folstein, S., & Maibach, E. (2015). *Views of allergy specialists on the health effects of climate change, key findings: Membership survey of the American Academy of Allergy, Asthma, Immunology, December 2015*. Retrieved from George Mason Center for Climate Change Communication website: https://www.climatechangecommunication.org/all/views-of-allergy-specialists-on-the-health-effects-of-climate-change-2/

Sarfaty, M., Kreslake, J., Casale, T., & Maibach, E. (2015). Views of AAAAI members on climate change and health. *Journal of Allergy and Clinical Immunology: In Practice, 4*, 333. https://doi.org/10.1016/j.jaip.2015.09.018

Sarfaty, M., Kreslake, J., Ewart, G., Guidotti, T., Thurston, G., Balmes, J., & Maibach, E. (2016). Views of American Thoracic Society international members on climate change and health. *Annals of the American Thoracic Society, 13*, 1808–1813. https://doi.org/10.1513/AnnalsATS.201604-229BC

Sarfaty, M., Mitchell, M., Bloodhart, B., & Maibach, E. (2014). A survey of African-American physicians on the health effects of climate change. *International Journal of Environmental Research and Public Health, 11*, 12473–12485. https://doi.org/10.3390/ijerph111212473

Schweizer, S., Davis, S., & Thompson, J. L. (2013). Changing the conversation about climate change: A theoretical framework for place-based climate change engagement. *Environmental Communication: A Journal of Nature and Culture, 7*, 42–62. https://doi.org/10.1080/17524032.2012.753634

Sciencetogo.org. (2017). *About the project*. Retrieved from the Sciencetogo.org website: http://sciencetogo.org/about/

Sears, D. O., & Freedman, J. L. (1967). Selective exposure to information: A critical review. *Public Opinion Quarterly, 31*, 194–213. https://doi.org/10.1086/267513

Slater, M. D. (2007). Reinforcing spirals: The mutual influence of media selectivity and media effects and their impact on individual behavior and social identity. *Communication Theory, 17*, 281–303. https://doi.org/10.1111/j.1468-2885.2007.00296.x

Somerville, R. C., & Hassol, S. J. (2011). The science of climate change. *Physics Today, 64*, 48. https://doi.org/10.1063/PT.3.1296?ver=pdfcov

Spence, A., Poortinga, W., & Pidgeon, N. (2012). The psychological distance of climate change. *Risk Analysis, 32*, 957–972. https://doi.org/10.1111/j.1539-6924.2011.01695.x

Tewksbury, D. (2005). The seeds of audience fragmentation: Specialization in the use of online news sites. *Journal of Broadcasting & Electronic Media, 49*, 332–348. https://doi.org/10.1207/s15506878jobem4903_5

Theel, S., Greenberg, M., & Robbins, D. (2013, October 10). *Media sowed doubt in coverage of UN climate report*. Retrieved from Media Matters for America website: https://www.mediamatters.org/research/2013/10/10/study-media-sowed-doubt-in-coverage-of-un-clima/196387

Trope, Y., & Liberman, N. (2011). Construal level theory. In P. Van Lange, A. Krugalanski, & E. T. Higgins (Eds.), *Handbook of theories of social psychology* (Vol. 1, pp. 118–134). Los Angeles, CA: Sage.

Valente, T. (2012). Network interventions. *Science, 337*, 49. https://doi.org/10.1126/science.1217330

van der Linden, S., Leiserowitz, A., Feinberg, G., & Maibach, E. (2014). How to communicate the scientific consensus on climate change: Plain facts, pie charts or metaphors? *Climatic Change Letters, 126*, 255. https://doi.org/10.1007/s10584-014-1190-4

van der Linden, S., Leiserowitz, A., Rosenthal, S., & Maibach, E. (2017). Inoculating the public against misinformation about climate change. *Global Challenges, 1*. https://doi.org/10.1002/gch2.201600008

van der Linden, S., Maibach, E., & Leiserowitz, A. (2015). Improving public engagement with climate change: Five "best practice" insights from psychological science. *Perspectives on Psychological Science, 10*, 758–763. https://doi.org/10.1177/1745691615598516

van der Linden, S. L., Leiserowitz, A. A., Feinberg, G. D., & Maibach, E. W. (2015). The scientific consensus on climate change as a gateway belief: Experimental evidence. *PLoS One, 10*, e0118489. https://doi.org/10.1371/journal.pone.0118489

Van Zomeren, M., Postmes, T., & Spears, R. (2008). Toward an integrative social identity model of collective action: A quantitative research synthesis of three socio-psychological perspectives. *Psychological Bulletin, 134*, 504. https://doi.org/10.1037/0033-2909.134.4.504

Walsh, J., Wuebbles, D., Hayhoe, K., Kossin, J., Kunkel, K., Stephens, G., … Somerville, R. (2014). Our changing climate. In J. Melillo, T. Richmond, & G. Yohe (Eds.), *Third national climate assessment* (pp. 19–67). Retrieved from http://nca2014.globalchange.gov/report/our-changing-climate/introduction

Weber, E. U. (2006). Experience-based and description-based perceptions of long-term risk: Why global warming does not scare us (yet). *Climatic Change, 77*, 103–120. https://doi.org/10.1007/s10584-006-9060-3

Wildavsky, A., & Dake, K. (1990). Theories of risk perception: Who fears what and why? *Daedalus, 119*, 41–60 Retrieved from http://www.jstor.org/stable/20025337

Witte, K. (1992). Putting the fear back into fear appeals: The extended parallel process model. *Communication Monographs, 59*, 329–349. https://doi.org/10.1080/03637759209376276

Wolsko, C., Ariceaga, H., & Seiden, J. (2016). Red, white, and blue enough to be green: Effects of moral framing on climate change attitudes and conservation behaviors. *Journal of Experimental Social Psychology, 65*, 7–19. https://doi.org/10.1016/j.jesp.2016.02.005

Zhao, X., Leiserowitz, A., Maibach, E., & Roser-Renouf, C. (2011). Attention to science/environment news positively predicts and attention to political news negatively predicts global warming risk perceptions and policy support. *Journal of Communication, 61*, 713–731. https://doi.org/10.1111/j.1460-2466.2011.01563.x

Zhao, X., Maibach, E., Gandy, J., Witte, J., Cullen, H., Klinger, B., … Pyle, A. (2014). Climate change education through TV weathercasters: Results of a field experiment. *Bulletin of the American Meteorological Society, 95*, 117–130. https://doi.org/10.1175/BAMS-D-12-00144.1

Index

D. A. Hope, R. A. Bevins (eds.), *Change and Maintaining Change*, Nebraska Symposium on Motivation 65, https://doi.org/10.1007/978-3-319-96920-6